BIOCHEMICAL ASPECTS OF NERVOUS DISEASES

BIOCHEMICAL ASPECTS OF NERVOUS DISEASES

edited by

J. N. CUMINGS

Professor of Chemical Pathology
The Institute of Neurology
The National Hospitals for Nervous Diseases
Queen Square
London, W.C.1

℗ PLENUM PRESS · London and New York · 1972

Plenum Publishing Company Ltd.
Davis House
8 Scrubs Lane
Harlesden
London NW10 6SE
Tel. 01-969-4727

U.S. Edition published by
Plenum Publishing Corporation
227 West 17th Street
New York New York 10011

ISBN-13: 978-1-4684-1958-0   e-ISBN-13: 978-1-4684-1956-6
DOI: 10.1007/978-1-4684-1956-6

Library of Congress Catalog Card Number: 70-178775

PREFACE

Within recent years basic knowledge concerning the chemistry, and the metabolic processes taking place in the brain, spinal cord, peripheral nerves and muscles has increased in a remarkable manner. As a consequence some very important books have been published both in America and in Europe in which some, at least, of this information has become available in an easily readable form to an ever increasing group of laboratory and scientific workers.

The application of such studies in a variety of neurological diseases can now be made, thus making possible an explanation of many of the clinical and pathological peculiarities that have been known for decades. Although a few small manuals have already been published, combining both biochemical and clinical aspects of such disorders and these have been studied by neurologists and chemical pathologists throughout the world, yet a volume devoted exclusively to the biochemistry of neurological diseases has not yet been readily available. The present volume is an attempt to remedy this omission in relation to just a few of the conditions. Individual writers of each of the six chapters have been chosen who are intimately concerned both with biochemistry and with its application to disease in man. Each author has been responsible for the accuracy of his chapter together with appropriate references from the literature, but the Editor does not necessarily concur with all the opinions expressed by the authors.

The Editor expresses his real thanks to each author, to the Plenum Press and to his secretary Miss S. Barkwell for their ready and most helpful assistance. In addition acknowledgement is given to Professor S. Granick, Dr. Atallah Kappas, Dr. Richard D. Levere, Dr. Daniel Steinberg, Grume & Stratton Inc., the Academic Press Inc. and the Annals of Internal Medicine for permission to use Tables and Figures in Chapter 1; to the Department of Medical Illustration, The Institute of Neurology for their help in providing the illustrations for Chapter 5, and to Blackwell Scientific Publications Ltd. for permission to use the illustrations in Chapter 6.

J. N. Cumings

v

CONTRIBUTORS

G. Curzon

Reader in Biochemistry,
Department of Chemical Pathology,
Institute of Neurology,
The National Hospital,
Queen Square,
London, W.C.1,
England.

Bruno Gerstl

Chief, Laboratory Service,
Professor (Emeritus) of Pathology,
Stanford University School of Medicine,
Veterans Administration Hospital,
Palo Alto,
California,
U.S.A.

R. J. T. Pennington

Member of External Scientific Staff,
Medical Research Council,
Honorary Reader in Neurochemistry,
University of Newcastle upon Tyne,
Regional Neurological Centre,
Newcastle General Hospital,
Newcastle,
England.

R. H. S. Thompson

Professor of Biochemistry,
Courtauld Institute of Biochemistry,
The Middlesex Hospital Medical School,
London, W.1,
England.

J. M. Walshe

Reader in Metabolic Disease,
University of Cambridge,
Honorary Consultant Physician,
Addenbrooke's Hospital,
The Department of Investigative Medicine,
University of Cambridge,
Cambridge,
England.

John Wilson

M.R.C. Clinical Genetics Research Unit,
Institute of Child Health,
Institute of Neurology,
Consultant Neurologist,
Hospital for Sick Children,
Great Ormond Street,
London, W.C.1,
England.

L. I. Woolf

Associate Professor (Neurochemistry),
Kinsmen Laboratory of Neurological
Research,
Department of Psychiatry,
University of British Columbia,
Vancouver, 8, B.C.,
Canada.

CONTENTS

CHAPTER 1

Metabolic Aspects of Some Diseases of Peripheral Nerves

J. WILSON and R. H. S. THOMPSON

1.1 INTRODUCTION

One of the most exciting developments in the past two decades has been the intimate study of the correlation of form and function at the ultrastructural level. Axonal and synaptic activities are now sufficiently well understood to allow an outline definition at molecular level, and it is possible to envisage an understanding of neuraxial function entirely in biochemical terms.

Although in clinical neurology the traditional aetiopathological classification which distinguishes between, for example, traumatic, infective, neoplastic, developmental, degenerative and metabolic causes of diseases, still dominates thinking, it is likewise possible (if still somewhat ambitious) to advance a similar holistic approach, and bring all conditions within the purview of the biochemist.

Nevertheless, for the purpose of this review we restrict ourselves to the conventional consideration of those toxic-nutritional-metabolic conditions which are of primary aetiological significance in the peripheral neuropathies.

Such factors are of special importance in relation to these diseases, and before considering in more detail specific abnormalities, it is worth while reflecting on the special structural characteristics of peripheral nerves which distinguish them from other neuraxial elements, and which may partly determine their characteristic responses to toxic-metabolic factors.

There is good evidence that not only is the structural integrity of an individual axon dependent on the vitality of the perikaryon, but also that there is nutritional dependence as well. As has been emphasized by Cavanagh [1], "The metabolic load imposed on their perikarya by the longest and largest fibres must be unequalled by that on any other type of cell in the body, for measurements have shown that the volume ratio of axon to perikaryon may be as great as a thousand to one."

Not only may this relationship confer a special susceptibility to metabolic derangements but so may also the endowment of certain axons with myelin sheaths. The intimate myelin investment of axons in segmental fashion by the specially differentiated cell membranes of Schwann cells serves to allow an increased rate of transmission of electrical impulses by virtue of "saltatory" conduction at the nodes of Ranvier. Since the rate of conduction of impulses in the absence of this segmental sheath is much slower, myelinated fibre function can be markedly altered by those diseases which damage Schwann cells and produce so-called segmental demyelination.

It is thus possible to distinguish between peripheral neuropathy predominantly due to axonal disease (with secondary Wallerian degeneration) and that due to so-called segmental demyelination following on Schwann cell damage (Table 1.1).

TABLE 1.

Wallerian Degeneration and Segmental Demyelination in the Polyneuropathies

Predominantly Wallerian degeneration	Predominantly segmental demyelination
Beri-beri	Diabetes
Porphyria	Leucodystrophies (metachromatic, globoid (cell))
Organo-phosphorus poisoning	Hypertrophic interstitial neuritis (Déjèrine-Sottas and Refsum)
Alcoholism	
Vitamin B_{12} deficiency	

Although in the conditions now to be discussed little is known of the precise mechanism of cell damage, it seems reasonable to conclude in each case that it is due to disruption of the normal metabolic activities of either neurones or Schwann cells, resulting in one or other of the above-mentioned types of degeneration.

1.1.1 Thiamine deficiency

The biochemical changes that are present in the polyneuropathy which can result from a deficiency of thiamine in the diet have been well worked out in the years that have elapsed since 1885 when the Japanese naval surgeon, Takaki, first claimed that beri-beri is a nutritional disease resulting from the ingestion of excessive quantities of polished rice [2]. Eijkmann in 1897 [3] carried out a classical nutritional experiment when he showed for the first time that fowls fed on a diet of polished rice developed weakness of the legs and opisthotonus. As a result of his observations he was able to conclude, and correctly, that the germ and the pericarp of rice contained an essential nutrient capable of protecting fowls from a disease resembling beri-beri. This nutrient, vitamin B_1 or thiamine, was synthesized [4], and its mode of action at the biochemical level defined in detail following the initial observations and experiments of Peters and his colleagues in Oxford on the changes in the metabolism of the brain in rice-fed pigeons. Peters was able to state that vitamin B_1 "is a catalyst needed for the oxidative removal of one of the lower degradation products of carbohydrate metabolism", and he added that "the biochemical lesion (in thiamine deficiency) is most closely related to the oxidation of pyruvic acid". [5]. It is now known that thiamine pyrophosphate is a part of the complex co-enzyme requirements needed for the conversion of pyruvate, by a process of oxidative decarboxylation, into acetyl-coenzyme A.

This conversion is carried out by a series of linked reactions. In the first of these pyruvate is decarboxylated by a reaction involving thiamine pyrophosphate which acts as an acceptor for the acetaldehyde which is produced

$$
\begin{array}{ccccc}
CH_3 & & & CH_3 \cdot CHO & \\
| & & & | & \\
C=O & + & ThPP \longrightarrow & ThPP & + CO_2 \\
| & & & & \\
COOH & & Thiamine & \text{"Active} & \\
& & pyrophosphate & acetaldehyde" &
\end{array}
$$

The "active acetaldehyde"-thiamine pyrophosphate complex then reacts enzymically with another co-factor lipoic acid (6,8-dithiooctanoic acid), or lipoamide, since in its active state inside the cells the acid exists in an amide linkage with a lysine residue of a specific protein

Lipoamide   Acetyl lipoamide

The acetyl lipoamide so formed is the immediate precursor of acetyl-coenzyme A

$$
\begin{array}{ccc}
\text{CH}_2\text{---SH} & & \text{CH}_2\text{---SH} \\
\text{CH}_2\qquad \text{CH}_3 & & \text{CH}_2 \\
\text{CH---S---C} \;+\; \text{CoA. SH} \longrightarrow & \text{CH----SH} + \text{CH}_3\,\text{COSCoA} \\
\quad\quad\;\; \text{O} & & \\
(\text{CH}_2)_4 & & (\text{CH}_2)_4 \\
\text{CONHR} & & \text{CONHR}
\end{array}
$$

Reduced   Acetyl
lipoamide   co-enzyme A

The reduced lipoamide is then re-oxidized by nicotinamide-adeninedinucleotide

$$
\begin{array}{ccc}
\text{CH}_2\text{---SH} & & \text{CH}_2\text{---S} \\
\text{CH}_2 & & \text{CH}_2 \\
\text{CH----SH} + \text{NAD}^+ \longrightarrow & \text{CH----S} + \text{NADH} + \text{H}^+ \\
(\text{CH}_2)_4 & & (\text{CH}_2)_4 \\
\text{CONHR} & & \text{CONHR}
\end{array}
$$

In thiamine deficiency, therefore, the formation from pyruvate of acetyl-coenzyme A, which is normally followed by the oxidation of the 2-C acetyl fragment to CO_2 and H_2O via the citric acid cycle is blocked, and the pyruvate formed by glycolysis consequently accumulates. In addition in its role in the oxidative decarboxylation of pyruvate, thiamine pyrophosphate is also needed as a co-enzyme in the similar decarboxylation of the closely related α-oxoglutarate, one of the intermediaries in the citric acid cycle.

It also plays an essential part in the alternative pathway of carbohydrate oxidation, the so-called "pentose phosphate pathway", where it is required as a co-enzyme of transketolase [6, 7]. This enzyme catalyses the interaction between xylulose-5-phosphate and ribose-5-phosphate, one of the steps in the series of metabolic transformations resulting from the initial conversion of glucose-6-phosphate to 6-phosphogluconic acid by glucose-6-phosphate dehydrogenase.

$$
\begin{array}{l}
\text{CH}_2\text{OH} \\
|\\
\text{C} = \text{O} \\
|\\
\text{HOCH} \\
|\\
\text{HCOH} \\
|\\
\text{H}_2\text{COPO}_3\text{H}_2
\end{array}
\; + \;
\begin{array}{l}
\text{CHO} \\
|\\
\text{HCOH} \\
|\\
\text{HCOH} \\
|\\
\text{HCOH} \\
|\\
\text{H}_2\text{COPO}_3\text{H}_2
\end{array}
\;\rightleftharpoons\;
\begin{array}{l}
\text{CH}_2\text{OH} \\
|\\
\text{C} = \text{O} \\
|\\
\text{HOCH} \\
|\\
\text{HCOH} \\
|\\
\text{HCOH} \\
|\\
\text{HCOH} \\
|\\
\text{H}_2\text{COPO}_3\text{H}_2
\end{array}
\; + \;
\begin{array}{l}
\text{CHO} \\
|\\
\text{HCOH} \\
|\\
\text{H}_2\text{COPO}_3\text{H}_2
\end{array}
$$

Xylulose-5-phosphate	Ribose-5-phosphate	Sedoheptulose-7-phosphate	Glycoaldehyde 3-phosphate

In its more severe forms thiamine deficiency can present as (1) wet beri-beri; with generalized oedema and tendency to heart failure, (2) dry beri-beri, a chronic polyneuropathy with degenerative changes in the peripheral nerves, (3) infantile beri-beri, a chronic marasmic state also frequently associated with sudden heart failure, and (4) Wernicke's encephalopathy, which may be seen in chronic alcoholics and may be regarded as a "cerebral beri-beri". Less severe states of thiamine deficiency usually manifest themselves as a chronic polyneuropathy. Problems of differential diagnosis from other forms of peripheral neuritis therefore arise, and it is in this connection that studies of pyruvate metabolism may be of help.

1.1.2 Pyruvate metabolism in peripheral neuritis

It has been known for many years that the block in pyruvate metabolism resulting from a deficiency of thiamine, as outlined above, results in an elevated level of pyruvate in the blood [8, 9]. A "pyruvate tolerance test" has, therefore, been devised in which a dose of glucose is given by mouth and the blood

pyruvate levels measured at 0, 30, 60 and 90 min [10, 11].
Under the conditions of the test, and it is important that the
subject be fasting and at rest in bed, thiamine-deficient patients
usually show a blood level greater than 1.4 mg pyruvic acid per
100 ml at 60 or 90 min.

It must be remembered, of course, that a number of factors
other than a deficiency of thiamine can also result in high blood
pyruvate levels. For example, there is evidence suggesting that
compounds of arsenic [12] and of antimony, gold and
mercury [13] owe their toxicity to their ability to react with
the −SH groups in reduced lipoamide (see above), and that the
therapeutic effect of dimercaprol (BAL) is due to this dithiol
competing effectively with the thiol groups of lipoamide and so
preventing the arsenic from interfering with the normal
functioning of this co-factor [14]. In view of the fact that
arsenicals inhibit pyruvate oxidation by this means it is of
interest to recall the many points of clinical resemblance that
have long been known to exist between arsenical neuritis and
the polyneuropathy of thiamine deficiency [15]. The blood
pyruvate level is also raised in patients with an untreated
vitamin B_{12} deficiency [16], and is rapidly returned to normal
after treatment with vitamin B_{12}. Exercise, anoxia and fever can
also cause raised levels. In order to differentiate between a
thiamine deficiency and these other conditions which may also
present with raised blood pyruvate levels it may be advisable to
carry out a second pyruvate tolerance test after a 14-day period
of parenteral thiamine therapy. If the high pyruvate level found
at the first test is restored to normal following such therapy it is
likely that the patient was thiamine-deficient prior to therapy.

The discovery of the function of thiamine as a co-factor for
transketolase activity had led to blood transketolase estimations
being used as a further test for thiamine deficiency [17, 18, 19,
20].

1.1.3 Alcoholic polyneuritis

Alcoholic polyneuritis has, for long, been held to be due
largely to an associated deficiency of thiamine brought about
by the unbalanced deficient diet consumed by the chronic
alcoholic, together with the chronic gastritis and associated

disturbances of gastro-intestinal function present in such patients.

Elevations of the blood pyruvate level in patients with alcoholic polyneuropathy were described by Beuding and Wortis in 1940 [21], and low levels of thiamine [22] and of thiamine pyrophosphate [23] in this condition were also reported. More recently Fennelly, Frank, Baker and Leevy [24] described the circulating levels of thiamine and of a number of other members of the vitamin B complex in healthy volunteers and in chronic alcoholics with and without evidence of peripheral neuropathy. Although the mean blood thiamine level was reduced in alcoholics without neuropathy, even lower levels were found in the group with neurological involvement. In a small proportion of cases some lowering of the levels of riboflavin, nicotinic acid, pyridoxine, folic acid, pantothenic acid and biotin were observed, but these levels did not, in general, appear to be correlated with the presence of neurological involvement, so that although deficiency of these other vitamins may contribute to the overall clinical picture, it is unlikely that they play a major part in the production of the neuropathy.

1.2 DIABETIC POLYNEUROPATHY

The underlying causes of the nervous changes that can occur in patients with diabetes mellitus present a challenge that is still with us. Symptoms of diabetic neuropathy may develop in mild, severe and controlled states of the disease, and with or without accompanying arteriosclerotic lesions.

Conflicting opinions have existed both as regards the nature of the changes that occur and as regards the aetiological factor or factors involved. The primary site of the disorder has for long been a matter of debate, some workers regarding the condition as being primarily a disturbance of the peripheral nerve fibre, and others regarding it as being primarily a neuronal degeneration affecting anterior horn and dorsal root ganglion cells, with secondary changes occurring in the peripheral nerves.

It is known that peripheral nerve conduction is slowed in patients with diabetic neuropathy, a finding which suggests that segmental demyelination is probably occurring [25]. Thomas and Lascelles [26, 27] have made observations on isolated nerve fibres and have obtained convincing evidence of segmental demyelination from which they have concluded that diabetic neuropathy is probably the result of a metabolic disorder of Schwann cells.

Turning to the aetiology of the condition, the three main hypotheses have been those of degenerative vascular disease, thiamine deficiency and the disordered metabolism of diabetes mellitus.

Apart from some conflicting therapeutic claims there is, however, little if any, convincing evidence of an associated thiamine deficiency in this condition. Goodhart and Sinclair [28] found that the levels of cocarboxylase in the blood were normal in four out of the five patients studied by them, the fifth patient, in whom a low level was found, being also an alcohol addict. Martin [29] carried out pyruvate tolerance tests following the intravenous injection of pyruvate to a series of diabetic subjects and concluded that pyruvate metabolism was normal. Thompson, Butterfield and Kelsey-Fry [30] reported on the blood pyruvate levels in glucose-insulin tests performed on a series of diabetic patients with and without neuropathy, and found that the levels were no higher in patients with neuropathy than in the other diabetics.

The view that the nerve lesions are the outcome of degenerative atheromatous changes in the vasa nervorum has been one that has been much debated and despite the repeated reports of poor correlation between occlusive vascular disease and neuropathy it would probably be premature to exclude this as a contributory, if not a causative, factor.

The third view, that the neuropathy is the result of a metabolic disturbance occurring in the Schwann cells, is difficult to assess because of our limited knowledge of the details and quantitative aspects of Schwann cell metabolism. It has been claimed that the Schwann cells are responsible for the major part of the resting respiration of peripheral nerve [31], and that the addition of insulin increases the rate of respiration of normal resting nerve *in vitro,* presumably by increasing the rate of glucose utilization [31, 32]. There are, therefore, some slight *a priori* grounds for the view that a metabolic disorder of these cells may represent the underlying biochemical lesion responsible for the development of diabetic neuropathy, but more must be known of the metabolism of the Schwann cell both in health and in the diabetic subject before we can safely regard this as the most likely explanation of this important diabetic complication.

1.3 WEST AFRICAN ATAXIC NEUROPATHY

Among the neurological syndromes reported in under-nourished prisoners in the 1939-45 war, a number included a more or less severe peripheral neuropathy. These conditions occurred mainly in tropical and sub-tropical zones and have some similarities with neuropathic disorders occurring endemically in these areas.

Neurological abnormalities are recognized in a number of nutritional syndromes such as beri-beri, pellagra, and in riboflavin deficiency, but since the accompanying malnourishment rarely, if ever, represents a "pure" deficiency of a single factor, the multifactorial character of the nutritional defects is widely acknowledged. Despite several common disease patterns throughout the tropics the degree of clinical variation is relatively wide, and it is, perhaps, just as misguided to equate syndromes which are clinically similar in different regions as it is to assume that one factor, viz.: thiamine or riboflavin deficiency, is the principal cause of peripheral neuropathy in these areas.

For these reasons it would be unwise to extrapolate too readily from the biochemical and nutritional data obtained from one part of Africa to the Caribbean or to Changi prison in Singapore. With these reservations, however, it is worth discussing some findings from Nigeria because of their possible relevance to neurological diseases of multifactorial toxic-nutritional aetiology seen elsewhere.

1.3.1 Historical review

In the last decade, a number of clinical and biochemical studies have been reported of a syndrome including sensory ataxia, optic atrophy and evidence of cord damage. Sensorineural deafness and dementia sometimes occur and are further evidence of what is manifestly a diffuse degenerative disease.

Unfortunately there is a dearth of pathological studies of this condition, but neurophysiological studies and nerve biopsies suggest that there is segmental demyelination of peripheral nerves as well as central components [33].

It has been suggested that this diffuse disease represents part of a spectrum which also includes some patients with visual failure alone—"tropical amblyopia" [34, 35].

This latter malady was studied clinically by Fitzgerald Moore and by Clark in Nigeria during their service as Colonial Medical Officers. Both agreed that the syndrome was seen in conditions of malnourishment, but whereas Moore emphasized that it coexisted with some clinical features of riboflavin deficiency and responded well to "Marmite" [36], Clark recognized that a major dietary component of sufferers was cassava in various forms [37, 38]. Knowing the high concentrations of the cyanogenetic glycoside linamarin that cassava contains, Clark suggested that tropical amblyopia was caused by subacute or chronic cyanide toxicity in patients who, because of their generally malnourished state, were unable to detoxicate it normally.

1.3.2 Recent studies

Epidemiological and biochemical data supporting this hypothesis have been obtained recently in Nigerian patients suffering from the more generalized degenerative disease, of which amblyopia, although prominent, was only a part [34, 35]. These studies also showed that the prevalence of the ataxic neuropathy is much greater and its severity more obvious in areas of very high cassava consumption than in other areas nearby where cassava is not the main source of carbohydrate in the diet. Moreover, there seems to be an occupational hazard, in that people concerned with production, harvesting and preparation of cassava are more commonly affected than others, and family studies [39] suggested that it is the common cooking pot rather than common genes which confers the familial incidence.

Cassava has a large farinaceous tuberous root which contains a high concentration of the cyanogenetic glycoside linamarin in its outer integument. The usual practice is to handle the tuber carefully and thus avoid activating the hydrolase which quickly liberates large amounts of cyanide. The outer skin contains the equivalent of 0.1% HCN as glycoside, whereas the central pulp contains an equivalent of 0.003% HCN [40].

The peeled tuber is steeped and then roasted after grating, and it has been suggested that although this must remove most of the free cyanide, heating also inactivates the hydrolase and may thus stabilize residual glycoside which may then be ingested and metabolized *in vivo* with the liberation of cyanide (Stanton, R.—personal communication).

The first systematic chemical studies of cyanide metabolism were reported in patients with Nigerian ataxic neuropathy [34]. The results obtained contrasted the very high mean concentration of thiocyanate in plasma of patients (12.6 μmoles/100 ml) with very low mean values in both Nigerian hospital controls and normal subjects (2.5 μmoles/100 ml and 2.9 μmoles/100 ml respectively). Similar high mean values (9.3 μmoles/100 ml in non-smokers, 11.6 μmoles/100 ml in smokers) were also found in another Nigerian population studied [35].

It was concluded that these high thiocyanate levels represented detoxicated cyanide or cyanide precursors since this is one of the principal detoxication pathways of cyanide.

1.3.3 Normal cyanide metabolic pathways

Lang demonstrated that an enzyme which he called rhodanese (thiosulphate : cyanide sulphurtransferase, E.C.-2.8.1.1.) accelerates the formation of thiocyanate from cyanide and thiosulphate, liver and kidney homogenates being particularly active [41].

Later studies showed that thiosulphate is derived enzymically from mercaptopyruvate (3-mercaptopyruvate : cyanide sulphurtransferase E.C.2.8.1.2.), the same enzyme also catalysing the formation of thiocyanate directly from cyanide and mercaptopyruvate [42]. Mercaptopyruvate is produced by the deamination of cysteine (Figure 1.1).

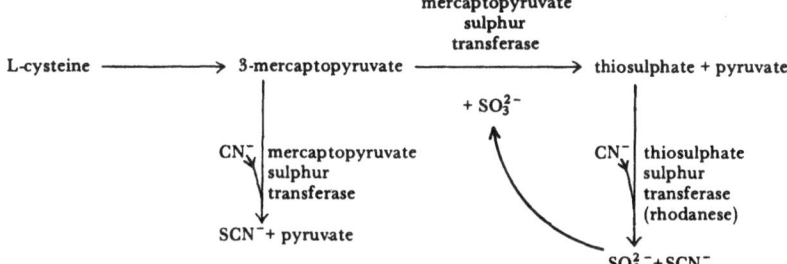

Figure 1.1. Pathways for the conversion of cyanide to thiocyanate.

In addition to that formed by the detoxication of cyanide, there are other sources of thiocyanate in body fluids, e.g. dietary thiocyanate in green vegetables and milk; in Europeans dietary thiocyanate probably accounts for mean plasma concentrations in non-smokers of 5.5 μmoles/100 ml. In healthy non-smoking Nigerians, however, dietary sources of thiocyanate are probably negligible, since Brassicae are not represented.

Although the high plasma concentrations of thiocyanate found in patients with ataxic neuropathy do not suggest a defect in cyanide detoxication, it is possible that the rate of cyanide detoxication may be diminished because of the relative deficiency of sulphur-containing substrate, and it is noteworthy that concentrations of the plasma sulphur-containing amino acids are markedly reduced [43]. In the areas where the disease occurs, there is other evidence of protein-calorie malnutrition, for example kwashiorkor, and animal protein tends to be lacking in the diet. Although other plasma amino acids tend to be low, aspartate levels were found to be contrastingly high in the studies mentioned above, and it has been suggested (Hammerschlag, R.—personal communication) that this not only may reflect an increased rate of transamination in substrate mobilization, but also may depress glutamic acid uptake in the brain, with deleterious effects on neuronal function [44, 45].

1.4 VITAMIN B$_{12}$ METABOLISM IN ATAXIC NEUROPATHY

There are clinical similarities between W. African ataxic neuropathy and subacute combined degeneration but absolute vitamin B_{12} levels in Nigerian patients and controls tend to be considerably higher than in normal European subjects [34], probably because of differences in binding to plasma proteins [46].

Nevertheless, abnormalities of vitamin B_{12} metabolism have been sought because of experimental evidence that vitamin B_{12} and cyanide are linked metabolically, and because of clinical evidence of these metabolic abnormalities in other amblyopic syndromes [47, 48, 49, 50, 51, 52, 53, 54]. The evidence relating cyanide and vitamin B_{12} can be summarized as follows:

The cyano-radical is an integral but labile component of the cyanocobalamin molecule, and studies using ^{14}C-labelled cyanide suggest that vitamin B_{12} may serve as an intermediary whereby the cyanide carbon can be incorporated into the 1-C metabolic pool [47]. The precise mechanism of this incorporation is unknown, but decyanase activity has been identified in liver [55] suggesting that the cyano-radical is removed in its entirety, with formation of hydroxocobalamin. On the other hand, it is possible that cyanocobalamin may be converted to methylcobalamin although this has never been specifically tested.

In normal subjects, there has been demonstrated an inverse relationship between the concentrations of cyanide and total vitamin B_{12}, inviting speculation on conditions that might prevail in vitamin B_{12}-deficient states [49].

With the refined chromatographic techniques now available for the identification of plasma cobalamins, it has been shown that two-thirds of normal subjects do not have any cyanocobalamin in plasma, and the remainder have only traces, most of the vitamin B_{12} being in the forms of hydroxocobalamin, methylcobalamin and 5'-deoxyadenosyl B_{12} ("co-enzyme B_{12}"). The low cyanocobalamin levels may reflect equilibrating mechanisms which prevent the total conversion of vitamin B_{12} to cyanocobalamin which would be expected from the exposure to large amounts of cyanide by tobacco smokers [56].

In another series of experiments, it was shown that normal smokers excrete larger amounts of vitamin B_{12} in the urine than non-smokers, probably because cyanocobalamin has a greater renal clearance than hydroxocobalamin [51].

Abnormalities suggestive of deranged cyanide and vitamin B_{12} metabolism have been demonstrated in Leber's disease (hereditary optic atrophy) and in dominantly inherited optic atrophy, and consist of significant elevations of plasma cyanocobalamin [56]. Similar changes have been reported in sporadic cases of bilateral optic atrophy occurring in Europeans, and in cases of so-called tobacco amblyopia.

Moreover, in the latter condition the therapeutic superiority of hydroxocobalamin over cyanocobalamin has been demonstrated [50], supporting the earlier suggestion that this condition represents the effects of chronic cyanide toxicity in conditions of relative vitamin B_{12} depletion [57].

As yet only preliminary findings have been reported in Nigerian patients [58], but in these too, despite high total levels of serum B_{12}, abnormally high concentrations of plasma cyanocobalamin have been found, but there is no evidence that the conversion of vitamin B_{12} is other than partial, or that secondary vitamin B_{12} deficiency ensues.

1.4.1 The role of other vitamin deficiencies

The clinical syndrome of beri-beri is seen sporadically in Nigeria, and an aetiological relationship to thiamine deficiency presumed from the therapeutic response to this vitamin. An implied relationship to the W. African ataxic neuropathy is sometimes suggested, but has been rejected because abnormalities of pyruvate metabolism are usually slight [39].

As mentioned earlier, Moore suggested that riboflavin deficiency was, in part, responsible for the occurrence of the syndrome, and certainly riboflavin intake tends to be low because of the limited intake of animal protein. The clinical signs of riboflavin deficiency—angular stomatitis and flexural dermatitis—are almost certainly non-specific effects of depressed tissue oxidation, and could be a direct or an indirect effect of cyanide itself. Although one report [39] suggested that riboflavin deficiency was slight in this area, more refined studies are required to decide whether or not coexisting riboflavin deficiency and delayed cyanide detoxication may not potentiate their adverse effect on neuronal metabolism.

1.5 Subacute Combined Degeneration of the Spinal Cord

The infrequent development of major neurological abnormalities in a small proportion of patients with vitamin B_{12} deficiency is still unexplained.

Early hopes that the identification of abnormalities of methyl malonic acid metabolism [59] might provide a clue to the pathogenesis of subacute combined degeneration have been unfulfilled, because similar abnormalities of methyl malonic acid and short-chain fatty acid excretion are seen in both uncomplicated pernicious anaemia and in subacute combined degeneration. Defective methylation has also been demonstrated by a reduction in the proportion of methylcobalamin present in plasma in vitamin B_{12}-deficient patients, the changes in patients with subacute combined degeneration being unexceptional [52].

Wilson and Langman suggested on clinical grounds that there was evidence to suggest that smoking was a contributory factor in some cases [60]. Arguing that the plasma studies in normal subjects suggested that in vitamin B_{12} deficiency cyanide levels might be abnormally high, they emphasized the reciprocal relationship between the degree of anaemia and the occurrence of subacute combined degeneration, suggesting that severe anaemia protects the subject from developing neurological complications. Conversely, neurological relapse sometimes follows a haematological remission induced by folate, and the following scheme was proposed:

Under normal conditions, there is an equilibrium between cyanide and thiocyanate in blood dependent on:

(1) The conversion of cyanide to thiocyanate in liver and kidney.
(2) The removal of cyanide to the 1-C metabolic pool by combination with hydroxocobalamin [47].
(3) The reconversion of thiocyanate to cyanide by the action of an enzyme thiocyanate oxidase present in red blood cells [61].

It has been suggested that the equilibrium is upset when vitamin B_{12} is deficient, but that the equilibrium is restored through the reduction in red cell mass as anaemia develops.

Although the separate identity of "thiocyanate oxidase" has

recently been questioned [62] there is evidence that cyanide is generated from thiocyanate by red blood cells, and this hypothesis would provide a neat explanation not only for the "protective" effect of anaemia, but also for the adverse effects of folate, and of tobacco smoking. The relationships are shown diagrammatically in Figure 1.2. Preliminary studies of cyanide concentration in patients with subacute combined degeneration

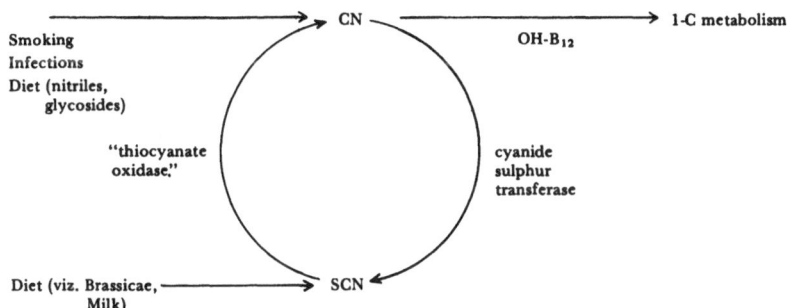

Figure 1.2. Metabolic interrelationships of cyanide, thiocyanate and Vitamin B_{12}.

have failed to substantiate this hypothesis, but it is acknowledged that present techniques of cyanide determination do not differentiate ionized from protein-bound cyanide.

1.6 PORPHYRIA

The porphyrias are a group of diseases in which disturbances of porphyrin metabolism occur either as inherited or acquired abnormalities. They are classified into the so-called erythropoietic and hepatic forms according to the chemical evidence of the primary site of the metabolic defect [63], and it is the second, hepatic group which mainly concerns us here in this discussion on neuropathies.

In three of the hereditary hepatic porphyrias, acute intermittent porphyria, porphyria variegata [64], and hereditary coproporphyria [65, 66] neurological abnormalities are recognized, of varying character and severity, and similar changes are described in a minority of cases of acquired hepatic porphyrias.

TABLE 1.2

Chemical Data in the Porphyrias[a]

(after Levere and Kappas [67])

Condition	Inheritance	Age of clinical onset	Organ primarily involved	Compounds[b] in urine per day	Compounds[b] excreted per gram of faeces (dry wt.)	Compounds[b] per 100 ml of red blood cells	Clinical
Normal	—	—	—	URO (15-30 µg) I > III; COPRO (60-250 µg) I > III; PBG-(< 2 mg); ALA-(< 3 mg)	COPRO I (~7 µg); PROTO IX (~23 µg)	COPRO I (1-2 µg); PROTO (10-60 µg)	—
Congenital erythro-poietic porphyria	Recessive	Birth to 5 years	Erythro-poietic	URO I, 3+ (~100 mg); COPRO I, 2+ (~10 mg)	URO, 2+ (~2 mg) I ≥ III; COPRO, 3+ (~130 mg) I > III	URO I, 3+; COPRO I, 2+; PROTO-N, to 1+	Severe photo-sensitivity
Erythro-poietic proto-porphyria	Dominant	Usually childhood	Erythro-poietic	URO III, N; COPRO III, (2+ (~500 µg))	PROTO-N; COPRO III 2+ (20-80 µg); PROTO- 2+ (20-100 µg)	URO-N; COPRO III, N to 1+; PROTO, 2 to 3+	Moderately severe photo-sensitivity
Acute inter-mittent porphyria	Dominant	15-40 years	Liver	Acute phase PBG, 3+ (40-200 mg); ALA, 2+ (20-40 mg); Remission PBG-N to 1+	Acute phase porphyrins, N to 1+; Remission, N	N	Neurological and psychiatric abnormalities. No cutaneous problems

Congenital cutaneous hepatic porphyrias	Dominant	20-50 years	Liver	(~20 mg) Acute phase PBG, 1 to 3+ (~20-200 mg) ALA, 1 to 2+ (~8-64 mg) URO 1 and III, N to 2+; COPRO, variable Remission PBG and ALA-N Porphyrins, N to 1+	Acute phase URO III-1 to 3+ COPRO III-2 to 3+ (~650 μg) PROTO-2 to 3+ (~900 μg) Remission URO III, 1 to 2+ COPRO III, 1 to 3+ (~400 μg) PROTO, 1 to 3+ (~650 μg)	N	Photosensitivity of varying severity. Neurological abnormalities unusual, but can occur— rarely severe
Hereditary copro-porphyria	Recessive	20-50 years	Liver	COPRO 2+ ALA, PBG URO, PROTO N or +	COPRO 2+	N	Cutaneous and neurological abnormalities of varying severity
Acquired hepatic porphyria	Acquired	—	Liver	ALA, N to 2+ (1-47 mg) PBG, N to 1+ (3-16 mg) COPRO, 2+ (1-2 mg) URO-1 to 3+ (up to 2.5 mg)	COPRO, 1 to 2+ PROTO, N to 2+	N	Photosensitivity of varying severity. Neurological involvement rare.

[a]N, normal amount; 1+, slightly increased amount; 2+, moderately increased amount; 3+, markedly increased amount.
[b]Porphyrins are expressed as total of porphyrins and porphyrinogens.

All of these conditions can be identified and differentiated by the estimation of urinary and faecal excretion of porphyrins, and comparative chemical data with salient clinico-pathological features are presented in Table 1.2.

For the neurologist, the main interest lies in acute intermittent porphyria in which psychotic features coexist with an acute or subacute peripheral neuropathy and abdominal pain. Similar features are less frequent and severe in the other forms of hepatic porphyria, both inherited and acquired.

1.6.1 Normal porphyrin synthesis

Before discussing the biochemical abnormalities in acute intermittent porphyria, present knowledge of normal porphyrin synthesis and utilization will be summarized. It is shown schematically in Figure 1.3, and has been well reviewed recently [67].

The classical studies of Shemin [68, 69] identified glycine as one of the precursors of haem, and led to the discovery that glycine and succinyl-coenzyme A are substrates for the enzymic synthesis of δ-aminolaevulinic acid (ALA). The mitochondrial enzyme concerned, ALA-synthetase, is present in both liver and in red cell precursors [70, 71] and requires the presence of pyridoxal phosphate [72].

The enzyme porphobilinogen synthetase is widespread in animal and plant tissues [73, 74] and is activated by sulphydryl compounds. It condenses two molecules of ALA to form the monopyrrole porphobilinogen (PBG) [75].

A succession of enzymically controlled steps leads to the formation sequentially of the tetrapyrrole isomers uroporphyrinogen I, uroporphyrinogen III, coproporphyrinogen III, and protoporphyrin IX, and finally ferrous iron is introduced into the molecule to yield haem.

1.6.2 Excretion of porphyrins

Under normal conditions mainly coproporphyrin I is excreted in the urine, with small amounts of uroporphyrin I, the total amounting to up to 200 μg per day [76, 77, 78], while the faeces contain an average of 23.5 μg protoporphyrin per g

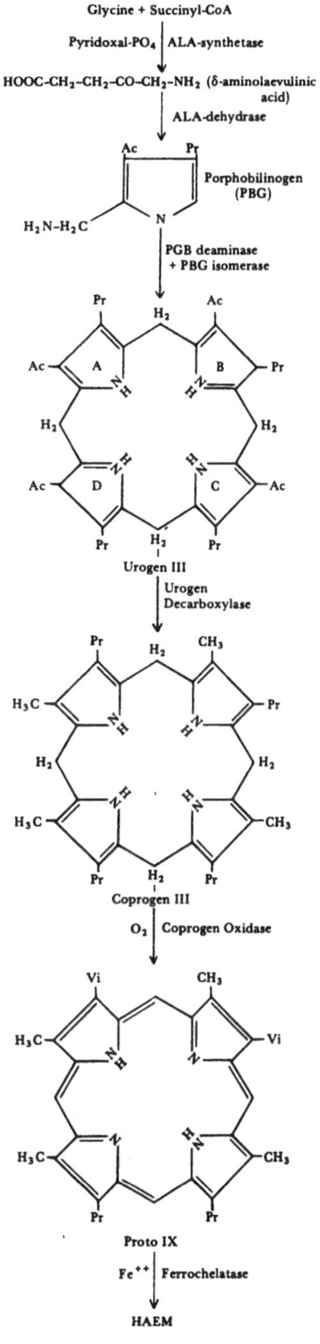

Glycine + Succinyl-CoA

Pyridoxal-PO$_4$ | ALA-synthetase

HOOC-CH$_2$-CH$_2$-CO-CH$_2$-NH$_2$ (δ-aminolaevulinic acid)

ALA-dehydrase

Ac   Pr

Porphobilinogen (PBG)

H$_2$N-H$_2$C   N

PGB deaminase + PBG isomerase

Urogen III

Urogen Decarboxylase

Coprogen III

O$_2$ | Coprogen Oxidase

Proto IX

Fe^{++} | Ferrochelatase

HAEM

Figure 1.3 Porphyrin synthesis. ALA = δ aminolaevulinic acid; PBG = porphobilinogen; Urogen = uroporphyrinogen; Coprogen = coproporphyrinogen; Proto = protoporphyrin; Ac = CH$_2$, COOH; Pr = CH$_2$, CH$_2$ —COOH; Vi = —CH = CH$_2$.

and 3.9 μg coproporphyrin per g [79]. Deuteroporphyrin, which is also present, is probably produced by the action of gut bacteria on porphyrins and haem. Although under normal circumstances most of these compounds are the end-products of endogenous metabolism, some apparently are derivatives of chlorophyll ingested in vegetables.

1.6.3 The metabolic abnormalities in porphyria

With the recognition that there is abnormal excretion of certain porphyrins in the hereditary porphyrias it was assumed that as in other metabolic errors, the abnormalities resulted from an enzyme block either in an associated pathway diverting more substrate to porphyrin synthesis or in porphyrin utilization leading to an accumulation of metabolic precursors. However, further observations showed that neither of these hypotheses was tenable.

Urata and Granick [70] demonstrated that in experimental porphyria induced in guinea pigs with 3,5-dicarbethoxydihydro-collidine, the only demonstrable abnormality among the porphyrin-synthesizing enzymes was a considerable increase in ALA-synthetase activity, an observation which has been repeatedly confirmed using other agents.

Later experiments with tissue cultures showed how substances producing porphyria in experimental animals could induce ALA-synthetase formation *de novo* [80, 81].

It seems likely that under normal conditions there is a mechanism for repression of this enzyme induction, and it has indeed been shown that haem and other metal-containing porphyrins repress ALA-synthetase induction in foetal liver cells [82].

This is the first example to be recognized of a genetically determined metabolic abnormality which is characterized by an *overproduction* of an enzyme. Granick [83] has proposed that the inherited defect resides in the operator of the structural gene for ALA-synthetase [84, 85].

The extrapolation to naturally occurring maladies of the experimental studies on which these hypotheses are based is justified, for example, by the demonstration of an increase of hepatic ALA-synthetase activity of seven times in a patient with acute intermittent porphyria [86]. Similar findings have been reported in other forms of porphyria [87, 88], and it is reasonable to conclude that this defect is present in red cell precursors in the erythropoietic forms, and in liver parenchyma in the hepatic forms.

The differing clinical and biochemical features of the various forms of porphyria could depend on which of the other enzymes concerned with porphyria biosynthesis are rate-limiting. For example, in acute intermittent porphyria, in which excretions of ALA and PBG are very much increased during acute episodes, PBG-deaminase may become rate-limiting as a result of increased ALA and PBG synthesis.

A scheme incorporating these features as proposed by Granick and Levere [84] is shown in Figure 1.4. Although the pathogenesis of the neurological abnormalities is not yet known, the correlation between certain clinical phenomena and experimental biochemical observations is striking. For example, it is almost unknown for attacks of acute intermittent porphyria to occur before puberty and they usually become less frequent in middle life, suggesting an endocrine component, a view which is supported by the observation that attacks are more common in women, and sometimes occur cyclically in relation to menstruation. These clinical observations are paralleled by the studies of Granick and Kappas [89] who have shown that a number of 5β-H steroids of the C_{19} and C_{21} series are potent inducers of ALA-synthetase activity in liver cell culture, and excessive urinary excretion of porphyrinogenic steroids in acute intermittent porphyria has been demonstrated [90]. Contraceptive steroids may have a similar effect clinically and experimentally [91, 92, 93].

In a clinical study it has been emphasized not only how the decreased food intake in for example slimming, induced attacks in 11% of patients with acute intermittent porphyria, but they also demonstrated how the urinary output of porphyrin precursors varied inversely with the amount of carbohydrate and protein in the diet [94]. The inhibitory effect of carbohydrate feeding on ALA-synthetase induction has also been demonstrated experimentally [95, 96, 97].

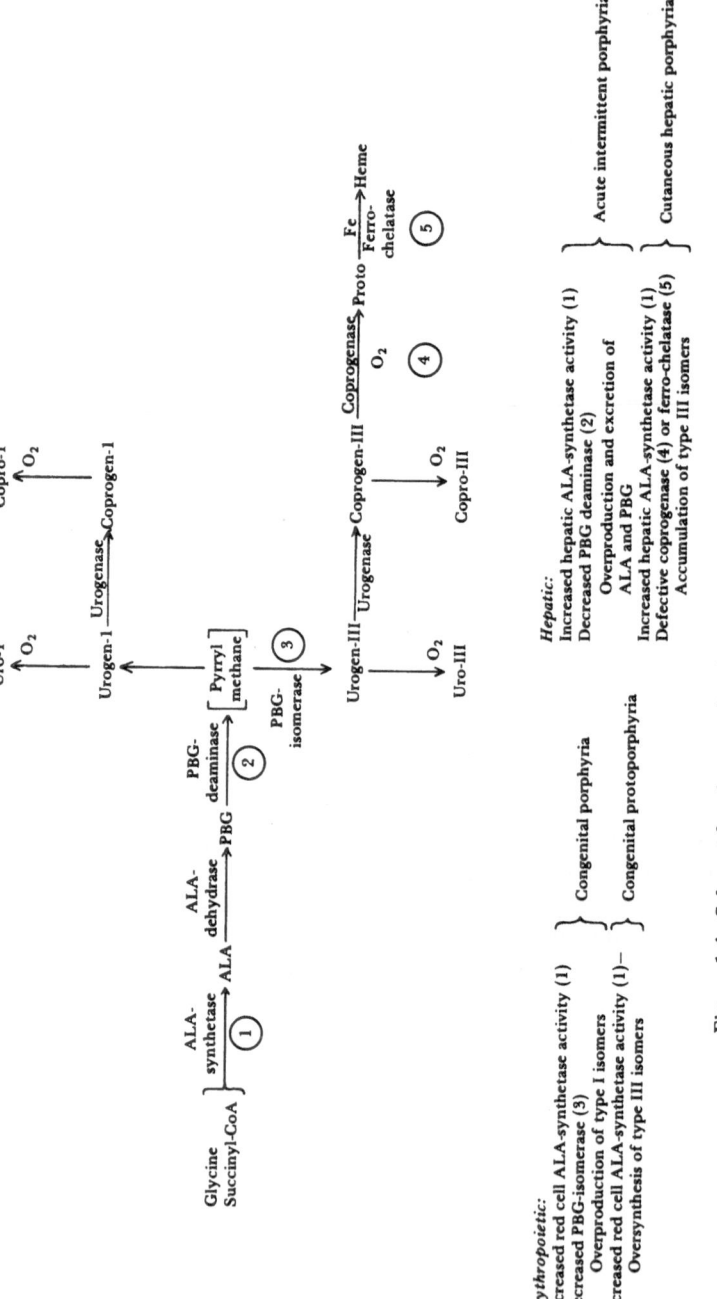

Figure 1.4. Scheme for the postulated enzymic lesions in the porphyrias (from Granick and Levere [84]).

1.6.4 Laboratory findings in acute intermittent porphyria

During an acute attack large amounts of ALA and PBG are excreted in the urine, together with a moderate increase in uroporphyrin. The presence of PBG can be easily demonstrated by the addition of Erhlich's aldehyde reagent, the red complex formed being insoluble in n-butanol (now used in preference to chloroform). The red colour which forms spontaneously in the urine of patients with acute intermittent porphyria during an attack is due to the formation of porphobilin and porphyrins from the spontaneous condensation of PBG. Faecal porphyrins are usually normal, or only very slightly elevated.

The liver, but not erythropoietic tissue, contains large amounts of PBG, and there is evidence of hepatocellular dysfunction in a proportion of patients; abnormal bromsulphthalein retention due to defective conjugation and excretion is occasionally seen [94], but elevation of serum bilirubin and alkaline phosphatase are more common.

An acute attack may be accompanied by hyponatraemia, hypochloraemia and oliguria, and this is almost certainly due to inappropriate antidiuretic hormone secretion [98, 99, 100, 101] which may also account for the hypomagnesaemia which has also been described [101, 102].

Increased levels of protein-bound iodine and thyroxine have been reported [103, 104], but their significance is not yet known.

The role of pyridoxal phosphate, the co-factor for ALA synthetase activity in the pathogenesis of peripheral neuropathy, has been extensively discussed. Although clinically the neuropathy of porphyria is different from that of pyridoxine deficiency [105], it has been suggested that an acute deficiency of vitamin B_6 might be the precipitating factor in the development of neuropathy in porphyrias [106]. Earlier studies [107] had shown that deliberate reduction of vitamin B_6 intake in a patient with porphyria in remission resulted in a reduction in urinary ALA and PBG, and although the experiment had to be terminated when the patient developed retrobulbar neuritis, there was no evidence of peripheral neuropathy. Later studies such as those of Hamfelt and Wetterberg [108] showed that although there was some evidence of incipient pyridoxal deficiency in their series of 21 patients, there was no correlation between plasma pyridoxal levels and clinical findings, and vitamin B_6 administration did not have any obvious therapeutic benefit.

The adverse effects of certain drugs, barbiturates, sulphonamides, alcohol excess, and phenytoin are well recognized, and probably act through the induction of ALA synthetase activity; prophylactic advice in known families is, therefore, essential. As mentioned in the Introduction, this is a good example of the gap between the characterization of the underlying biochemical defect and our understanding of pathogenesis, but it is to be hoped that just as the careful study of patients with these rare conditions has considerably advanced our understanding of normal biochemical mechanisms, so the further study of the neurological abnormalities will advance our neurobiological understanding.

1.7 POLYNEUROPATHY DUE TO ORGANO-PHOSPHORUS COMPOUNDS

The delayed neurotoxic action of a number of organo-phosphorus compounds is now well recognized. The earliest reported example of nerve damage caused by compounds of this type to be extensively investigated was the outbreak of a severe motor neuritis in the United States in 1930, which was shown to have been produced by the drinking of a beverage containing triorthocresylphosphate (TOCP), present as an adulterant [109, 110]. Numerous other outbreaks of polyneuropathy due to the ingestion of this compound have since been described.

A very similar delayed polyneuropathy has also been reported following intoxication by certain of the organo-phosphorus anti-cholinesterase compounds which have been studied because of their potential insecticidal activity. In 1953 for example a detailed report appeared of two cases following poisoning by mipafox (N,N'-di-isopropylphosphorodiamidic (fluoride)) [111]. Barnes and Denz [112] succeeded in producing delayed neurotoxic effect in hens after the administration of single doses of either mipafox, DFP (di-isopropylphosphorofluoridate) or TOCP, and both they and Cavanagh [113] have described the pathology of the lesions. In the experimentally induced condition in the hen these neurotoxic effects manifest themselves clinically as an ataxia coming on after 10 to 14 days, and histologically as a degeneration of both axis cylinders and myelin sheaths, i.e. as a dying-back process of certain of the long axons in both the central nervous system and the peripheral nerves.

Compounds that produce these delayed neurotoxic effects are all esters of phosphorus-containing acids, and they are all inhibitors of esterases, including cholinesterases, or are converted *in vivo* into inhibitors of these enzymes [114], but not all organo-phosphorus inhibitors of esterases are neurotoxic. Examples of some of these neurotoxic compounds are shown in Figure 1.5. It should be pointed out, however, that TOCP itself is not the neurotoxic principle, but first undergoes conversion *in vivo* into a neurotoxic metabolite [115].

The interactions of organo-phosphorus compounds such as DFP and related substances with esterases have been most fully worked out in relation to the cholinesterases, and it is clear that the early, acute phases of intoxication by these compounds are associated with a profound inhibition of cholinesterase activity. Inhibition of these enzymes is thought to be the result of the phosphorylation of the enzyme protein by the toxic agent:

$$\text{Enz} + \text{PX} \rightleftharpoons (\text{Enz} \ldots \text{PX}) \rightarrow \text{Enz} -\text{P} + \text{X}.$$

The enzyme reacts with the agent, PX, as if it was an ester substrate, to form the stable, phosphorylated enzyme, Enz $-$P, liberating the group X. Following on the inhibition of this enzyme acetylcholine accumulates at cholinergic nerve-endings, and the acute symptoms of intoxication by these anti-cholinesterase organo-phosphorus compounds can, therefore, in mild cases, be relieved by the injection of atropine. Re-activation of the inhibited cholinesterase can also be brought about by certain oximes such as pralidoxime which are, therefore, also of therapeutic value in the relief of the acute cholinergic effects.

When we turn, however, to the delayed neurotoxic effects of these organo-phosphorus compounds the position is more complex since not all esterase inhibitors of this type are neurotoxic. It would seem, therefore, that cholinesterase

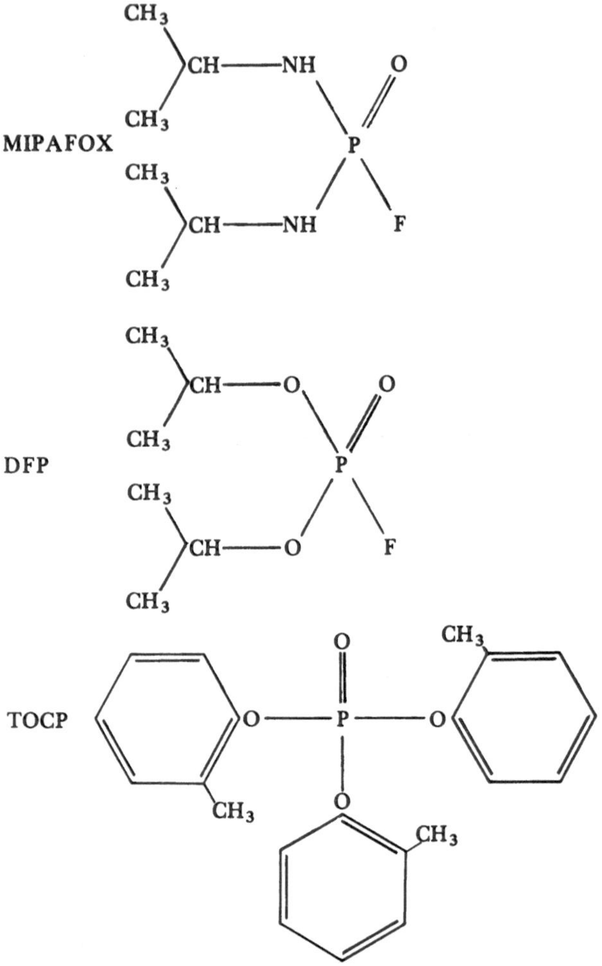

Figure 1.5. Structures of some neurotoxic organo-phosphorus compounds.

inhibition *per se* cannot account for these delayed changes in the nervous system. In recent years Johnson has investigated this problem in detail, and has shown that the nervous system contains an enzyme which he has called the "neurotoxic esterase". He has further shown that neurotoxicity can be correlated with phosphorylation of this enzyme, with consequent loss of activity, but that the "neurotoxic effect is a result of phosphorylation as such and not a consequence of prolonged deficiency of the esterase activity" [116].

1.8 REFSUM'S DISEASE (HEREDOPATHIA ATACTICA POLYNEURITIFORMIS)

Hereditary ataxic polyneuropathy is a rare but well-recognized genetically determined degenerative disease characterized by hemeralopia with atypical retinitis pigmentosa, peripheral neuropathy, gross ataxia, deafness and ichthyosis, first described by Refsum in 1945, and amplified by an English-language account in the following year [117, 118]. Electrocardiographic abnormalities are common and sudden death may result from cardiac involvement.

Klenk and Kahlke [119] discovered that patients with Refsum's disease accumulate large amounts of a branched-chain fatty acid (3, 7, 11, 15-tetramethylhexadecanoic acid, phytanic acid) (Figure 1.6) in serum and in tissues, identifying the condition as another lipid-storage disease.

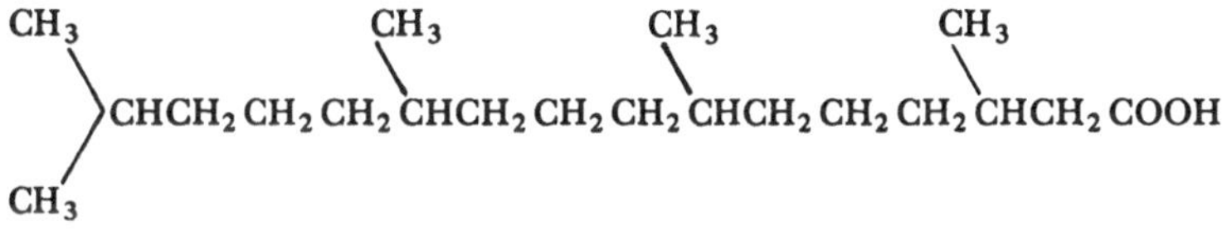

$$CH_3 \quad CH_3 \quad CH_3 \quad CH_3$$
$$CH_3\big\rangle CHCH_2\,CH_2\,CH_2\,CHCH_2\,CH_2\,CH_2\,CHCH_2\,CH_2\,CH_2\,CHCH_2\,COOH$$

Figure 1.6. 3, 7, 11, 15-tetramethylhexadecanoic acid (phytanic acid)

These observations have been confirmed in a number of other patients [120, 121, 122] but it has recently been suggested that there may be another disease clinically similar to Refsum's in which phytanic acid does not apparently accumulate (Gumbinas, M., 1970—personal communication).

In patient's with Refsum's disease, phytanic acid is deposited in large amounts in liver and kidneys [119, 123] and in heart, but not in brain [124]. Although it was recognized that phytanic acid is a normal metabolite, it was concluded that there must be an enzymic basis for its relatively enormous visceral accumulation.

Two possibilities have been investigated:
(1) that phytanic acid is synthesized endogenously in abnormally large amounts, and
(2) that the assimilated fatty acid is not degraded.

Thanks to the important systematic studies of Steinberg's group at the National Institutes of Health, Bethesda, in collaboration with Norwegian workers, the metabolic abnormality has been elucidated, and their observations will be briefly outlined.

Concerning the first possibility, there is a theoretical metabolic pathway by which phytanic acid could be

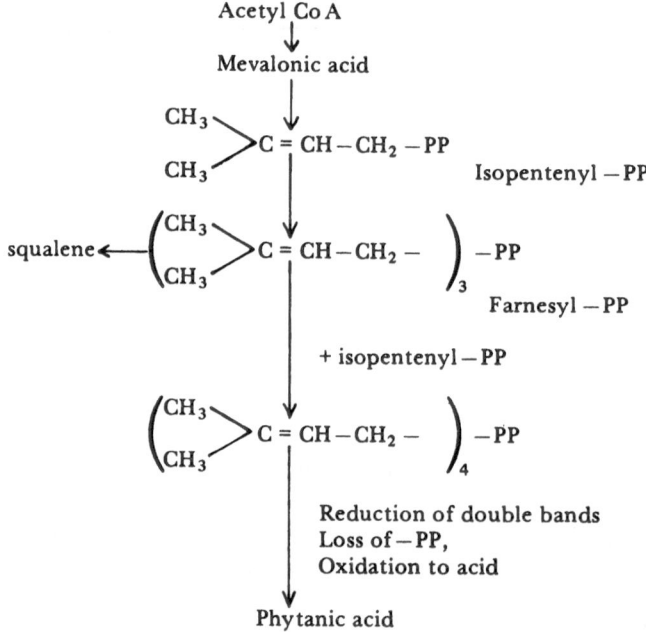

Figure 1.7. Possible biosynthetic pathway of phytanic acid from Acetyl CoA.

synthesized endogenously from simple precursors as shown in Figure 1.7.

Structurally, phytanic acid is related to farnesyl pyrophosphate, a precursor of steroid biosynthesis. If a molecule of farnesyl pyrophosphate, formed by the condensation of three molecules of isopentenyl pyrophosphate condensed with a fourth molecule of isopentenyl pyrophosphate, geranyl-geranylpyrophosphate (GGPP) would be produced, a reaction which has been shown to occur in pig liver [125]. The formation of phytanic acid from GGPP is then a relatively simple matter, involving oxidation and removal of pyrophosphate.

The possible contribution of this pathway to phytanic acid synthesis in Refsum's disease was investigated in a Norwegian patient who was given 25 μc mevalonic acid-2-^{14}C intravenously. Although there was normal uptake of radioactivity into plasma cholesterol there was little radioactivity in the plasma fatty acids, suggesting that if any biosynthesis of phytanic acid occurred, it must be at a very slow rate. Confirmation was provided by extended studies of the uptake of deuterium oxide over four months in the same patient. Although after this time 91% of the expected equilibration occurred between body water and cholesterol, there was minimal incorporation of deuterium in the phytanic acid, and this occurred unevenly, mainly concentrated in the first three carbon atoms of the molecule [121, 126, 127, 128].

Subsequently it has been convincingly demonstrated that the primary metabolic lesion is in the degradative pathway of phytanic acid, and not on the synthetic chain.

In considering the results of studies of oxidative metabolism of phytanic acid it must be recognized that the presence of a methyl group in the β position effectively prevents degradation by the normal method of β-oxidation.

Eldjarn [121] and his colleagues [129] considered first the possibility that ω-oxidation, i.e. step-wise degradation from the opposite end of the molecule, might be blocked in Refsum's disease. Their early results did indeed suggest that there was such a defect; they showed that in patients with Refsum's disease there was a reduction in the excretion of sebacic acid (αC_{10}-dicarboxylic acid) after a loading dose of tricaprin [121]. However, these preliminary results were of uncertain significance because their patients did not show defects in ω-oxidation of other substrates [130]. Later they showed that in patients whose serum phytanic acid was reduced by dietary treatment, the tricaprin test became normal [131], and in fact there is no direct evidence that ω-oxidation is of importance in phytanic acid metabolism.

Instead, from Steinberg's laboratory has come convincing evidence of the importance of α-oxidation of phytanic acid in normal subjects and their results point to a defect in this degradative pathway in patients [131], which has since been well reviewed [133].

Using fibroblast cultures, the metabolic pathways have been delineated more clearly [134, 135]. In control cells it has been confirmed that the major pathway of phytanate degradation is by α-oxidation initially, followed by successive β-oxidation steps shown diagrammatically in Figure 1.8. Cultured fibroblasts from skin biopsies of patients did not contain elevated levels of phytanic acid, but the rate of ^{14}C-phytanate oxidation was less than 3% of that seen in cells from normal controls. Nevertheless, these cells were able to oxidize pristanic acid, the η-1 homologue of phytanic acid at normal, or near-normal rates.

Interestingly, cell cultures from eight heterozygotes oxidized phytanic acid at a rate approximately half that in controls, providing elegant support for genetic theory at cellular level.

These findings disclose what seems to be the site of a primary enzymic defect underlying the disease, but do not indicate the pathogenetic mechanisms. These are still largely a matter for speculation, but there is some biochemical evidence suggesting that a defect in myelin formation and structure does not cause the recurrent segmental demyelination which gives the distinctive "onion skin" hypertrophic interstitial neuropathy of peripheral nerves. Most of the chemical changes in nervous tissue described by MacBrinn and O'Brien [136] were those of severe demyelination rather than of abnormal myelin synthesis. It is possible that as in metachromatic and globoid (cell) leucodystrophy segmental demyelination could result from focal disturbances of glial function arising from the disrupting physico-chemical effects of phytanic acid accumulation.

From the therapeutic standpoint, the most promising development has been the recognition that most, if not all, phytanic acid accumulating in patients with Refsum's disease is of exogenous, dietary origin [129, 133]. It occurs naturally in various dairy products [137, 138, 139] and its precursor phytol occurs in chlorophyll. Most dietary experiments have strictly limited the amounts of chlorophyll phytol ingested, but

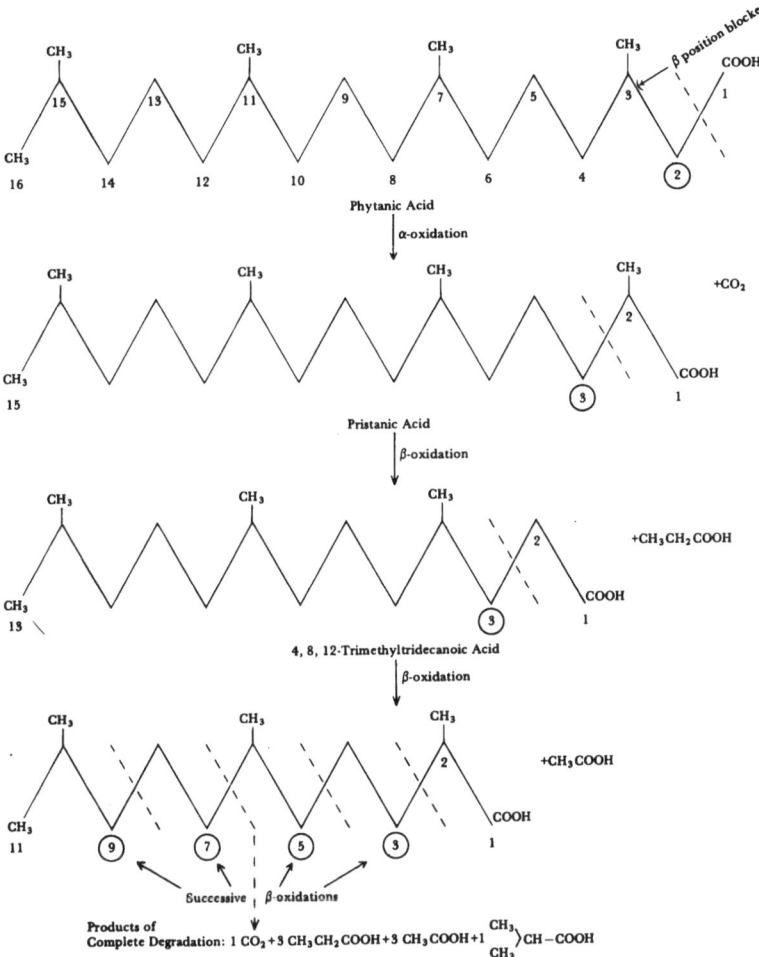

Figure 1.8. Proposed pathway for degradation of phytanic acid in mammals. The three degradation products shown have been identified as products of phytanic acid in animals. The circled locations indicate the methylene groups that are converted to carboxyl groups in each successive oxidative step (after Steinberg et al., [127].

Baxter [140] has shown that chlorophyll phytol is hardly absorbed at all, probably because of the stability of the ester linkage [140, 141] and therefore further dietary trials may not require the stringent exclusion of green vegetables, although the possibility of other phytanic acid precursors from vegetable sources has not been excluded.

Several studies have confirmed that restriction of phytanic acid and phytol intake is accompanied not only by a fall in serum phytanic acid concentration, but also by limited clinical and electrophysiological improvement [128, 130, 133]. The steady fall in serum levels of phytanic acid suggests that patients with Refsum's disease can slowly eliminate phytanic acid, although the mechanism is as yet undetermined.

Unfortunately since two of the most incapacitating problems, poor vision and deafness, have not so far improved on treatment one suspects that tissue damage is irremediable, and prophylactic dietary measures begun in the pre-morbid phase offer the best hope of avoiding these severe clinical manifestations.

One puzzling and unexplained facet of the disease is the wide clinical variation which exists, particularly in respect of age of presentation. Although it is customary to explain such variation in genetic terms, it is also possible to explain it on the basis of exogenous, i.e. dietary, variation.

In recognizing that phytanic acid can occur in diastereomeric forms, it has been pointed out that although asymmetries exist at the 3,7 and 11 carbon atoms, it is likely that naturally occurring material has methyl groups in the D-configuration at the 7- and 11-positions, and both L- and D-forms at position 3 [142]. In patients with Refsum's disease, both LDD and DDD forms accumulate in widely varying proportions in different patients. Curiously, the slow degradation of phytanic acid which occurs even in these patients removes the two forms at similar rates despite the different kinetics of several acyl activating systems and acyl transferases for the respective isomers present in serum. It has also been suggested that differences in distribution of the DDD and LDD isomers may be of pathogenetic significance and could account for part at least of the clinical variation [142].

1.9 HYPERTROPHIC INTERSTITIAL NEUROPATHY

Although the names of Déjèrine and Sottas are linked in a clinically and pathologically well-defined genetically determined disease in which hypertrophic interstitial neuropathy is an outstanding finding, this distinctive pathological abnormality is now considered to represent a non-specific response to repeated segmental demyelination, and the typical microscopic appearance is seen in other conditions, e.g. Refsum's disease.

It is somewhat difficult to be sure of the precise diagnostic criteria included in some published reports, but since some at least of the reported conditions are genetically determined, it is reasonable to assume that they may be the clinical expression of inborn metabolic errors, as in Refsum's disease. There have been at least two reports describing abnormalities of pyruvate metabolism in Déjèrine-Sottas disease [143, 144]. The latter authors concluded that at least in some of their patients abnormal pyruvate tolerance was secondary to dietary thiamine deficiency.

More recently Dyck and his colleagues [145] have reported lipid abnormalities in peripheral nerve in patients apparently suffering from Déjèrine-Sottas disease. Although they acknowledge that the marked decrease in cerebroside concentration in peripheral nerve could be secondary to demyelination, the relative preservation of sulphatide concentrations seems to be anomalous. Because there is a marked increase in ceramide monohexoside sulphates and decrease of ceramide dihexoside sulphates in the liver of one patient, the same authors suggested that there may be a systemic defect in ceramide hexoside and ceramide hexoside sulphate metabolism. Obviously there must be caution in the interpretation of chemical abnormalities in liver obtained terminally in an illness characterized in inanition, but these findings are interesting especially since an underlying metabolic defect is presumed to exist because of its hereditary nature.

REFERENCES

1. J. B. Cavanagh (ed.), G. Payling Wright and W. St. C. Symmers, Systemic Pathology, Vol. 2, p. 1299, Longmans Green & Co. (1966)
2. K. Takaki, Lancet, i, 1369, 1451, 1520 (1906)
3. C. Eijkmann, Virchows Archiv. Path. Anat., 149, 1504 (1897)
4. R. R. Williams and J. K. Cline, J. Amer. Chem. Soc., 75, 1009 (1936)

5. R. A. Peters, *Lancet*, i, 1161 (1936)
6. D. L. Horecker and P. Z. Smyrniotis, *J. Amer. Chem. Soc.*, 75, 1009 (1953)
7. E. Racker, G. de la Haba and I. G. Leder, *J. Amer. Chem. Soc.*, 75, 1010 (1953)
8. R. H. S. Thompson and R. E. Johnson, *Biochem. J.*, 29, 694 (1935)
9. B. S. Platt and G. D. Lu, *Biochem. J.*, 33, 1525 (1939)
10. R. D. Williams, H. L. Mason, M. H. Power and R. M. Wilder, *Arch. Intern. Med.*, 71, 38 (1943)
11. C. L. Joiner, R. H. S. Thompson and B. McArdle, *Brain*, 73, 431 (1950)
12. R. A. Peters, H. M. Sinclair and R. H. S. Thompson, *Biochem. J.*, 40, 516 (1946)
13. R. H. S. Thompson and V. P. Whittaker, *Biochem. J.*, 41, 342 (1947)
14. L. A. Stocken and R. H. S. Thompson, *Biochem. J.*, 40, 535 (1946)
15. R. Ross and E. S. Reynolds, *Brit. med. J.*, 2, 979 (1901)
16. R. M. Buckle, *Proc. Roy. Soc. Med.*, 60, 48 (1967)
17. S. J. Wolfe, M. Brin and C. S. Davidson, *J. clin. Invest.*, 37, 1467 (1958)
18. P. M. Dreyfus, *New Engl. J. Med.*, 267, 596 (1962)
19. P. M. Dreyfus, *in* Thiamine Deficiency (G. E. W. Wolstenholme and M. O'Connor, eds), p. 103, Churchill, London (1967)
20. M. Brin, *Ann. N.Y. Acad. Sci.*, 98, 528 (1962)
21. E. Bueding and H. Wortis, *Proc. Soc. exp. Biol.* (N.Y.), 44, 245 (1940)
22. H. M. Sinclair, C. R. IIIme Congrs. Neurol. Internat. Copenhagen, p. 885 (1939)
23. R. Goodhart and H. M. Sinclair, C. R. IIIme Congrs. Neurol. Internat. Copenhagen, p. 885 (1939)
24. J. Fennelly, O. Frank, H. Baker and C. M. Leevy, *Brit. med. J.*, 2, 1290 (1964)
25. R. W. Gilliatt *in* Biochemical Aspects of Neurological Disorders (J. N. Cumings and M. Kremer, eds), p. 117, Blackwell Scientific Publications, Oxford (1965)
26. P. K. Thomas and R. G. Lascelles, *Lancet*, i, 1355 (1965)
27. P. K. Thomas and R. G. Lascelles, *Quart. J. Med.*, 35, 489 (1966)
28. R. Goodhart and H. M. Sinclair, *J. biol. Chem.*, 132, 11 (1940)
29. M. M. Martin, *Brain*, 76, 594 (1953)
30. R. H. S. Thompson, W. J. H. Butterfield and I. Kelsey-Fry, *Proc. Roy. Soc. Med.*, 53, 149 (1960)
31. I. H. Heller and S. Hesse, *Exp. Neurol.*, 1, 117 (1959)
32. R. A. Field and L. C. Adams, *Medicine (Baltimore)*, 43, 275 (1964)
33. A. O. Williams and B. O. Osuntokun, *Archs. Neurol* (Chicago), 21, 475 (1969)
34. G. L. Monekosso and J. Wilson, *Lancet*, i, 1062 (1966)
35. B. O. Osuntokun, G. L. Monekosso and J. Wilson, *Brit. med. J.*, 1, 547 (1969)
36. D. G. F. Moore, *W. Afr. med. J.*, 9, 35 (1937)

37. A. Clark, *J. trop. Med. Hyg.*, 39, 269 (1936)
38. A. Clark, *J. trop. Med. Hyg.*, 39, 285 (1936)
39. B. O. Osuntokun, *Brain*, 91, 215 (1968)
40. H. M. Sinclair and D. B. Jelliffe, Tropical nutrition and dietetics, 4th ed. Baillière, Tindall & Cassell, London (1961)
41. K. Lang, *Biochem. Z.*, 259, 243 (1933)
42. H. Fiedler and J. L. Wood, *J. biol. Chem.*, 222, 387 (1956)
43. B. O. Osuntokun, J. E. Durowoju, H. McFarlane and J. Wilson, *Brit. med. J.*, 3, 647 (1968)
44. Y. Tsukada, Y. Nagata, S. Hirano and T. Matsutani, *J. Neurochem.*, 10, 241 (1963)
45. R. Blasberg and A. Lajtha, *Brain Res.*, 1, 86 (1966)
46. A. F. Fleming, *W. Afr. med. J.*, 17, 25 (1968)
47. G. E. Boxer and J. C. Rickards, *Archs. Biochem.*, 39, 7 (1952)
48. J. M. Heaton, A. J. A. McCormick and A. G. Freeman, *Lancet*, ii, 286 (1958)
49. J. Wilson and D. M. Matthews, *Clin. Sci.*, 31, 1 (1966)
50. I. A. Chisholm, J. Bronte-Stewart and W. S. Foulds, *Lancet*, ii, 450 (1967)
51. J. C. Linnell, A. D. M. Smith, C. L. Smith, J. Wilson and D. M. Matthews, *Brit. med. J.*, 2, 215 (1968)
52. J. C. Linnell, H. M. Mackenzie, J. Wilson and D. M. Matthews, *J. clin. Path.*, 22, 545 (1969)
53. E. J. Watson-Williams, A. C. Bottomley, R. G. Ainley and C. I. Phillips, *Brit. J. Ophthal.*, 53, 549 (1969)
54. D. M. Matthews and J. Wilson, The Cobalamins, Churchill, London (1971)
55. P. Reizenstein, *Blood*, 29, 494 (1967)
56. J. Wilson, J. C. Linnell and D. M. Matthews, *Lancet*, i, 259 (1971)
57. F. Wokes, *Lancet*, ii, 526 (1958)
58. B. O. Osuntokun, Ph.D. Thesis, University of Ibadan (1969)
59. E. V. Cox and A. M. White, *Lancet*, ii, 853 (1962)
60. J. Wilson and M. J. S. Langman, *Nature (Lond.)*, 212, 787 (1966)
61. F. Goldstein and F. Rieders, *Am. J. Physiol.*, 167, 47 (1951), and 173, 287 (1953)
62. J. Chung and J. L. Wood, *J. biol. Chem.*, 246, 555 (1971)
63. R. Schmid, S. Schwartz and C. J. Watson, *A.M.A. Archs. int. Med.*, 93, 167 (1954)
64. G. Dean, *Brit. med. Bull.*, 25, 48 (1969)
65. H. Berger and A. Goldberg, *Brit. med. J.*, 2, 85 (1955)
66. A. Goldberg, C. Rimington and A. C. Lockhead, *Lancet*, i, 632 (1967)
67. R. D. Levere and A. Kappas, *Ann. Rev. Med.*, 18, 325 (1968)
68. D. Shemin, *Harvey Lectures*, 50, 258 (1955)
69. D. Shemin, *Ergels Physiol. Biol. Chem. Exptl. Pharmakol.*, 49, 299 (1957)
70. G. Urata and S. Granick, *J. biol. Chem.*, 238, 811 (1963)
71. K. D. Gibson, W. G. Laver and A. Neuberger, *Biochem. J.*, 70, 71 (1958)

72. M. P. Schulman and D. A. Rickert, *J. biol. Chem.*, 226, 181 (1957)
73. K. D. Gibson, A. Neuberger and J. J. Scott, *Biochem. J.*, 61, 618 (1955)
74. L. Bogorad, *Science*, 121, 878 (1955)
75. S. Granick and D. Mauzerall, *J. biol. Chem.*, 232, 1119 (1958)
76. L. Zieve, E. Hill, S. Schwartz and C. J. Watson, *J. Lab. clin. Med.*, 41, 663 (1953)
77. C. J. Watson, *Adv. int. Med.*, 6, 235 (1954)
78. C. Rimington, *Panminerva Med.*, 4, 307 (1962)
79. C. Rimington, P. N. Morgan, I. Nicholls, J. D. Everall and R. R. Davies, *Lancet*, ii, 318 (1963)
80. S. Granick, *J. biol. Chem.*, 238, 2247 (1963)
81. S. Granick, *J. biol. Chem.*, 241, 1359 (1966)
82. S. Granick, The Biochemistry of Chloroplasts (T. W. Goodwin, ed.), p. 373, Academic Press, New York (1967)
83. S. Granick, Proc. 9th Congr. Europ. Soc. Haematol., Lisbon (Karger, Basel) (1963)
84. S. Granick and R. D. Levere, *Prog. Hematol.*, 4, 1 (1964)
85. C. J. Watson, W. Runge, L. Taddeini, I. Bossenmaier and R. Cardinal, *Proc. nat. Acad. Sci., U.S.*, 52, 478 (1964)
86. D. P. Tschudy, M. G. Perlroth, H. S. Marver, A. Collins, G. Hunter, Jr. and M. Rechcigl, Jr., *Proc. nat. Acad. Sci., U.S.*, 53, 841 (1965)
87. E. B. Dowdle, P. Mustard and L. Eales, *S. Afr. J. Lab. Clin. Med.*, 41, 1093 (1967)
88. N. McIntyre, A. J. G. Pearson, D. J. Allan, S. Craske, G. M. L. West, M. R. Moore, A. D. Beattie, J. Paxton and A. Goldberg, *Lancet*, i, 560 (1971)
89. S. Granick and A. Kappas, *Proc. nat. Acad. Sci., U.S.*, 57, 1463 (1967)
90. A. Goldberg, M. R. Moore, A. D. Beattie, P. E. Hall, J. McCallum and J. K. Grant, *Lancet*, i, 115 (1969)
91. F. H. Welland, E. S. Hellman, A. Collins, G. W. Hunter and D. P. Tschudy, *Metabolism*, 13, 251 (1964)
92. T. S. Zimmerman, J. M. McMillin and C. J. Watson, *Archs. intern. Med.*, 118, 229 (1966)
93. J. Koltra and A. Kappas, *Ann. Rev. Med.*, 18, 325 (1967)
94. J. A. Stein and D. P. Tschudy, *Medicine (Baltimore)*, 49, 1 (1970)
95. F. H. Welland, E. S. Hellman, E. M. Goddes, A. Collins, G. W. Hunter and D. P. Tschudy, *Metabolism*, 13, 232 (1964)
96. D. P. Tschudy, F. H. Welland, A. Collins and G. Hunter, *Metabolism*, 13, 396 (1964)
97. B. F. Felsher and A. G. Redeker, *Medicine (Baltimore)*, 46, 217 (1967)
98. G. D. Ludwig, *Clin. Res.*, 9, 340 (1961)
99. E. S. Hellman, D. P. Tschudy and F. C. Bartler, *Amer. J. Med.*, 32, 734 (1962)
100. G. D. Ludwig and M. Goldberg, *Ann. N.Y. Acad. Sci.*, 104, 710 (1963)

101. B. Nielsen, *Acta Endocrinol.*, **45**, 151 (1964)
102. B. Nielsen and N. A. Thorn, *Amer. J. Med.*, **38**, 345 (1965)
103. E. S. Hellman, D. P. Tschudy, J. Robbins and J. E. Rall, *J. clin. Endocrinol.*, **23**, 1185 (1963)
104. C. S. Hollander, R. L. Scott, D. P. Tschudy, M. G. Perlroth, A. Wakman and K. Sterling, *New Engl. J. Med.*, **277**, 995 (1967)
105. A. Ridley, *Quart. J. Med.*, **38**, 307 (1969)
106. J. B. Cavanagh and A. R. Ridley, *Lancet*, ii, 1023 (1967)
107. T. D. Elder and C. E. Mengel, *Amer. J. Med.*, **41**, 369 (1966)
108. A. Hamfelt and L. Wetterberg, *Lancet*, i, 50 (1968)
109. M. I. Smith and E. Elvove, *Publ. Hlth. Rep (Wash).*, **45**, 1703 (1930)
110. M. I. Smith, E. Elvove and W. H. Frazier, *Publ. Hlth. Rep. (Wash.)*, **45**, 2509 (1930)
111. P. L. Bidstrup, J. A. Bonnell and A. G. Beckett, *Brit. med. J.*, **1**, 1068 (1953)
112. J. M. Barnes and F. A. Denz, *J. Path. Bact.*, **65**, 598 (1953)
113. J. B. Cavanagh, *J. Neurol. Neurosurg. Psychiat.*, **17**, 163 (1954)
114. W. N. Aldridge, *Biochem. J.*, **56**, 185 (1954)
115. M. Eto, J. E. Casida and T. Eto, *Biochem. Pharmacol.*, **11**, 337 (1962)
116. M. K. Johnson, *Biochem. J.*, **120**, 523 (1970)
117. S. Refsum, *Nord. Med.*, **28**, 2682 (1945)
118. S. Refsum, *Acta psychiat. neurol. scand. Suppl.*, **38**, 1 (1946)
119. E. Klenk and W. Kahlke, *Hoppe Seylers Z. Physiol. Chem.*, **333**, 133 (1963)
120. W. Kahlke, *Klin. Wschr.*, **42**, 1011 (1964)
121. L. Eldjarn, *Scand. J. clin. Lab. Invest.*, **17**, 178 (1965)
122. W. S. Alexander, *J. Neurol. Neurosurg. Psychiat.*, **29**, 412 (1966)
123. R. P. Hansen, *Biochim. Biophys. Acta*, **106**, 304 (1965)
124. T. R. Skrbic and J. N. Cumings, *Clin. chim. Acta*, **23**, 17 (1969)
125. D. L. Nandi and J. W. Porter, *Archs. Biochem.*, **7**, 105 (1964)
126. D. Steinberg, J. Avigan, C. Mize, L. Eldjarn, K. Try and S. Refsum, *Biochem. Biophys. Res. Commun.*, **19**, 783 (1965)
127. D. Steinberg, F. Q. Vroom, W. K. Engel, J. Cammermeyer, C. E. Mize and J. Avigan, *Ann. intern. Med.*, **66**, 365 (1967)
128. D. Steinberg, C. E. Mize, J. H. Herndon, H. M. Fales, W. K. Engel and F. Q. Vroom, *Arch. intern. Med.*, **125**, 75 (1970)
129. L. Eldjarn, K. Try, O. Stokke, A. W. Munthe-Kaas, S. Refsum, D. Steinberg, J. Avigan and C. Mize, *Lancet*, i, 691 (1966)
130. L. Eldjarn, K. Try and O. Stokke, *Scand. J. clin. Lab. Invest.*, **18**, 141 (1966)
131. K. Try and L. Eldjarn, *Scand. J. clin. Lab. Invest.*, **20**, 294 (1967)
132. J. Avigan, D. Steinberg, A. Gutman, C. E. Mize and G. W. A. Milne, *Biochem. Biophys. Res. Commun.*, **24**, 838 (1966)
133. D. Steinberg, C. E. Mize, J. Avigan, H. M. Fales, L. Eldjarn, K. Try, O. Stokke and S. Refsum, *J. clin. Invest.*, **46**, 313 (1967)
134. J. H. Herndon, D. Steinberg and B. W. Uhlendorf, *New Engl. J. Med.*, **281**, 1034 (1969)

135. J. H. Herndon, D. Steinberg, B. W. Uhlendorf and H. M. Fales, *J. clin. Invest.*, **48,** 1017 (1969)
136. M. C. MacBrinn and J. S. O'Brien, *J. Lipid Res.*, **9,** 552 (1968)
137. W. Sonneveld, P. Haverkamp Begemann, G. J. Van Beers, R. Keuning and J. C. M. Schogt, *J. Lipid Res.*, **3,** 351 (1962)
138. R. P. Hansen, *N.Z. J. Sci.*, **8,** 158 (1965)
139. R. P. Hansen, *Chem. Industr.*, **7,** 303 (1965)
140. J. H. Baxter, *J. Lipid Res.*, **9,** 636 (1968)
141. J. H. Baxter and D. Steinberg, *J. Lipid Res.*, **8,** 615 (1967)
142. L. Eldjarn, K. Try, R. G. Ackman and S. N. Hooper, *Biochim. Biophys. Acta*, **164,** 94 (1968)
143. F. Andermann, D. L. Lloyd-Smith, H. Mavor and G. Mathieson, *Neurology, (Minneap.)*, **12,** 712 (1962)
144. J. Gilroy, J. S. Meyer, R. B. Bauer, M. Vulpe and D. Greenwood, *Amer. J. Med.*, **40,** 368 (1966)
145. R. J. Dyck, R. D. Ellefson, A. C. Lais, R. C. Smith, W. F. Taylor and R. A. Van Dyke, *Mayo Clinic Proc.*, **45,** 286 (1970)

CHAPTER 2

Biochemistry of Muscle Diseases

R. J. T. PENNINGTON

A considerable amount of information on biochemical changes in muscle diseases has been amassed during the past two decades or so, and reference may be made to several reviews and to the published proceedings of a number of meetings concerned with the subject [1-5]. In this chapter an attempt is made to deal concisely with some aspects and, since this book is concerned primarily with the nervous system, to pay particular attention to the possible role of the latter in muscle diseases. In recent years important new developments in the study of nerve-muscle interactions have appeared, although knowledge of the underlying mechanisms is still scanty, and this new knowledge may prove to be very important in the understanding of some muscle diseases. It is pertinent, therefore, first of all to review briefly the existing knowledge and hypotheses in this field.

2.1 NERVE AND MUSCLE

The skeletal muscles are innervated by the motor neurones, the anterior horn cells, the axon of each of which branches extensively and innervates a large number of individual muscle fibres. The muscle fibres and the controlling motor neurone together form the motor unit. The area of contact between the terminus of the motor neurone`branch and the muscle fibre is the motor end-plate, and within this structure the terminal nerve branches lie within hollows (the synaptic gutters) in the muscle fibre. There is structural discontinuity between the axoplasm and the sarcoplasm but, as shown by the electron microscope, the plasma membranes of the nerve and muscle are in close proximity. The arrival of the nerve impulse liberates acetylcholine at the motor nerve ending; the acetylcholine molecules diffuse across the narrow synaptic space and combine with specific receptor sites on the post-synaptic membrane. This leads to an increased ionic permeability of the muscle membrane which sets off a local change in potential, the end-plate potential; the latter, in turn, generates the muscle action potential which activates the contractile mechanism. The liberated acetylcholine is subsequently destroyed by cholinesterase, which is present in high concentration in the motor end-plate.

2.1.1 Denervation atrophy

As has been known for a century or so, the importance of the motor nerve to the muscle extends beyond its function in initiating contraction. If the nerve is severed or incapacitated by disease the muscle undergoes a profound atrophy. There is a progressive decrease in the diameter of the fibres, with loss of both myofibril and sarcoplasmic protein; there appears, however, to be no decrease in the number of nuclei in the fibres. The first effects of experimental denervation have been reported to occur within 24 hours and commonly the weight of the muscle may be reduced to about one-quarter within a few months. An extensive review of the effects of denervation was provided by Gutmann's monograph [6].

2.1.2 Disuse atrophy

Atrophy of muscle will occur even in the presence of an intact motor nerve if inactivity is induced by other means. Tower [7] and others have accomplished this by section of the spinal cord and division of dorsal roots to the isolated spinal segment. Tenotomy or immobilization of limbs have also been commonly used to study this process. As pointed out by Guth [8] there are hazards in all these procedures; it is difficult, for example, to control the degree of inactivity induced by plaster casts, whilst contraction of muscle fibres after tenotomy may complicate the effects of the latter. Evidently, therefore, some caution is required in the interpretation of experiments on disuse atrophy. With this proviso, a comparison of the detailed changes resulting from denervation and disuse is of interest in relation to the mechanism by which the nerve maintains the muscle fibre in a healthy state. Helander [9] found quantitative differences in the relative changes in myofibril and sarcoplasmic proteins among the different types of experimental atrophy. More recently Klinkerfuss and Haugh [10] have reported histochemical differences between disuse and denervation atrophy, whilst Brooks [11] concluded from electromyographic studies that changes in muscle membrane characteristics occasioned by denervation were not simply a consequence of disuse.

2.1.3 Embryonic muscle

It is clear from histology of embryonic or regenerating muscle and from growth of muscle in culture that the requirement for a nerve influence appears only at a certain stage in the development of the muscle fibre. Muscle fibres originate from myoblasts, single elongated cells which multiply by mitosis. These fuse to form binucleate cells and further fusion gives rise to syncytia containing numerous nuclei—the myotubes [12]. Myofibrils are formed, the nuclei move to the periphery and eventually the mature fibre results. The earlier stages in this sequence occur readily in the absence of a nerve supply. Current attempts in some laboratories to demonstrate interaction between nerve and muscle in tissue culture, if successful, may help to define the precise stage at which the nerve influence becomes important.

2.1.4 Innervation and muscle type

Muscles are classified as fast (e.g. flexor hallucis longus) or slow (e.g. soleus) depending on their speed of contraction; this distinction is associated with certain other differences in response characteristics. In early life, at least in some species, the contraction times of all muscles are slow. There are differences also in the properties of the nerves which supply fast and slow muscles, thus the nerves supplying fast muscles have higher conduction velocity and thicker fibres. Of particular interest, in respect to nerve-muscle relationships, is that the contraction time of the muscle is influenced by the nerve which supplies it. Thus fast muscle becomes slower after cutting its nerve whilst, more strikingly, it has been shown by Buller and his colleagues [13] that cross-union of the nerves to fast and slow muscles results in a lengthening of the contraction time of the fast muscle, whilst the contraction time of the slow muscle is decreased.

Roughly speaking, slow muscles are red muscles whilst fast muscles are white, although exceptions are known (see, for example, [14]). Muscle redness or whiteness is determined by the predominating fibre type; most muscles contain a mixture of fibre types. Histochemical studies have shown the existence of two main types of fibre, the red (Type I) and white (Type II) fibres. (A third intermediate type is also recognized [15] and others have been reported.) The Type I fibres, which are usually smaller, have more numerous mitochondria and thus a high content of oxidative enzymes such as cytochrome oxidase and succinate dehydrogenase; the myoglobin concentration is high and fat droplets tend to be common. In contrast, they are poor in glycolytic enzymes, and thus stain weakly for phosphorylase, for example. Type II fibres are distinguished, on the other hand, by high levels of enzymes of the glycolytic pathway, whilst being relatively poor in oxidative enzymes. Quantitative enzyme studies on typical red and white muscle have been published [16, 17, 18]. Furthermore, there are differences in the myosin from red and white muscle [19, 20]; that from the latter has higher adenosine triphosphatase activity. The calcium-binding activity of the sarcoplasmic reticulum is also higher in white muscle [21]; this property is responsible for the relaxation of contracted muscle (see below). The specific biochemical features of white muscle clearly provide the basis for the shorter contraction time, together with a more rapid production of the necessary energy by breakdown of glycogen.

It is now clear, from the results of several workers, that the biochemical characteristics of a muscle fibre are also profoundly influenced by the nature of the associated nerve. Several years ago Gutmann's group [22] reported that the concentration of glycogen and potassium is higher in fast muscles and that reinnervation of the soleus muscle (slow) with nerve fibres which normally supplied a fast muscle led to an increase in these constituents in the soleus. A marked tendency towards interconversion of the enzyme pattern in red and white fibres following cross-innervation of the soleus and flexor hallucis longus (fast) muscles was demonstrated histochemically by Romanul and Van der Meulen [23] and by Dubowitz and Newman [24], and other workers have described similar effects of cross-innervation on other biochemical activities which differ in red and white muscle.

2.1.5 Mechanism of regulatory influence of nerve upon muscle

From the above it is evident that the influence of the nerve upon the composition of the muscle fibres is more complex than was once supposed. Not only does the cessation of nerve impulses have a profound effect upon the metabolism of the fibres, but it appears also that the nature of the nerve has a highly discriminating effect upon the synthesis of numerous proteins by the muscle fibres. (The alternative possibility that the changed protein concentrations following cross-innervation are the result of alterations in the rates of degradation is less plausible, for various reasons.)

2.1.6 Nature of nerve influence

The means by which the nerve exerts such detailed control is an intriguing problem and at the present time the subject of much discussion and controversy; well-established and unambiguous experimental evidence is lacking, however. The problem cannot be discussed fully here and an excellent critical account is given in Guth's review [8]. A central question is whether this activity of the nerve is mediated by the pattern of nerve impulses and release of acetylcholine, or whether other substances (the hypothetical "trophic" factor(s)) pass from nerve to muscle and regulate protein synthesis in the latter. (It is also conceivable, of course, that the rate of transfer of trophic factors could be increased by nerve impulses.) It is not easy to accept that variations in the frequency of acetylcholine release could alone account for the complexity of the biochemical differences between Type I and Type II fibres. If such is the case, however, it may be conjectured that the chemical changes in the muscle which accompany contraction (e.g. alterations in the levels of glycolytic intermediates), the pattern of which will vary among the fibre types, can differentially affect the synthesis of cell proteins. However, in the virtual absence of knowledge of the mechanisms of control of the synthesis of individual proteins in mammalian cells, this is mere speculation. In support of the trophic factor hypothesis Korr and co-workers [25, 26] have provided some elegant evidence for the direct passage of nerve components into muscle; labelled inorganic phosphate and amino acids were applied directly to the hypoglossal nucleus and the passage of radioactivity was traced down the hypoglossal nerve and into the tongue muscles. Control studies were included to attempt to show that this was the result of direct passage. The possible importance of such experiments and the potentialities of this approach in investigating the nature of trophic substances is obvious, and confirmation of these studies is awaited with interest. Other direct evidence for trophic substances is scanty. The evidence for "axoplasmic flow", the passage of material along the nerve axon [27], perhaps makes it easier to accept a trophic function of the nerve.

Indirect evidence for or against trophic factors has tended to be equivocal. Comparison of the effects of denervation and disuse atrophy should be considered cautiously since, as mentioned above, disuse atrophy is difficult to control. Observations, largely by Gutmann and his colleagues [28], that changes in the muscle after nerve section are more rapid if the nerve is cut close to the muscle, have been taken to indicate that trophic factors may be transmitted from the distal nerve stump. However, as pointed out by my colleague, Dr. J. B. Harris, nerve section close to the muscle may not denervate adjoining muscles, hence the denervated muscle may be subject to stretching and the effects of this would have to be taken into account.

2.1.7 Relevance to muscle diseases

Because of the necessity of the nerve supply for the normal maintenance of muscle fibres many diseases originating in the nervous system are manifested, sometimes predominantly, by muscle weakness and wasting. The muscle atrophy may be diffuse, as in poliomyelitis, or focal, as in motor neurone disease. Apart from such well-recognized neurogenic atrophies, however, there are other muscle diseases, in particular the muscular dystrophies, the biochemistry of which has been most often studied, where the involvement of a neural factor, although postulated by some, is not so well established. Several types of muscular dystrophy are recognized [29] although some uncertainties in classification still exist. They include the Duchenne form (see below) which is the most severe and appears at an early age, and the limb-girdle and facioscapulo-humeral varieties, which usually commence at a later age. Myotonic dystrophy is a separate form which manifests the additional phenomenon of myotonia, a delay in muscle relaxation. The recognition from the cross-innervation studies, of the complexity of the nerve-muscle relationship and the possible existence of multiple trophic factors, facilitates the concept that muscular dystrophy may result from subtle changes in the nerve which cannot be detected by histopathologists. Recently McComas and his colleagues [30, 31] have obtained electrophysiological evidence for the loss of activity of motor neurones in the various kinds of human muscular dystrophy. Tissue culture studies may be relevant to this problem, since normal and dystrophic muscle can be compared in a situation where the nerve is not involved. Earlier experiments [32] indicated that culture of human dystrophic muscle behaved abnormally, suggesting a defect in the muscle independent of the nerve. More recent work, however [33], has not confirmed this, and more studies are required.

The possibility of nerve involvement must also be taken into account in certain inherited myopathies in animals. Some of these conditions are being widely studied in the hope that the results will throw light on the nature of the human muscular dystrophies, and it is important to establish whether they are neurogenic myopathies or whether the primary lesion is in the muscle. The best-known animal myopathies were the subject of a symposium [34] and mention is made below of many investigations involving these conditions. Probably the most studied has been the hereditary myopathy in the mouse (strain 129/Re, discovered at the Jackson Laboratory, Bar Harbor, Maine, in 1955) [35]. This disease is inherited recessively and is characterized by the smaller size of the animal, progressive weakness, particularly in the hind legs, muscle atrophy, and a reduced life-span. A number of workers [36, 37, 38] have demonstrated differences between the growth of normal and dystrophic mouse muscle in tissue culture, suggesting the existence of a genetic defect in the muscle fibres. Electrophysiological experiments [39], however, have been taken to implicate the motor neurones in this disease. Studies of the behaviour of muscle transplanted between dystrophic and normal animals should provide useful evidence bearing on this question, but the results have not been consistent [40, 41].

Below are reviewed some of the biochemical differences which have been found to exist between normal and diseased muscle, with particular reference to the muscular dystrophies, to which the most research has been directed. Inevitably, it has been necessary to exercise a degree of selection. Where possible, comparison has been made with studies of experimentally denervated muscle; although any nerve changes which may occur in the muscular dystrophies might not be very comparable with the immediate removal of the nerve influence resulting from section of the nerve, nevertheless a close comparison of the biochemical changes in denervation and the so-called primary myopathies might help to indicate the extent of nerve involvement in the latter.

2.2 MORPHOLOGICAL CHANGES IN DISEASED MUSCLE

Chemical and enzymic measurements on dystrophic muscle clearly cannot be considered without reference to the extensive structural changes which can be seen with the light and electron microscope. These include vacuolization and hyalinization of fibres, and inward migration of nuclei. Many fibres show severe atrophy and necrosis although some hypertrophied fibres may be seen. Small regenerating fibres are also observed, becoming less common as the disease progresses. Macrophages appear and the disappearing muscle fibres are gradually replaced by fat cells and fibrous tissue. The relative importance of these pathological features may vary, for example, between different types of human dystrophy. The loss of true muscle tissue and the appearance and proliferation of other cell types will, of course, profoundly influence the results of gross analysis of muscle samples. These are commonly expressed in relation to the "non-collagen" protein of the sample, which is taken as an approximate measure of the true muscle protein; this is a reasonably satisfactory way of recording changes in concentration of constituents of the muscle fibres, since the latter contribute most of the protein, other than collagen, of the samples.

In denervation atrophy, on the other hand, a much simpler change is seen, consisting merely of a progressive reduction in size of the muscle fibres. In diseases where the motor units are affected one at a time, the remaining healthy fibres may markedly increase in size, probably as a result of work hypertrophy. In the later stages, some of the other pathological changes mentioned above will occur [42] and the histological picture becomes less distinguishable from that of the muscular dystrophies. It is generally accepted, however, that regeneration is absent.

It was a reasonable hope that application of the electron microscope would provide structural clues pointing to the site of the initial lesion in dystrophic muscle, but studies by many workers during the past decade have not revealed any sufficiently specific changes [43]. However, a number of rare congenital myopathies have shown certain changes in ultrastructure which have assisted classification and which may help in their understanding; for example, some manifest particular abnormalities in the mitochondria.

2.3 MUSCLE GLYCOLYSIS

Among the quantitative biochemical changes recorded in human dystrophic muscle, one of the most striking is a decline in the activity of enzymes of the glycolytic pathway [44, 45]. The rate of lactate production by muscle homogenates (referred to non-collagen protein) from patients with Duchenne-type muscular dystrophy may be reduced to a small fraction of normal in advanced cases, and most of the individual enzymes of glycolysis have been shown to be considerably diminished. It is certain that such changes are not specific for Duchenne muscular dystrophy, since a comparable result has been seen in neurogenic muscle disease [46] and aldolase activity was shown to decrease markedly in denervated rat muscle [47]. Nevertheless, it was reported by Vignos and Lefkowitz [48] that glycolysis was normal in muscle from adult forms of muscular dystrophy, whilst Mayers and Epstein [49] found this to be true of the mouse dystrophy; aldolase, in fact, may be elevated in older dystrophic mice [50].

2.3.1 Developmental changes

It is of interest and probably relevant to compare these changes in the activity of glycolytic enzymes with their variation which occurs during the development of normal muscle. There is a considerable increase during development [51, 52], so that in this respect the composition of the dystrophic muscle more nearly represents that of foetal muscle. This similarity has been observed also in relation to other enzymes. The relation between other changes in muscle during development and atrophy has been recently reviewed by Perry [53]. Such changes, as would be expected, concern primarily the white fibres, which are the richer in glycolytic enzymes; thus the increase in glycolytic enzymes during development of the chicken was much the higher in white muscle [51], whilst Romanul and Hogan [54] observed that, after denervation, the more rapid decrease of a particular enzyme was observed in the fibre type which was richer in that enzyme.

A partial cause of the changes in glycolytic enzymes during development and atrophy of muscle fibres may be the variation in physical activity undergone by the muscle. The rate of increase in the activity of muscle enzymes during development can be influenced by the use of the muscles [52, 55], and short-term exercise or stimulation was shown to increase the activity of muscle creatine kinase [56]. Whether such effects are mediated solely through increased acetylcholine release or whether trophic factors are also involved, is an open question (see above). Exercise does not seem to be entirely responsible, however, for the increase in levels of glycolytic enzymes during development since this occurs in white muscle even if totally immobilized [57].

2.3.2 Isoenzymes

A related alteration in enzyme pattern occurring in many types of diseased muscle is a change in the relative amounts of lactate dehydrogenase isoenzymes, first noted by Wieme and Lauryssens in 1962 [58, 59, 60]. Electrophoresis reveals five separate isoenzymes of lactate dehydrogenase in most tissues. The most abundant one in the majority of normal muscles is LDH5, the least negatively charged under the usual conditions of electrophoresis. In Duchenne dystrophy and many other muscle diseases, irrespective of recognized nerve involvement, there is a striking change in the LDH isoenzyme pattern, marked by a considerable reduction in the proportion of LDH5. Again, the altered pattern seen in disease resembles the pattern in normal foetal muscle [61]. In Duchenne dystrophy it has been observed in the preclinical stage [62] and it is even possible that the normal adult pattern is never attained; this has been shown to be the case in muscular dystrophy in the chicken [55] another inherited animal myopathy which has been widely studied, particularly in its developmental aspects. It is of considerable interest that the abnormal muscle LDH isoenzyme pattern is sometimes seen in female carriers of Duchenne dystrophy [63].

The significance of the existence of several isoenzymes of lactate dehydrogenase has been the subject of much discussion [64]. LDH5 is commonly thought to function predominantly in the reduction of pyruvate to lactate during glycolysis whereas LDH1, for example, might be more important in the oxidation of lactate, in tissues where this occurs. Thus it is reasonable to suppose that changes in the proportion of LDH5 may be engineered by the same mechanisms which bring about the changes in the levels of other glycolytic enzymes.

2.3.3 AMP deaminase

An enzyme which undergoes a particularly sharp fall in activity in dystrophic muscle (human and mouse) [65, 66], which may be related to the changes in glycolysis, is AMP deaminase. The significance of the presence of a high level of this enzyme in normal muscle (it is almost absent from liver and some other tissues) is not known for certain. It has recently been suggested [67] that the production of ammonia from AMP by this enzyme may be important in the regulation of glycolysis.

2.4 PROTEIN METABOLISM

The progressive loss of muscle proteins which characterizes muscle atrophy may be considered in relation to the continual replacement process which involves proteins of muscle as of other tissues. In the normal adult tissues there is a balance of degradation and resynthesis, which maintains the intracellular proteins at constant levels. Many workers have attempted to assess the speed of breakdown and resynthesis of proteins in normal muscle by measuring the rates of incorporation and release of labelled amino acids [68]. Refinement of the techniques used has led to higher estimates of these rates, and recent estimates of a few days for the half-life (i.e. the time required for replacement of 50% of a protein) of the mixed muscle proteins have been obtained [69, 70]. Evidence was put forward that myosin, the major muscle protein, is not randomly degraded but has a definite life-span [71] (as does haemoglobin, for example) but this has been recently questioned [70]. Evidently, in principle, the disturbance of the protein balance in atrophying muscle could result from either a moderate decrease in the synthesis rate or a moderately increased degradation. The latter might involve accelerated activity of the normal breakdown processes or new degradative mechanisms may come into action. The former question can readily be answered in the animal by experiments with labelled amino acids. Simon *et al.* [72], and subsequently other workers, have found an accelerated incorporation of amino acid and a shortened half-life for muscle proteins in muscular dystrophy in the mouse, indicating that there is, overall, an accelerated breakdown of protein but actually an increase also in the rate of synthesis (evidently insufficient to match the increased breakdown). Confirmation of this finding with the newer procedure for measuring protein turnover is desirable. *In vitro* studies with cell-free preparations of dystrophic mouse muscle [73] have also demonstrated an increased rate of protein synthesis, and a similar result has been obtained with polyribosome preparations from human dystrophic (Duchenne) muscle [74].

The situation in experimentally denervated muscle, however, appears to be somewhat different. The turnover studies of Slack [75] and more recently of Goldberg [76] have indicated that whilst again there is an increase in the rate of protein breakdown there is, in this case, a decrease in the rate of synthesis. The significance of these findings can emerge only after much more research, since many fundamental questions have yet to be answered. Although the mechanism of protein synthesis is known in outline, little is known of the factors which control its rate and how these operate.

2.4.1 Proteolytic enzymes

The mechanism and control of intracellular protein breakdown has not been established and the manner in which its rate is normally synchronized with that of protein synthesis is obscure. Muscle, like other tissues, contains enzymes which are capable of attacking proteins. The best characterized is a proteolytic enzyme with maximum activity at an acid pH (cathepsin D) [77], which may be present in lysosomes [78]. Such an intracellular localization, together with its low pH optimum, tends to suggest that it may not be involved in the normal turnover of protein in muscle but is perhaps important in pathological processes. Other proteolytic enzymes, with optimal activity at an alkaline pH, are also present in muscle [66, 79, 80], but have not yet been well characterized. A proteolytic inhibitor was found in muscle homogenates [81], and this may well obscure the presence of some proteinases. Its intra- or extra-cellular location and its possible role in the regulation of protein breakdown in muscle remains to be explored.

Both muscular dystrophy (human and animal) and denervation atrophy are associated with increased concentrations of proteolytic enzymes in muscle. The likelihood that this is related to the enhanced protein turnover is clear, but evidence is scanty. Both acid [65, 82, 83] and alkaline [66, 83, 84] cathepsin activity increase in dystrophic muscle and either or both may be important in this respect.

Some attempt has been made to investigate in detail the increased protein synthetic activity in dystrophic muscle [74, 85, 86], but no clear answer has emerged as to which stage in the pathway is primarily involved. A separate question, still to be answered, is to what extent the faster turnover results from the presence of regenerating fibres.

2.5 MEMBRANE CHANGES

2.5.1 Sarcolemma

The electron microscope has shown that muscle fibres are surrounded by an inner plasma membrane and an outer basement membrane. The latter is not observed in myoblasts or developing muscle and its function may be one of structural support. The former shows the characteristic unit-membrane structure of other plasma membranes; it is considered that the electric potential of the muscle fibre is maintained across it and that its characteristics influence the passive and active transport of substances in and out of the muscle fibre. It is continuous with the membranes which constitute the transverse tubular system (T-system) of the muscle fibres; hence the compartments of the T-system are continuous with the extracellular space. The ability of a large molecule (ferritin) to pass into the T-system from outside the fibre has been demonstrated [87]. Whether any proteins can normally pass in and out of the true intracellular space of muscle fibres is not certain.

2.5.2 Enzyme leakage

The suspicion that muscular dystrophy (in particular, the Duchenne type) might result from an inherited structural defect in the sarcolemma originated largely from the increased level of certain enzymes in the plasma in this disease (first noted by Sibley and Lehninger in 1949 [88]), and the realization that this is due to leakage from muscle tissue. As mentioned in more detail below, although this phenomenon is far from specific for any kind of muscle disease, the plasma enzymes are particularly high in Duchenne type dystrophy. The leakage is clearly not simply a predictable consequence of muscular wasting since experimental denervation has little or no effect on plasma enzymes; in Kwashiorkor (protein deficiency with extreme wasting) the serum creatine kinase level tends actually to be lower than normal [89].

Attempts have been made to understand this phenomenon by studying the leakage of enzymes from intact isolated muscles held in a suitable medium. It was observed [90] that there was a markedly higher rate of leakage of aldolase from muscle from dystrophic mice than from normal mouse muscle under these conditions. However, the use of such a model to give information on the protein permeability of fibres in vivo must be treated with some caution. The rate of leakage in the experiments quoted was almost certainly of a higher order than occurs in the body. Also, as shown by this author, it is very readily increased by unfavourable conditions such as mechanical treatment or insufficiency of oxygen. Subsequent studies [91, 92], moreover, have shown that denervated muscle displays a greatly increased rate of enzyme leakage *in vitro*, although this is not reflected by any marked increase in the level of blood enzymes following denervation of muscles in an animal.

The elevation of plasma enzyme levels in several types of muscle disease, and indeed the common occurrence of this phenomenon in disease of other tissues, makes it very unlikely that the leakage of enzymes signifies a primary membrane defect in Duchenne dystrophy. The demonstration that leakage of enzymes *in vitro* is readily enhanced by interference with cellular energy production [90] makes it easier to accept that increased leakage *in vivo* might result from metabolic changes in the fibres. To what extent such factors can explain the vastly different rates of leakage in Duchenne dystrophy and denervation atrophy is not known; the necrosis and rupture of individual fibres is probably also important. A further unanswered question is why widely varying amounts of different muscle proteins are detectable in the blood in muscular dystrophy, an observation which cannot always be explained by their different concentrations in muscle. Thus the level of AMP deaminase, one of the most abundant muscle enzymes, is barely raised in the blood in Duchenne dystrophy, and phosphofructokinase and myoglobin, also abundant in muscle, could not be detected in the blood by immunochemical tests [93]. Many factors, including possible intracellular binding of sarcoplasmic enzymes [94], are probably responsible for these differences.

2.5.3 Uptake of amino acids

Muscle fibres have the ability to accumulate amino acids, a property which may be important in the regulation of muscle protein metabolism. There is evidence that several mechanisms for transporting amino acids into cells exist, and the amino acids can be classified into transport groups; the transport of some into muscle is stimulated by insulin. It is speculated that there is a separate carrier protein for each group within the sarcolemma. An increased accumulation of amino acids into muscle has been reported in hereditary muscular dystrophy in the mouse [95], in muscular dystrophy resulting from a deficiency of vitamin E [96] and in denervated muscle [96]. It appears, therefore, that changes in the uptake of amino acids into the fibres do not necessarily parallel changes in the rate of protein synthesis since, as mentioned above, there is evidence that the latter is decreased in denervated muscle. Diehl *et al.* [96] interpreted their results to show that the increased accumulation of amino acids was due to an increase in active transport, not a change in the passive permeability of the membrane.

2.5.4. Membrane chemistry

Methods of isolating intact sarcolemma free from admixture with other cell structures are necessary for precise study of its chemical and enzymic composition and for the investigation of possible changes in these in disease. A number of procedures have been devised to this end [97, 98], but it appears that there are difficulties still to be overcome. The sarcolemma may be expected to be rich in phospholipids which are important constituents of cell membranes. Changes have been reported in the fatty acid composition of phospholipids in muscle in human muscular dystrophy [99], in the autosomal dominant form of myotonia congenita [100], after denervation [101], and in muscular dystrophy in the mouse [102, 103]. Further work will be required to show whether the phospholipids of the sarcolemma are concerned in these abnormalities. The increased turnover of proteolipids [104] and increased biosynthesis of gangliosides [105] in denervated muscle may also represent changes in the characteristics of the sarcolemma.

Isolated sarcolemmal fragments have been shown by a number of workers to contain a Na^+, K^+-stimulated ATP-ase. It has recently been shown [106] that in such preparations from the dystrophic hamster this activity is much higher than normal.

2.5.5 Calcium uptake by sarcoplasmic reticulum

The tubular network seen in muscle fibres under the electron microscope comprises the T-system, mentioned above, and the longitudinal tubules of the sarcoplasmic reticulum, the compartments of which appear to have no connections with the extracellular space. A detailed account of the structure is given by Peachey [107]. Fragmented sarcoplasmic reticulum, in the form of small vesicles, is the main constituent of the "microsome" fraction which is sedimented by high-speed centrifuging of muscle homogenates after removal of other cellular organelles by centrifuging at a lower speed. At the present time very few enzymic activities have been shown to be associated with the sarcoplasmic reticulum (unlike the analogous endoplasmic reticulum of liver cells). Its most clearly-established function is in the control of muscle contraction, by release of calcium following excitation of the sarcolemma and T-system and its subsequent reaccumulation. The latter process, which terminates contraction, requires energy in the form of ATP and is thought to involve a calcium-activated ATP-ase which has been found in the microsome fraction. Termination of muscle contraction was formerly thought to be the property of a soluble "relaxing factor".

A decreased ability of the sarcoplasmic reticulum to accumulate calcium has been reported in muscular dystrophy in both human [108] and mouse [109] and in some other human muscle diseases [108], although not in myotonic dystrophy [110]; the slow relaxation rate in the latter condition appears, therefore, to be due to other causes. After experimental denervation in the rat an increase in calcium-accumulating ability has been reported [111] both in fast and slow muscle, particularly the latter.

2.6 BIOCHEMICAL DIAGNOSIS OF MUSCLE DISEASE

As will be clear from what has been said above, the recognized biochemical changes in muscle diseases are, in general, rather non-specific, although there are often quantitative differences in the degree of abnormality between the various disorders. (In a small number of rare inherited defects of glycogen metabolism, described in the next section, the defect is sufficiently marked and unique to be identifiable.) A number of changes in the composition of blood and urine may be seen in muscle diseases [1] and, of these, the creatinuria was commonly utilized as a diagnostic test but this is an almost completely non-specific consequence of muscle wasting and is observed in a wide variety of conditions in which wasting occurs [112]. Increased amino aciduria is variable and non-specific, and none of the reported changes in the main plasma protein and lipid constituents have been shown to have diagnostic value. The increase in plasma enzymes already mentioned, particularly creatine kinase, has proved by far the most useful test. It is sufficiently discriminating to assist often in differentiation of muscle disorders and its high sensitivity is valuable in the detection of carriers of Duchenne dystrophy, in which muscle atrophy may be minimal.

The highest levels of serum creatine kinase are found in boys with Duchenne dystrophy. Values up to several hundred times normal may be recorded in the early stages, but the amount decreases as the disease progresses [113]. Elevation of serum enzymes precedes the clinical signs; in a boy studied by Heyck and co-workers [114] (the younger brother of a patient) the levels were increased at birth, reached a peak at 14-22 months and then began to decline before clinical signs appeared, although diagnosis was confirmed by histopathology.

Generally a much more limited increase in serum creatine kinase is encountered in the adult form of muscular dystrophy and in myotonic dystrophy. It is normally raised in untreated cases of polymyositis, and the level may be very high. Typical data are provided by Pearce et al. [113] and other workers. It was at one time considered that little or no rise in serum creatine kinase occurred in muscle diseases of recognized neurogenic origin, but modest increases have been recorded in Kugelberg-Welander disease and spastic spinal paralysis [115] and in motor neurone disease [116]. Elevated values may occur also in hyperkalaemic and hypokalaemic myopathies [117, 118].

Probably the most valuable application of serum creatine kinase measurements is in the detection of the female carriers of Duchenne dystrophy. Apart from a relatively infrequent autosomal recessive form, this disease is inherited by an X-linked gene. Consequently there would be an even chance that any son born to a carrier would have the disease, and it is therefore of the utmost importance to be able to test all females whose family relationship with patients would indicate as possible carriers. Serum creatine kinase is the best available test [119], although all published results indicate that a minor proportion (one-third or less) of carriers have normal levels. The majority of the others have slightly raised levels although a few are much higher [120]. The reason for these differences is not clear; the degree of elevation cannot, for example, be clearly related to the extent of pathological changes in the muscles [121].

Normal values for serum creatine kinase published from various laboratories have differed widely owing to the multiplicity of procedures available for its determination. The chemical reaction catalysed by the enzyme is freely reversible and can be readily measured in either direction. The reaction of creatine phosphate with ADP (to form creatine and ATP) is several times faster than the reverse reaction and is therefore to be preferred on grounds of sensitivity. The addition of a sulphydryl reagent such as cysteine to the reaction mixture [122] to protect the enzyme has often been omitted, which usually leads to lower values. The inclusion of cysteine is particularly important in the case of serum samples which are not perfectly fresh, since it serves to restore the enzyme to its original activity. Under these conditions samples that have been posted the previous day or stored frozen for two or three weeks are satisfactory. Slight haemolysis of samples is unimportant since red cells contain little of the enzyme.

A further practical consideration in the application of serum creatine kinase measurements is the possible effect of physical exercise upon the levels of this enzyme. Exercise of sufficient intensity and duration can substantially increase serum creatine kinase in normal individuals, and it is particularly important that this should be avoided in suspected carriers before testing (since the expected elevations may be small).

A possibility that the serum creatine kinase level in carriers might be more susceptible to enhancement by exercise than that in normals, has been investigated; if true, it would provide a means of increasing the sensitivity of the test. However, in spite of earlier indications [123] that this might be the case,

Hudgson and colleagues [124] found that the slight rise in creatine kinase induced by everyday activity or by a long walk was, on average, no higher in carriers than in normal women.

2.7 GLYCOLYTIC ENZYME DEFICIENCIES

As outlined above, muscle diseases may be accompanied by a rather non-specific fall in the activity of the glycolytic pathway in muscle. Aside from this, however, a small number of conditions have been described in which there is a specific deficiency in one of the enzymes concerned in the breakdown of muscle glycogen. Although rare, such cases are of much theoretical interest and eminently suited to biochemical investigation, and a brief discussion of these will conclude this chapter. Detailed accounts are available in several good reviews, e.g. [125, 126].

The classic example is that of a deficiency of muscle phosphorylase (McArdle's disease) and much has been written of this since its first description. This inherited enzyme deficiency appears to be confined to muscle. The resulting inability to break down glycogen gives rise to a raised muscle glycogen (usually 2-5%) and the absence of a rise in blood lactate following ischaemic exercise; diagnosis can be established by measuring the activity of phosphorylase in a muscle biopsy. Clinically the main feature is muscular pain on exercise and a minority of cases have some degree of myopathy. Presumably direct utilization of glucose from the blood can mitigate the effects of phosphorylase lack, except when energy demands are high.

More recently a case was described [127] in which the total activity of phosphorylase in both muscle and liver was normal, but the enzyme was in the inactive form. Evidence was obtained for a deficiency of the cyclic $3', 5'$-AMP-dependent kinase which phosphorylates phosphorylase kinase which, in turn, converts inactive phosphorylase b to active phosphorylase a.

A deficiency of amylo-1,6-glucosidase (the "debrancher enzyme") has also been recognized for a considerable time. This results in the accumulation of an abnormal glycogen with short outer chains. Both muscle and liver may be affected and there is a low activity of the enzyme in leucocytes.

In 1965 Japanese workers [128] identified a deficiency in muscle of phosphofructokinase, another glycolytic enzyme; the symptoms were quite similar to those of muscle phosphorylase deficiency. The enzyme was also low in erythrocytes. Inheritance is probably autosomal recessive and a small number of other cases have since been reported. A late-onset muscle disorder in two brothers associated with a low activity of phosphohexoseisomerase in the muscle has been reported in another Japanese family [129].

In all these conditions it is clear how the disturbance in glycogen breakdown can result from the recognized enzyme deficiency. Another type of glycogen storage disease (Pompe's disease) is associated with a deficiency of amylo-1 : 4 glucosidase (acid maltase) [130] and is less easy to understand. This enzyme breaks down glycogen independently of the phosphorylase pathway and is present in lysosomes. Nevertheless, in this condition much of the glycogen is extra-lysosomal, hence it would have been anticipated that it would be subject to breakdown by phosphorylase, which is normal. In the usual form the deficiency is general and the life expectation is normally less than two years. However, a few cases [131, 132] have been described of a much milder form, characterized by myopathy, in which the deficiency may have been confined to muscle, although in other such mild forms the deficiency was shown also in the liver [133]. Recently [134] a low activity of this enzyme in muscle was reported in a case of hypothyroidism; the activity was restored by treatment with thyroxin.

The success in identifying the site of the metabolic defect in these diseases contrasts with the failure, so far, to discover the congenital absence of a specific enzyme or other protein in the muscular dystrophies. As the latter are also inherited diseases it can be expected that such will eventually be found, although whether in muscle or nerve or both is as yet uncertain. It may be hoped, however, that effective treatment of muscular dystrophy may not be conditional upon finding the underlying genetic defect. A study of the secondary and less specific biochemical changes associated with muscle wasting may indicate a rational approach to therapy, and it is here that the investigation of the animal myopathies may be of most value.

REFERENCES

1. R. J. Pennington, *In* Disorders of Voluntary Muscle (J. N. Walton, ed.), p. 385. Churchill, London (1969)
2. R. J. Pennington, *In* Biochemical Aspects of Neurological Disorders (J. N. Cumings and M. Kremer, eds), p. 28. Blackwell, Oxford (1965)
3. G. Schapira, J. C. Dreyfus and F. Schapira, *Enzym. biol. clin.*, 11, 8 (1970)
4. J. N. Walton, N. Canal and G. Scarlato (eds), Muscle diseases: Proceedings of an International Congress, Milan, 19-21 May, 1969, Excerpta Medica, Amsterdam (1970)
5. A. T. Milhorat (ed.), Exploratory concepts in muscular dystrophy. Excerpta Medica, Amsterdam (1967)
6. E. Gutmann, The Denervated Muscle, Czechoslovak Academy of Science, Prague (1962)
7. S. S. Tower, *J. comp. Neurol.*, 67, 241 (1937)
8. L. Guth, *Physiol. Rev.*, 48, 645 (1968)
9. E. Helander, *Acta. physiol. Scand.*, 41, Suppl. 141 (1957)
10. G. H. Klinkerfuss and M. J. Haugh, *Arch. Neurol.*, 22, 309 (1970)
11. J. E. Brooks, *Arch. Neurol.*, 22, 27 (1970)
12. K. F. A. Ross and P. Hudgson, *In* Disorders of Voluntary Muscle (J. N. Walton, ed.), p. 319, Churchill, London (1969)
13. A. J. Buller, J. C. Eccles and R. M. Eccles, *J. Physiol. (London)*, 150, 417 (1960)
14. W. Fiehn and J. B. Peter, *J. clin. Invest.*, 50, 570 (1971)
15. J. M. Stein and H. A. Padykula, *Amer. J. Anat.*, 110, 103 (1962)
16. D. M. Dawson and F. C. A. Romanul, *Arch. Neurol.*, 11, 369 (1964)
17. A. Bass, D. Brdiczka, P. Eyer, S. Hofer and D. Pette, *Europ. J. Biochem.*, 10, 198 (1969)
18. D. F. Goldspink, J. B. Harris, D. C. Park and R. J. Pennington, *Enzym. biol. clin.*, 11, 481 (1970)
19. F. A. Sreter, J. C. Seidel and J. Gergely, *J. biol. Chem.*, 241, 5772 (1966)
20. W. M. Kuehl and R. S. Adelstein, *Biochem. biophys. Res. Comm.*, 39, 956 (1970)
21. S. Harigaya, Y. Ogawa and H. Sugita, *J. Biochem. (Tokyo)*, 63, 324 (1968)
22. Z. Drahota and G. Gutmann, *Physiol. Bohemoslov.*, 12, 339 (1963)
23. F. C. A. Romanul and J. P. Van Der Meulen, *Nature (Lond.)*, 212, 1369 (1966)
24. V. Dubowitz and D. L. Newman, *Nature (Lond.)*, 214, 840 (1967)

25. I. M. Korr, P. M. Wilkinson and F. W. Chornock, *Science*, **155**, 342 (1967)
26. I. M. Korr and G. S. L. Appeltauer, *Fed. Proc.*, **30**, 665 (1971)
27. S. H. Barondes and F. E. Samson, Jr. *Neurosciences Res. Prog. Bull.*, **5**, 307 (1967)
28. I. Hajek, E. Gutmann and I. Syrovy, *Physiol. bohemoslov.*, **13**, 32 (1963)
29. J. N. Walton and D. Gardner-Medwin, *In* Disorders of Voluntary Muscle (J. N. Walton, ed.), p. 455, Churchill, London (1969)
30. A. J. McComas, R. E. P. Sica and S. Currie, *Nature (Lond.)*, **226**, 1263 (1970)
31. A. J. McComas, R. E. P. Sica and M. J. Campbell, *Lancet*, i, 321 (1971)
32. R. S. Geiger and J. S. Garvin, *J. Neuropath. exp. Neurol.*, **16**, 532 (1957)
33, B. Gallup, Abstr. IImes Journees Internationales de Pathologie Neuro-musculaire, Marseille (1970)
34. E. Bajusz (ed.), *Ann. N.Y. Acad. Sci.*, **138** (Art. 1), 1 (1966)
35. A. M. Michelson, E. S. Russell and P. J. Harman, *Proc. Nat. Acad. Sci.*, **41** 1079 (1955)
36. G. W. Pearce, *In* Research in Muscular Dystrophy, p. 75. Pitman, London (1963)
37. W. K. O'Steen, *Texas Rep. Biol. Med.*, **21**, 369 (1963)
38. K. F. A. Ross, *In* Research in Muscular Dystrophy, p. 119. Pitman, London (1965)
39. J. Harris and P. Wilson, *Nature (Lond.)*, **229**, 61 (1971)
40. J. L. Laird and R. F. Timmer, *Arch. Path.*, **80**, 442 (1965)
41. B. Salafsky, *Nature (Lond.)*, **229**, 270 (1971)
42. D. B. Drachman, S. R. Murphy, M. P. Nigam and J. R. Hills, *Arch. Neurol.*, **16**, 14 (1967)
43. P. Hudgson and G. W. Pearce, *In* Disorders of Voluntary Muscle (J. N. Walton, ed.), p. 277. Churchill, London (1969)
44. J. C. Dreyfus, G. Schapira, F. Schapira and J. Demos, *Clin. chim. Acta*, **1**, 434 (1956)
45. H. Heyck, G. Laudahn and C.-J. Luders, *Klin. Wschr.*, **41**, 500 (1963)
46. S. Di Mauro, C. Angelini and C. Catani, *J. Neurol. Neurosurg. Psychiat.*, **30**, 411 (1967)
47. G. L. A. Graff, A. J. Hudson and K. P. Strickland, *Canad. J. Biochem.*, **43**, 699 (1965)
48. P. J. Vignos and M. Lefkowitz, *J. clin. Invest.*, **38**, 873 (1959)
49. G. L. Mayers and N. Epstein, *Proc. Soc. exp. Biol. (N.Y.)*, **111**, 450 (1962)
50. U. Srivastava and L. Berlinguet, *Canad. J. Biochem.*, **42**, 1301 (1964)
51. A. Bass, G. Lusch and D. Pette, *Europ. J. Biochem.*, **13**, 289 (1970)
52. J. Kendrick-Jones and S. V. Perry, *Biochem. J.*, **103**, 207 (1967)
53. S. V. Perry, *J. Neurol. Sci.*, **12**, 289 (1971)

54. F. C. A. Romanul and E. L. Hogan, *Arch. Neurol.*, **13**, 263 (1965)
55. D. M. Dawson and N. O. Kaplan, *J. biol. Chem.*, **240**, 3215 (1965)
56. J. Kendrick-Jones and S. V. Perry, *Nature (Lond.)*, **208**, 1068 (1965)
57. W. S. Mann and B. Salafsky, *J. Physiol.*, **208**, 33 (1970)
58. R. J. Wieme and M. J. Lauryssens, *Lancet*, i, 433 (1962)
59. I. A. Brody, *Neurology (Minneap.)*, **14**, 1091 (1964)
60. A. E. H. Emery, *J. Neurol. Sci.*, **7**, 137 (1968)
61. J. C. Dreyfus, J. Demos, F. Schapira and G. Schapira, *C.R. Acad. Sci. (Paris)*, **254**, 4384 (1962)
62. C. M. Pearson, N. C. Kar, J. B. Peter and T. L. Munsat, *Amer. J. Med.*, **39**, 91 (1965)
63. A. E. H. Emery, *Nature (Lond.)*, **201**, 1044 (1964)
64. A. L. Latner and A. W. Skillen, Isoenzymes in Biology and Medicine, p. 80. Academic Press, London (1968)
65. R. J. Pennington, *Proc. Ass. clin. Biochem.*, **2**, 17 (1962)
66. R. J. Pennington, *Biochem. J.*, **88**, 64 (1963)
67. J. Lowenstein and K. Tornheim, *Science*, **171**, 397 (1971)
68. R. J. Pennington, *In* Muscle diseases: Proceedings of an International Congress, Milan, 19-21 May, 1969 (J. N. Walton, N. Canal and G. Scarlato, eds), p. 252. Excerpta Medica, Amsterdam (1970)
69. J. C. Waterlow and J. M. L. Stephen, *Clin. Sci.*, **35**, 287 (1968)
70. D. J. Millward, *Clin. Sci.*, **39**, 577 (1970)
71. J. C. Dreyfus, J. Kruh and G. Schapira, *Biochem. J.*, **75**, 574 (1960)
72. E. J. Simon, C. S. Gross and I. M. Lessell, *Arch. Biochem.*, **96**, 41 (1962)
73. U. Srivastava and L. Berlinguet, *Arch. Biochem. Biophys.*, **114**, 320 (1966)
74. G. Monckton and T. Nihei, *Neurology (Minneap.)*, **19**, 415 (1969)
75. H. G. B. Slack, *Clin. Sci.*, **13**, 155 (1954)
76. A. L. Goldberg, *J. biol. Chem.*, **244**, 3223 (1969)
77. A. A. Iodice, V. Leong and I. M. Weinstock, *Arch. Biochem. Biophys.*, **117**, 477 (1966)
78. N. Stagni and B. de Bernard, *Biochim. Biophys. Acta*, **170**, 129 (1968)
79. T. R. Koszalka and L. L. Miller, *J. biol. Chem.*, **235**, 665 (1960)
80. T. Noguchi and M. Kandatsu, *Agric. Biol. Chem.*, **34**, 390 (1970)
81. R. J. Pennington and K. Fitzpatrick, *Muscle Notes*, 47 (1969)
82. I. M. Weinstock, S. Epstein and A. T. Milhorat, *Proc. Soc. exp. Biol. (N.Y.)*, **99**, 272 (1958)
83. T. R. Koszalka, K. E. Mason and G. Krol, *J. Nutrit.*, **73**, 78 (1961)
84. R. J. Pennington and J. E. Robinson, *Enzymol. biol. Clin.*, **9**, 175 (1968)
85. U. Srivistava, *Arch. Biochem. Biophys.*, **135**, 236 (1969)
86. D. C. Watts and J. C. Reid, *In* Research in Muscular Dystrophy, p. 336. Pitman, London (1968)
87. H. E. Huxley, *Nature (Lond.)*, **202**, 1067 (1964)
88. J. A. Sibley and A. L. Lehninger, *J. nat. Cancer Inst.*, **9**, 303 (1949)
89. S. Reindorp and R. G. Whitehead, *Brit. J. Nutrit.*, **25**, 273 (1971)

90. K. Zieler, *Bull. Johns Hopk. Hosp.*, 108, 208 (1961)
91. C. Pellegrino and C. Bibbiani, *Nature (Lond.)*, 204, 483 (1964)
92. D. M. Dawson, *Arch. Neurol.*, 14, 321 (1966)
93. L. P. Rowland, R. B. Layzer and L. J. Kagan, *Arch. Neurol.*, 18, 272 (1968)
94. W. R. Amberson, F. J. Roisen and A. D. Bauer, *J. Cell. comp. Physiol.*, 66, 71 (1965)
95. R. D. Baker, *Texas Rep. Biol. Med.*, 22, (Suppl. 1), 880 (1964)
96. J. F. Diehl and R. R. Jones, *Amer. J. Physiol.*, 210, 1080 (1966)
97. D. L. McCollester, *Biochim. Biophys. Acta*, 57, 427 (1962)
98. T. Kono, F. Kakuma, M. Homma and S. Fukuda, *Biochim. Biophys. Acta*, 88, 155 (1964)
99. A. Takagi, Y. Muto, Y. Takahashi and K. Nakao, *Clin. chim. Acta*, 20, 41 (1968)
100. E. Kuhn and D. Seiler, *Klin. Wschr.*, 48, 1134 (1970)
101. P. Patriarca, M. Zatti and D. Gompertz, *Biochem. J.*, 115, 1079 (1969)
102. Y. Furukawa, I. Yano, K. Fukuama and J. Tani, *Proc. Symp. chem. Physiol. Path.*, 9, 68 (1969)
103. K. Owens, *In* Research in Muscular Dystrophy: Proceedings of the Fourth Symposium on Current Research in Muscular Dystrophy, p. 286. Pitman, London (1968)
104. G. G. Lunt, E. de Robertis and E. Stefani, *Biochem. J.*, 121, 23P (1971)
105. S. E. Max, P. G. Nelson and R. O. Brady, *J. Neurochem.*, 17, 1517 (1970)
106. P. V. Sulakhe, M. Fedelesova, D. B. McNamara and N. S. Dhalla, *Biochem. Biophys. Res. Comm.*, 42, 793 (1971)
107. L. D. Peachey, *In* The Physiology and Biochemistry of Muscle as a Food (E. J. Briskey, R. G. Cassens and B. B. Marsh, eds), p. 273. Univ. of Wisconsin Press (1970)
108. H. Sugita, K. Okimoto and S. Ebashi, *Proc. Jap. Acad.* 42, 295 (1966)
109. A. Martonosi, *Proc. Soc. exp. Biol. (N.Y.)*, 127, 824 (1968)
110. F. J. Samaha and J. Gergely, *New Engl. J. Med.*, 280, 184 (1969)
111. A. Margreth, S. Di Mauro, G. Salviati and G. F. Turati, Abstr. IImes Journees Internationales de Pathologie Neuro-musculaire, Marseille (1970)
112. J. F. Van Pilsum and E. A. Wolin, *J. Lab. clin. Med.*, 51, 219 (1958)
113. J. M. S. Pearce, R. J. Pennington and J. N. Walton, *J. Neurol. Neurosurg. Psychiat.*, 27, 96 (1964)
114. H. Heyck, G. Laudahn and P. M. Carsten, *Klin. Wschr.*, 44, 695 (1966)
115. H. Iwashita and Y. Ohta, *Lancet* i, 621 (1967)
116. E. R. Williams and A. Bruford, *Clin. chim. Acta*, 27, 53 (1970)
117. B. McArdle, *In* Muscle Diseases: Proceedings of an International Congress, Milan, 19-21 May, 1969 (J. N. Walton, N. Canal and G. Scarlato, eds), p. 205. Excerpta Medica, Amsterdam (1970)
118. G. V. Horn, J. B. Drori and F. D. Schwartz, *Arch. Neurol.*, 22, 335 (1970)

119. J. N. Walton and R. J. T. Pennington, *Ann. N.Y. Acad. Sci.*, **138** (Art. 1), 315 (1966)
120. J. M. S. Pearce, R. J. Pennington and J. N. Walton, *J. Neurol. Neurosurg. Psychiat.*, **27**, 181 (1964)
121. B. P. Roy, J. F. Laws and A. R. Thomson, *Biochem. J.*, **120**, 177 (1970)
122. B. P. Hughes, *Clin. chim. Acta*, **7**, 597 (1962)
123. J. Stephens and E. Lewin, *J. Neurol. Neurosurg. Psychiat.*, **28**, 104 (1965)
124. P. Hudgson, D. Gardner-Medwin, R. J. T. Pennington and J. N. Walton, *J. Neurol. Neurosurg. Psychiat.*, **30**, 416 (1967)
125. B. McArdle, *In* Disorders of Voluntary Muscle (J. N. Walton, ed.), p. 607. Churchill, London (1969)
126. K. Steinitz, *In* Advances in Clinical Chemistry, (H. Sobotka and C. P. Stewart, eds), Vol. 9, p. 227. Academic Press, New York (1967)
127. G. Hug, W. K. Schubert and G. Chuck, *Biochem. Biophys. Res. Comm.*, **40**, 982 (1970)
128. S. Tarui, G. Okuno, Y. Okura, T. Tanaka, M. Suda and M. Nishikawa, *Biochem. Biophys. Res. Comm.*, **19**, 517 (1965)
129. E. Satoyoshi and H. Kowa, *Arch. Neurol.*, **71**, 248 (1967)
130. H. G. Hers, *Biochem. J.*, **86**, 11 (1963)
131. H. Zellweger, B. Illingworth Brown, W. E. McCormick and T. Jun-Bi., *Ann. paediat.*, **205**, 413 (1965)
132. P. Hudgson, D. Gardner-Medwin, M. Worsfold, R. J. T. Pennington and J. N. Walton, *Brain*, **91**, 435 (1968)
133. A. G. Engel, *Brain*, **93**, 599 (1970)
134. L. J. Hurwitz, D. McCormick and I. V. Allen, *Lancet*, i, 67 (1970)

CHAPTER 3

The Biochemistry of Demyelination and Demyelinating Diseases

B. GERSTL

Part I

Prototypes of Demyelination and Their Biochemical Aspects

3.I.1 WALLERIAN DEGENERATION

Wallerian degeneration was the first experimental model of demyelination devised and has been widely investigated both structurally and biochemically. After severing a peripheral nerve there is increasing loss of cerebrosides, sphingomyelin, cholesterol and phospholipids, that of the cephalins starting earlier and exceeding that of lecithin [1]. During the first 14 days after neurotomy the decrease of fatty aldehydes exceeds that of phosphatides and of fatty acid esters [2]. The fatty acids of the total lipids [3] decrease at different rates: C16 : 1

69

and C18 : 2 starting earlier, the PUFA at 16 days. PI remains constant until the 32nd day after injury. Cholesterol esters are found in significant amounts as early as eight days [3]. Loss of lipids, as well as increased neutral proteinase activity [4, 5, 6], proceed until approximately the 32nd day. Then resynthesis of lipids starts and continues up to the 132nd day but the quantity synthesized does not reach the amount seen in the controls [1, 7]. There is overlapping of these processes, and the phagocytosis and catabolism of myelin by the Schwann cells, and esterification of cholesterol. Sequential study [8] reveals that myelin formed last is the first to fall prey to the degenerative process, progressing toward the one laid down first. ^{14}C-labelled choline, ethanolamine or serine administered during the phase of remyelination in rats are incorporated in greater amounts into the lipids of the regenerating nerve than into the intact control. This is noted up to eight weeks after the injury [7].

The chemical analysis, by necessity, includes all the structures of the peripheral nerve. For separation of the changes in axons and Schwann cells resort has been taken to histochemistry and electron microscopy. In the axon, as in the myelin, there is a continuum of changes, the earliest (24 h) consisting of increase in number and density of neuro-filaments [9], in addition to accumulation of axonal mito-chondria which soon swell and fragment. This accumulation is particularly noted in the perinodal axoplasm of large myelinated fibres [10]. Within 48 h a large number of "bodies" of different morphology replace the entire axis cylinder. As early as 12 h after neurotomy there is activation of acid phosphatase and proteinase, probably of lysosomal origin [5, 9, 11]. Almost simultaneously there is decrease of trypanophilic protein [6]. Both the phosphatase and proteinase activity increase during the degenerative period while alkaline phosphatase activity becomes more prominent during regenera-tion [5, 12]. From the fourth day on, labelled thymidine is increasingly incorporated into the Schwann cells, apparently paralleling their enhanced metabolic activity and increase of ribosomes [11] considered a preliminary to augmented protein synthesis.

In the CNS the degenerative process proceeds slower and

somewhat differently [13, 14, 15]. Here, the myelin fragments retain their staining characteristics, and cholesterol esters are not demonstrable until 7-8 weeks after severance of the posterior roots [16]. This also has been observed on the dorsal columns of the spinal cord of the cat with phagocytes containing remnants of myelin present up to 6-8 weeks after sectioning [17]. The slower rate may be due to the myelin-forming oligodendroglia cells not behaving like Schwann cells, and myelin digestion depending on the arrival of macrophages. In the optic nerve, after enucleation of the homolateral eye [18], a marked increase of the S-100 acidic protein occurs, while other soluble proteins remain stable.

The data presented indicate that axonal lysosomal enzymes, which, in addition to the demonstrated proteinases and phosphatases are likely to include phospholipases [19], play a primary role in the destruction of myelin. Digestion of phagocytosed myelin by macrophages follows soon in the instance of the peripheral nerve, later in the CNS. There is preferential catabolism of plasmalogens and certain fatty acids, followed by resynthesis.

3.1.2 DEMYELINATION DUE TO INGESTION OR INHALATION OF TOXIC SUBSTANCES

3.1.2.1 Cyanide intoxication

This prototype of demyelinating disorder is of interest in view of the particular susceptibility of the corpus callosum when small protracted doses of cyanide are given [20, 21]. Recent EM studies [22] corroborate earlier light microscopic findings [23] that the axon is not the locus of the primary injury. In acute poisoning, separation of the myelin lamellae and intramyelinic vacuolization takes place and membranous fragments are seen in the spaces thus formed. The ensuing myelin degeneration is frequently asymmetric. The oligodendrocytes show swelling of the endoplasmic reticulum in the perikarion. Phagocytosis of myelin fragments starts 2-3 days later [22].

Histochemical and biochemical data furnish only partial explanation of the morphologic changes. The increased activity of oxidative enzymes [24, 25] probably represents attempts at repair and would correspond to the remyelination usually beginning at 10 days [26]. When larger doses of cyanide are used, oxidative enzyme activity is depressed [27].

In the areas of damage, cerebrosides and DNA are decreased [28]. *In vitro* experiments reveal decreased uptake of acetate into lipids and of leucine into proteins [29] of both myelin and non-myelin structures of brain but not of spinal cord, suggesting a difference in susceptibility. The concentration of cyanide in *in vitro* experiments, however, is probably much higher than occurs *in vivo*.

Cyanide ions form complexes with metallo-enzymes such as cytochrome oxidase [30], and also have a depressive effect upon acetyl-Coenzyme A synthetase and ATP-citrate lyase [31]. Also, an unknown cyanide-sensitive factor is involved in the desaturation of fatty acids [32, 33]. These effects may be part of the mechanism leading to structural alterations.

Furthermore, cyanide causes, *in vitro*, a marked efflux of calcium from the unmyelinated squid axon [34]. Calcium in the axon is assumed to be held in mitochondria and other intracellular membranes [34] and has been considered essential for their stability [35]. Whether cyanide is instrumental in removing it therefrom or from myelin has not been tested.

3.1.2.2 Carbon monoxide

Several comprehensive reviews of the anatomical lesions caused by CO poisoning are available [36, 37, 38, 39]. After intermittent exposure there is extensive demyelination in the CNS with gliosis, but preservation of the U fibres [40, 36, 37]. Whenever demyelination is incomplete, the axons, by light microscopic criteria, are intact [36]. Leucoencephalopathy, however, following acute CO poisoning also has been reported [41]. Part of the pathology of the white matter in human cases appears to be contributed by the destructive changes of venules and capillaries described as focal disintegration, partial necrosis and obliteration [36] or endothelial swelling [37] leading to impairment of the BBB.

The greater sensitivity of white matter to CO has been corroborated by EM studies on experimental animals [42].

There, neurones in both acute and subacute poisoning reveal only slight and infrequent fragmentation of endoplasmic reticulum and Golgi apparatus, while nucleus and mitochondria remain intact. In contrast, oligodendroglia cells show marked dilatation and fragmentation of the endoplasmic reticulum. The tissues surrounding the capillaries in these experiments are intact and no evidence of oedema is found, suggesting that, at least in experimental animals, impairment of the BBB does not play a major role. The myelin reveals exfoliation and disappearance of the lamellar structure. In the axons, both myelinated and unmyelinated, enlarged mitochondria with their cristae fragmented or having disappeared, and only their limiting double membrane remaining, are seen. These changes progress to complete degeneration of the mitochondria.

The biochemical findings in a human case with relapsing symptoms after CO poisoning [43] include reduction of total phospholipids, cerebrosides and of total cholesterol to about 40-50% of the amount in the controls. Lipid hexosamines and total hexosamines are not markedly different from controls. In the grey matter, however, biochemical changes are practically absent.

In non-lethal experimental CO poisoning there is marked decrease of glycogen with concomitant increase of lactate, indicating accelerated carbohydrate catabolism [44]. Glycogen phosphorylase which catabolizes the transformation into glucose-1-phosphate does, however, not show any increased activity. AMP which activates phosphorylase B (dephosphorylase) is increased by 50%. Cyclic AMP, which stimulates the conversion of phosphorylase B to A in liver preparations [45] and is one of the controlling factors in phosphorylase activation in liver and skeletal muscle, has not been investigated as to its involvement in the control of brain phosphorylase action [46].

The structural changes of the mitochondria mentioned may be related to the great affinity of haemoprotein P-450 to CO. This cytochrome is known to be present in subcellular structures of liver [47, 48] and adrenals [49]. Thus, the primary damage may be that to the mitochondria of oligodendrocytes and axons with the described ultrastructural changes ensuing. The assumption that CO poisoning effect in brain is largely independent of ischaemia is suggested by the

CNS damage in foetuses after CO exposure of the mother [50]. It is well known that the foetal brain is rather resistant to anoxia, and thus the severe alterations occurring in the foetus point to a specific damage incurred by the CO exposure of the mother.

3.I.2.3 Lead

Although the neuropathological effect of lead poisoning has been known for almost a century [51], and is of no less actuality today than then [52], the pathomechanism of this intoxication has been only partly elucidated. There is also lack of correlation between sequelae of lead poisoning such as anaemia or renal lesions and the onset of neuropathy [53, 54]. Likewise, the disturbance of the porphyrin metabolism expressing itself in urinary excretion of coproporphyrin, porphobilinogen and 5-amino laevulinic acid, although a reliable criterion for lead poisoning in humans [55, 56], far antecedes neurological damage.

The amount of lead found in the CNS is small compared with that in liver (150 vs 700-3,000 μg/100 g wet wt) [57] and, therefore, a direct toxic effect has been questioned. A postulated increase of permeability of the BBB [58] has been ascribed to alterations of the pericapillary structures [59].

In the peripheral nerve, the primary damage seems to occur in Schwann cells [60]. Electron dense granules in these cells observed in unstained preparations have been interpreted as lead particles [61]. The segment of myelin that is related to the degenerating Schwann cell shows splitting of the major and minor dense lines, and membranous blebs formation interpreted as a hydration effect [60]. In addition, accumulation of acid phosphatases in the nodal part of the axoplasm [61] point to abnormal lysosomal activity.

The changes described are considered insufficient to account for the demyelinating effect of lead, and a specific chemical pathology has been sought for. Porphyrin and porphobilinogen, when injected into experimental animals, do not cause neuropathy [62, 63]. It has been suggested, therefore, that a substance for which porphobilinogen serves as precursor is essential for maintenance of myelin. The synthesis of this precursor in the liver is assumedly blocked by lead and, therefore, not available [64].

Lead could exert an effect upon myelin maintenance also by its combination with sulph-hydryl groups, inhibiting enzymes where this group is essential for activity. This has been demonstrated for haem synthetase and delta-amino-laevulinic acid dehydrase [65, 66]. Acyl carrier protein (ACP) which binds acyl intermediates in the course of formation of long chain fatty acids [67] contains one free —SH group per mole which is the substrate binding group. Although ACP has not been isolated as yet from animal tissues [68, 69], the —SH group is similarly essential in the synthetase multi-enzyme complex and obliteration of this —SH group by lead causing insufficient fatty acid synthesis or elongation and, thereby, destabilization of myelin [70] could well be part of the pathomechanism in lead intoxication. Regrettably, fatty acid data on CNS or PNS in this condition are not available.

3.1.3 DIPHTHERITIC NEUROPATHY

Diphtheritic neuropathy [71, 72] varies in its morphology depending on the animal species. It is segmental in character. In the guinea pig diphtheria toxin appears to exert a selective damage upon the Schwann cell [73, 74], while the axon remains unaffected if small amounts of toxin are used. After parenteral injection of the toxin into chicken, electron dense bodies containing acid phosphatase and probably representing abnormal lysosomes appear in a few Schwann cells close to the axon, while only a very occasional myelin lamina shows fragmentation. At 6-9 days, these dense bodies become slightly more numerous and fragmentation is more frequent. Then phagocytosis of myelin by, and digestion in, Schwann cells starts [75]. Biochemically, acid phosphatase, and histochemically, activity of this enzyme as well as of acid protease are markedly increased [76, 77].

A nutritional disturbance as part of the pathomechanism of this lesion is suggested by the interference by diphtheria toxin with protein synthesis [78, 79]. Inhibition of ^{14}C glycine incorporation into proteins of peripheral nerve of rats by diphtheria toxin [80], a phenomenon also observed in various other tissues [81, 82], correlates to the decreased protein synthesis and indicates damage to metabolic processes in the Schwann cells which are responsible for maintaining the myelin.

3.I.4 DEMYELINATING CONDITIONS DUE TO INBORN METABOLIC ERRORS

3.I.4.1 Sudanophilic leucodystrophy (Jimpy mice)

The genetically determined defective development of myelin in Jimpy mice is a prototype most promising for elucidation of demyelination since the pathological process is limited to the central nervous system, axons are spared and inflammatory or gliotic response is absent [83]. The availability of littermates free of the genetic defect as controls enhances the value of this model.

It is well established now that the most striking biochemical deviation from the control values is the almost complete failure of the cerebrosides and sulphatides to increase during development, the former at 29 days being only 2-10% of the amount in the controls [84, 85, 86, 87]. Glucocerebrosides represent about 20% of the total glycolipids in contrast to trace amounts in the controls [88]. The deficit of phosphatides is considerably less than that of cerebrosides [87, 89]. The amount of sphingomyelin and the distribution of the individual phospholipids are similar to those in controls [87] with the exception of plasmalogens, which, at 22 days, are only 50% of the amount in the littermates [87, 90].

Reports on cholesterol are at variance. In two series it was found in normal amounts [89, 91], while in two others [84, 90] it was decreased. Cholesterol esters are absent [87]. Gangliosides are quantitatively and qualitatively similar to those in controls [91, 92].

The inadequacy of cerebroside formation is associated with a deficit of lignoceric and nervonic acid [91]. Increased activity of cerebroside galactosidase after sonication of brain homogenate [86] is one of the enzymatic abnormalities demonstrated. Another is the greatly reduced activity of the galactosyl-sphingosine transferase, the enzyme catalyzing the synthesis of psychosine from sphingosine and UDP-galactose [88].

Additional enzymatic defects have to be postulated including one of epimerase; one of the synthesis of the fatty acyl moiety, possibly of the elongation process, and a defect in synthesis, or a specific catabolism of plasmalogens. Tissue culture experiments establish that the enzymatic disturbances are not due to a diffusible factor [93].

Cyclic AMP has been reported to be one-eighth at 18 days, and one-tenth that in controls at 25 days [94]. It is unknown at present whether this is due to inadequate synthesis by adenyl cyclase or increase of the specific phosphodiesterase [95]. The former is localized in particulate fractions [96] derived from membranous structures [97, 98].

It is noteworthy that the Quaking mutant with a normal or near normal longevity and resembling the Jimpy mutant by their body tremor is devoid of sudanophilic deposits in the central nervous system though showing a deficit of cerebrosides which is of a lower degree [87]. The decrease of the long chain fatty acids is, however, present here as in the Jimpy mutant [91, 99].

These findings would suggest that the concentration of cerebrosides in mice may be lowered to about 30% of normal causing clinical symptoms but allowing the animal an almost normal life span. Cerebrosides below that level, however, are incompatible with CNS function essential for life.

Another mutant reported recently in which death occurs even earlier than in Jimpy mice shows also marked reduction of galactolipids and cholesterol and normal amounts of gangliosides, but a deficiency of hexaenes and absence of fatty acids of 24 carbon chain length [100].

3.1.4.2 Globoid (cell) leucodystrophy in dogs

This familial canine disease, first reported in 1963 [101], is characterized by bilateral symmetrical loss of myelin in white matter with sparing of the arcuate fibres, demyelination of the spinal cord, and by presence of globoid cells containing PAS positive, non-metachromatic material [102]. Biochemically, total lipids in white matter are 31-45% and sulphatides 50-60%

of normal, while cerebrosides are slightly increased. The most striking change is a 160-300% increase of sphingomyelin. The fatty acids of the latter show a shift toward shorter chain length [103]. An enzymatic abnormality, namely a beta-galactosidase deficiency, found also in liver and kidney, appears to be the same as in human globoid (cell) leuco-dystrophy [104], and will be discussed there. Also, a slight reduction of the sulphotransferase is noted in the cerebellum, but not elsewhere in the CNS.

3.1.5 EXPERIMENTAL ALLERGIC ENCEPHALITIS

This experimental disease is of interest in view of its close resemblance to rabies vaccine induced encephalitis in humans [105, 106, 107] and its possible role as a model for studying other demyelinating diseases, including MS. Its biochemical aspects include:

(a) Chemical alterations preceding the infiltration of the CNS by haematogenous cells and at the time of the fully developed disease.
(b) The chemical-structural properties of the EAE inducing-protein and its biologically active fragments responsible for the exceedingly powerful antigenicity and,
(c) Attempts at their modification for the purpose of preventing the disease.

The first change occurring in the brain antecedent to cellular infiltration and demyelination appears to be increase of vascular permeability, as demonstrated by fluorescent micro-scopy [108], by intravenous injection of dyes [109], of labelled albumin [110, 111], or of labelled homologous gamma globulins [112]. The increase in permeability is, however, not regularly observed [112]. It is noteworthy that emigration of inflammatory cells occurs sometimes from vessels that appear to be impermeable to labelled gamma globulins suggesting two different mechanisms.

In guinea pigs, there is also exudation of autologous proteins containing gamma globulins, as demonstrated by specific flourescent labelled anti-sera [113, 114, 115].

The increased permeability of the BBB has been shown also in rats by intravenous injection of Thorotrast (colloidal thorium dioxide) [116]. In this species, the passage of Thorotrast and of protein takes place concomitantly with the infiltration by haematogenous mononuclear cells. Clefts seen between endothelial cells appear to be the anatomical correlate of this [116].

At the early stage of EAE (day 1-10), the myelin, by EM criteria, is intact [117] and the axons are free of change. Demyelination which usually occurs 10 days or more after sensitization shows two distinct patterns: (a) focal vesiculation with extracellular lysis, often preceded by separation of myelin lamellae, and (b) invasion of the myelin sheath by haematogenous mononuclear cells, with peeling off of myelin laminae [116, 117].

During the early stage there is increased proteinase activity, as demonstrated histochemically [118, 119]. This may result from increased permeability of lysosomal membranes allowing release of lysosomal enzymes [120]. There is also depression of myelin and non-myelin lipid synthesis as demonstrated by ^{14}C glucose uptake into slices of spinal cord [121].

At a later stage (10-18 days) cellular infiltration is usually extensive and clinical symptoms of the disease are overt. Lysosomal permeability, and hydrolase, and neutral proteinase activity are markedly accentuated [120]. Soluble brain proteins at this stage are decreased [122]. Myelin lipid synthesis, as measured by ^{14}C glucose uptake, remains below normal while that of protein increases. In the non-myelin fraction, however, both of these metabolic activities are intensified [121]. The latter may be ascribed to the invading inflammatory cells. These changes, as well as the loss of myelin seen at this stage in microscopic sections, correlate with reduction of the amount of phospholipids and cholesterol, and the appearance of cholesterol esters [123].

Although the encephalitogenic effect of brain or spinal cord homogenate had been known for many years, it was the separation of two proteins, homogeneous by ultracentri-fugational and electrophoretic criteria, that promoted further research. These were a collagen-like protein with low EAE activity [124], and a basic protein obtained by a different extraction procedure but antigenically active in guinea pigs at a dosage as low as 8 μg [125]. The molecular weight of this basic protein has been variously estimated from 10,000 to 50,000 [126]. It is remarkable that the biological activity of this protein remains intact after heating to 100° C for one hour or treatment with 8 M urea [126]. Neither an alpha helix nor a beta-structure has been found in it [127]. Fragments of this cathodic protein have been isolated that, although only of peptide size, are effective in inducing EAE [128, 129, 130]. The active fragment is derived from the carboxyl terminus of the basic protein [128].

The amino acid sequence of an active peptide obtained from the basic protein has been established [131], and several active polypeptides [132] also have been synthesized. The most active one contains only nine amino acid residues. It appears that the encephalitogenic region can be reduced to the following sequence of nine residues: Phe-Ser-Try-Gly-Ala-Glu-Gly-Gin-Lys [132], with the NH_2 terminal phenylalanine and the carboxyl terminal lysine surrounding a single tryptophan residue which is essential for the activity in guinea pigs. Modification of the basic protein with 2-hydroxy-5-nitrobenzyl bromide or with 2-nitrophenylsulphenyl, which reacts with the tryptophan residue, eliminates its encephalitogenic activity for guinea pigs but not for rabbits [133, 134]. Results of guinea pig inoculation with other chemical or enzymic degradation products of the basic protein, or with polypeptides derived therefrom [135], indicate that the amino acid carboxyl-terminal ends of the chain can be removed without loss of activity. These and other data [130] suggest that there are two species-specific determinants present in the basic protein.

REFERENCES

1. N. S. Burt, A. R. McNabb and R. J. Rossiter, *Biochem. J.*, 47, 318 (1950)
2. J. Domonkos and L. Heiner, *J. Neurochem.*, 15, 87 (1968)
3. J. F. Berry, W. H. Cevallos and R. R. Wade, Jr., *JAOCS.*, 42, 492 (1965)
4. G. Porcellati and B. Curti, *J. Neurochem.*, 5, 277 (1960)
5. J. F. Hallpike, C. W. M. Adams and O. B. Bayliss, *Histochem. J.*, 2, 209 (1970)

6. J. F. Hallpike, C. W. Adams and O. B. Bayliss, *Histochem. J.*, 2, 323 (1970)
7. D. Nicholls and R. J. Rossiter, *J. Neurochem.*, 11, 813 (1964)
8. R. G. Simon, R. R. Wade, J. E. DeLarco and M-L. Baker, *J. Neurochem.*, 16, 1435 (1969)
9. H. Cravioto, *Los Angeles Neurol. Soc. Bull.*, 34, 233 (1969)
10. H. DeF. Webster, *J. Cell Biol.*, 12, 361 (1962)
11. E. Holtzman and A. B. Novikoff, *J. Cell Biol.*, 27, 651 (1965)
12. T. Samorajski, *J. Histochem. Cytochem.*, 5, 15 (1957)
13. S. A. Luse and R. E. McCaman, *Amer. J. Path.*, 33, 586 (1957)
14. R. E. McCaman and E. Robins, *J. Neurochem.*, 5, 18 (1959)
15. P. M. Daniel and S. J. Strich, *Acta neuropath. (Berlin)*, 12, 314 (1969)
16. P. W. Lampert and M. R. Cressman, *Amer. J. Path.*, 49, 1139 (1966)
17. A. Bignami and H. J. Ralston, *Brain Res.*, 13, 444 (1969)
18. V. J. Perez, J. W. Olney, T. J. Cicero, B. W. Moore and B. A. Bahn, *J. Neurochem.*, 17, 511 (1970)
19. M. Waite, G. L. Scherphof, F. M. G. Boshouwers and L. L. M. Van Deenen, *J. Lipid Res.*, 10, 411 (1969)
20. C. E. Lumsden, *J. Neurol. Neurosurg. Psychiat.*, 13, 1 (1950)
21. S. Levine and W. Stypulkowski, *Arch. Path.*, 67, 306 (1959)
22. A. Hirner, *Acta neuropath. (Berlin)*, 13, 350 (1969)
23. E. W. Hurst, *Aust. J. exp. Biol. Med. Sci.*, 18, 201 (1940)
24. W. H. Houten and R. L. Friede, *Exp. Neurol.*, 4, 402 (1961)
25. M. Z. M. Ibrahim, P. B. Briscoe, O. B. Bayliss and C. W. M. Adams, *J. Neurol. Neurosurg. Psychiat.*, 26, 479 (1963)
26. A. Hirano, S. Levine and H. M. Zimmerman, *J. Neuropath. exp. Neurol.*, 26, 200 (1967)
27. Adolfo F. Fernandez, J. Gonzalez-Quintana and M. Russek, *Am. J. Physiol.*, 204, 314 (1963)
28. N. H. Bass, *Neurology, Minneap.*, 18, 167 (1968)
29. M. E. Smith, *Trans. amer. Soc. Neurochem.*, 1, 111 (1970)
30. H. R. Mahler and E. H. Cordes (eds), Biological Chemistry, p. 256. Harper & Row, New York and London (1966)
31. S. Serra, G. Amore and V. Bonavita, *Riv. Pat. nerv. ment.*, 90, 69 (1969)
32. N. Oshino, Y. Imai and R. Sato, *Biochim. Biophys. Acta*, 128, 13 (1966)
33. W. Stoffel and H. G. Schiefer, *Hoppe Seyler Z. Physiol. Chem.*, 345, 41 (1966)
34. M. P. Blaustein and A. L. Hodgkin, *J. Physiol., Lond.*, 200, 497 (1969)
35. F. A. Vandenheuvel, *JAOCS*, 42, 481 (1964)
36. C. B. Courville, *J. nerv. ment. Dis.*, 125, 534 (1957)
37. F. Seitelberger and K. Jellinger, *Wien. klin. Wschr.*, 74, 422 (1960)
38. H. Shiraki, *Advances Neurol. Sci. (Tokyo)*, 12, 389 (1968)
39. H. Garland and J. Pearce, *Quart. J. Med.*, 36, 445 (1967)
40. A. Meyer, *Z. ges. Neurol. Psychiat.*, 112, 172 (1928)

41. K. Jellinger, *Acta neuropath. (Berlin)*, 1, 411 (1962)
42. T. Miyagishi and N. Suwa, *Acta neuropath. (Berlin)*, 14, 118 (1969)
43. M. Wender, *Acta neuropath. (Berlin)*, 2, 371 (1963)
44. C.-J. Estler, H. P. T. Ammon and V. Zimmerman, *Naunyn-Schmiedebergs Arch. Pharmak. exp. Path.*, 263,204 (1968)
45. T. W. Rall and E. W. Sutherland, *J. biol. Chem.*, 232, 1065 (1958)
46. G. I. Drummond, J. Keith and M. W. Gilgan, *Arch. Biochem. Biophys.*, 105, 156 (1964)
47. M. Klingenberg, *Arch. Biochem. Biophys.*, 75, 376 (1958)
48. D. Garfinkel, *Arch. Biochem. Biophys.*, 77, 493 (1958)
49. L. D. Wilson and B. W. Harding, *Biochemistry*, 9, 1621 (1970)
50. H. Bankl and K. Jellinger, *Beitr. Path. Anat.*, 135, 350 (1967)
51. M. Gombault, *Arch. Neurol., Paris*, 1, 11 (1880)
52. Editorial, *Lancet*, 1, 704 (1970)
53. P. M. Fullerton, *J. Neuropath. exp. Neurol.*, 25, 214 (1966)
54. S. S. Schochet, Jr. and J. C. Harkin, Lead Neuropathy in Rats. Unpublished data
55. K. Cramer and S. Selander, *Brit. J. indust. Med.*, 22, 311 (1965)
56. S. Selander and K. Cramer, *Brit. J. indust. Med.*, 27, 28 (1970)
57. N. Popoff, S. Weinberg and I. Feigen, *Neurology, Minneap.*, 13, 101 (1963)
58. A. Pentschew and F. Garro, *Acta neuropath. (Berlin)*, 6, 266 (1966)
59. A. J. Raimondi, F. Beckman and J. P. Evans, *Trans. amer. Neurol. Assoc.*, 9, 322 (1966)
60. P. W. Lampert and S. S. Schochet, Jr., *J. Neuropath. exp. Neurol.*, 27, 527 (1968)
61. W. W. Schlaepfer, *J. Neuropath. exp. Neurol.*, 28, 401 (1969)
62. A. Goldberg, *Quart. J. Med.* 28, 183 (1959)
63. J. B. Gibson and A. Goldberg, *J. Path. Bact.*, 71, 495 (1956)
64. M. Kreimer-Birnbaum and M. Grinstein, *Biochim. Biophys. Acta*, 111, 110 (1965)
65. M. Grinstein, R. M. Bannerman and C. V. Moore, *Blood*, 14, 476 (1959)
66. J. J. Chisholm, Jr., *J. Pediat.*, 64, 174 (1964)
67. P. W. Majerus and P. R. Vagelos, *Adv. Lipid Res.*, 5, 1 (1967)
68. A. R. Larrabee, E. G. McDaniel, H. A. Bakerman and P. R. Vagelos, *Proc. natn. Acad. Sci. U.S.A.*, 54, 267 (1965)
69. C. J. Chesterton, P. H. W. Butterworth, A. S. Abramovitz, E. J. Jacob and J. W. Porter, *Arch. Biochem. Biophys.*, 124, 386 (1968)
70. J. S. O'Brien, *Science*, 147, 1099 (1965)
71. P. Meyer, *Virchow Arch. Path. Anat.*, 85, 181 (1881)
72. E. Stransky, *J. Psychol. Neurol.*, 1, 169 (1902)
73. B. H. Waksman, R. D. Adams and H. C. Mansmann, Jr., *J. exp. Med.*, 105, 591 (1957)
74. J. B. Cavanagh and J. M. Jacobs, *Brit. J. exp. Path.*, 45, 309 (1964)
75. R. O. Weller, *J. Path. Bact.*, 89, 591 (1965)
76. R. O. Weller and R. S. Mellick, *Brit. J. exp. Path.*, 47, 425 (1966)

77. J. F. Hallpike and C. W. M. Adams, *Histochem. J.*, 1, 559 (1969)
78. N. Strauss, *J. exp. Med.*, 112, 351 (1960)
79. I. Kato and A. M. Pappenheimer, Jr., *J. exp. Med.*, 112, 329 (1960)
80. D. F. Matheson, *J. Neurochem.*, 15, 179 (1968)
81. I. Kato and H. Sato, *Japan J. exp. Med.*, 32, 495 (1962)
82. R. I. Collier and A. M. Pappenheimer, *J. exp. Med.*, 120, 1019 (1964)
83. R. L. Sidman, M. M. Dickie and S. H. Appel, *Science*, 144, 309 (1964)
84. J. L. Nussbaum, N. M. Neskovic, D. M. Kostic, P. Mandel, *Bull. Soc. Chim. Biol.*, 50, 2194 (1968)
85. C. Galli, D. re Cecconi Galli, *Nature (Lond.)*, 220, 165 (1968)
86. D. M. Bowen and N. S. Radin, *J. Neurochem.*, 16, 457 (1969)
87. E. L. Hogan, K. C. Joseph and G. Schmidt, *J. Neurochem.*, 17, 75 (1970)
88. N. Neskovic, J. L. Nussbaum and P. Mandel, *Brain Res.*, 21, 39 (1970)
89. C. Galli, G. M. Kneebone and R. Paoletti, *Life Sciences*, 8, 911 (1969)
90. C. M. Jacque, M. L. Harpin and N. A. Baumann, *Europ. J. Biochem.*, 11, 218 (1969)
91. N. A. Baumann, C. M. Jacque, S. A. Pollet and M. L. Harpin, *Europ. J. Biochem.*, 4, 340 (1968)
92. D. Kostic, J. L. Nussbaum and P. Mandel, *Life Sciences*, 8, 1135 (1969)
93. M. K. Wolf and A. B. Holden, *J. Neuropath. exp. Neurol.*, 28, 195 (1969)
94. T. Kurihara, J. L. Nussbaum and P. Mandel, *Brain Res. (Amst.)*, 13, 401 (1969)
95. G. A. Robison, R. W. Butcher and E. W. Sutherland, *Ann. Rev. Biochem.*, 37, 149 (1968)
96. E. DeRobertis, G. Rodriguez de Lores Arnaiz and M. Alberici, *J. biol. Chem.*, 242, 3487 (1967)
97. P. R. Davoren and E. W. Sutherland, *J. biol. Chem.*, 238, 3016 (1963)
98. M. Rubinowitz, L. Desalles, J. Meisler and L. Lorand, *Biochim. Biophys. Acta*, 97, 29 (1965)
99. N. A. Baumann, M. L. Harpin and J. M. Bourre, *Nature (Lond.)*, 227, 960 (1970)
100. H. Meier and A. D. MacPike, *Exp. Brain Res.*, 10, 512 (1970)
101. R. Fankhauser, H. Luginbuhl and W. Hartley, *Schweiz. Arch. Tierheilk.*, 105, 198 (1963)
102. B. Jortner and A. Jonas, *Acta neuropath. (Berlin)*, 10, 171 (1968)
103. J. D. Austin, D. Armstrong and G. Margolis, *Trans. amer. Neurol. Ass.*, 93, 181 (1968)
104. Y. Suzuki, J. Austin, D. Armstrong, K. Suzuki, J. Schlenker and T. Fletcher, *Exp. Neurol.*, 29, 65 (1970)
105. I. Uchimura and H. Shiraki, *J. Neuropath. exp. Neurol.*, 16, 139 (1957)

84 B. GERSTL

106. S. Lackermeier, *Schweiz. Arch. Tierheilk.*, **108**, 581 (1966)
107. K. Jellinger and F. Seitelberger, *Dtsch. Z. Nervenheilk.*, **184**, 508 (1963)
108. M. Serban and M. Matei, *Stud. Cercet. Neurol.*, 14, 279 (1969)
109. B. H. Waksman, *Int. Arch. Allergy*, Suppl. to Vol. 14, 1 (1959)
110. J. Olszewski, *In* Allergic Encephalomylelitis (M. W. Kies, ed.), p. 172. Charles C. Thomas, Springfield, Illinois (1952)
111. M. Vulpe, A. Hawkins, B. Rozdilsky, *Neurology (Minneap.)*, 10, 171 (1960)
112. R. W. P. Cutler, A. V. Lorenzo and C. F. Barlow, *J. Neuropath. exp. Neurol.*, 26, 558 (1967)
113. A. Ridley, *Z. Immun. Forsch.*, 125, 173 (1963)
114. E. Frick, *Zbl. ges. Neurol.*, 180, 218 (1965)
115. H. C. Rauch and S. Raffel, *Ann. N.Y. Acad. Sci.*, 122, 297 (1965)
116. P. Lampert, *Acta neuropath. (Berlin)*, 9, 99 (1967)
117. P. W. Lampert and M. W. Kies, *Exp. Neurol.*, 18, 210 (1967)
118. G. Benetato and E. Gabrielescu, *Ann. histochim.*, 9, 295 (1964)
119. G. Benetato, E. Gabrielescu and I. Boros, *Rev. Rouman. Physiol.*, 2, 379 (1965)
120. E. Gabrielescu, *Wien. Z. Nervenheilk.*, Suppl. 11, 70 (1960)
121. M. E. Smith, *J. Neurochem.*, 16, 1099 (1969)
122. Gr. Benetato, St. Secăreanu, E. Neumann, V. Vasilescu and G. Schmidt, *St. cerc. med. Cluj.*, 10, 17 (1959)
123. M. Wender, T. Wróblewski, Z. Adamczewska, M. Owsianowski and B. Zgorzalewicz, *Neuropat. pol.*, 7, 311 (1969)
124. E. Roboz, N. Henderson and M. W. Kies, *J. Neurochem.*, 2, 254 (1958)
125. E. R. Einstein, D. M. Robertson, J. M. DiCaprio and W. Moore, *J. Neurochem.*, 9, 353 (1962)
126. E. H. Eylar and M. Thompson, *Arch. Biochem. Biophys.*, 129, 468 (1969)
127. F. B. Palmer and R. M. C. Dawson, *Biochem. J.*, 111, 629 (1969)
128. L-P. Chao and E. R. Einstein, *J. biol. Chem.*, 234, 6050 (1968)
129. E. R. Einstein, J. Csejtey, W. J. Davis, A. Lajtha and N. Marks, *Int. Arch. Allergy*, 36, 363 (1969)
130. R. Kibler, R. Shapira, S. McKneally, S. Jenkins, P. Selden, F. Chou, *Science*, 164, 577 (1969)
131. E. H. Eylar and G. Hashim, *Proc. nat. Acad. Sci.*, 61, 644 (1968)
132. E. H. Eylar, J. Caccam and J. J. Jackson, *Science*, 168, 1220 (1970)
133. L-P. Chao and E. R. Einstein, *J. biol. Chem.*, 245, 6397 (1970)
134. R. J. Swanborg, *Fed. Proc.*, 29, 726 (1970)
135. L-P. Chao and E. R. Einstein, *J. Neurochem.*, 17, 1121 (1970)

Part II

Biochemical Aspects of Human Demyelinating Diseases

3.II.1 DEMYELINATION SECONDARY TO BRAIN OEDEMA

Brain oedema in humans may be a sequelae to a variety of conditions such as tumour, injuries, hypertension, infarct or hypercapnic hypoxia. In some instances there is overlapping of mechanisms, such as tumour causing increased intracranial pressure followed by haemorrhage. Brain oedema may be focal or diffuse, frequently occurring with exclusion of the arcuate fibres. It is now recognized by most authors that two types of brain oedema can be differentiated: vasogenic and cytoxic [1]. Their chemical parameters can be elucidated better in experimental models and tend to differ with the type of the oedema. The term "demyelination" in this condition refers to the pallor of white matter seen in sections stained for demonstration of myelin.

Vasogenic oedema affecting predominantly white matter results from vascular injury and ensuing increased capillary permeability. It can be produced experimentally by stab wounds, cold application, or insertion of space occupying substances, e.g., pellets, balloons, psyllium seeds. The oedema seen at the periphery of intracranial tumours belongs in this category.

In vasogenic oedema of white matter the fluid content, tissue sodium chloride and sodium : potassium ratio are increased. Total proteins, albumins and alpha fractions are also augmented [2, 3]. Incorporation of labelled amino acids into proteins and of uridine into RNA is enhanced [4]. PC and gangliosides are markedly decreased but PE and sphingomyelin do not show any change [5]. In oedematous areas of white matter in cases of brain tumour, increase of water content, decrease of cholesterol, cerebrosides and of total phospholipids, with relative increase of ethanolamine plasmalogens and of cholesterol esters, have been reported [6]. These areas stained by the Loyez method show pallor when compared with controls, confirming earlier observations [7]. In oedema of areas adjacent to haemorrhage there is reduction in the amount of ethanolamine plasmalogen, as well as diacyl-ethanolamine phosphatide [8].

There is impairment of oxidative phosphorylation [9] and of mitochondrial ATP formation. Increase of free fatty acids has been suggested as part of the mechanism leading to these enzymatic alterations [9]. By histochemical methods, SDH, a mitochondrial enzyme and acid phosphatase, a lysosomal enzyme, show enhanced activity [10]. The latter may be an antecedent to regressive astrocytic changes [11] but is not distinctive of vasogenic oedema since it is also seen after TET implantation [12].

Cytoxic oedema resulting from damage to the parenchymal cells in either grey or white matter is characterized by cellular swelling. Permeability of the vascular channels remains largely unimpaired, and the accumulated fluid resembles an ultrafiltrate of serum. Experimental models for this can be obtained by intravenous administration of distilled water, by hypercapnic hypoxia, or TET poisoning. Fluid, sodium and chloride are significantly increased but the BBB is intact, as indicated by tracer studies, and the extracellular space is of normal size [13]. LDH is increased in oedema produced by water intoxication, but not after triethyltin (TET) [12].

Ultrastructural studies in acute cytotoxic oedema obtained by TET application [14, 15] reveal separation of myelin lamellae and splitting of the intraperiod line but no evidence of destruction of myelin. In contrast, in brain oedema induced by insertion of PPD (vasogenic type), [16] there is myelin damage, and macrophages with phagocytosed myelin are found.

An hypothesis on the mechanism of production and spread of vasogenic brain oedema has been advanced based upon elevated serotonin levels in brain after injury and beneath subdural haematoma [17] as well as after hypothermia [18]. Increased 5-hydroxy tryptophan hydroxylase and diminished amino oxidase activity in the latter condition [18], resulting in both augmented formation and decreased catabolism of serotonin, are in line with this suggestion.

Two less frequent types of brain oedema merit mentioning: in cases of severe hypoglycaemia, due to insulin shock, oedema associated with pallor of white matter in corresponding myelin stains has been demonstrated [19]. This may find its explanation in the decrease of cerebral phospholipids demonstrated in rats subjected to experimental hypoglycaemia [20]. Brain oedema has also been observed in children afflicted with galactosaemia. In these cases, it is ascribed to osmotic action of the accumulated galactitol (dulcitol) [21, 22].

3.II.2 GLOBOID (CELL) LEUCODYSTROPHY

The hallmark of this inherited autosomal recessive disease is globoid cells which appear to be engorged with cerebrosides [23, 24, 25, 26, 27]. Experimental production of globoid cells by intracerebral injection of bovine cerebrosides into rats [28] corroborate this interpretation. Ultrastructurally, tubular [29, 30], randomly oriented pyramidal structures [31], slightly curved inclusion bodies [32] and laminated crystals [33] suggestive of crystals of cerebrosides are present within the globoid cells. Early in the disease granular changes are seen in the axons and myelin-like bodies in the oligodendroglia [34]. It is noteworthy that globoid cells may form also due to storage of sphingomyelin as seen in GLD in dogs.

Chemical analyses of white matter reveal decrease of total phospholipids, cholesterol, cerebrosides and sulphatides, increase of water content and near absence of cholesterol esters, as well as a ratio of cerebrosides : sulphatides almost double that in controls [35]. Decrease of hydroxy fatty acids [36, 37] has been reported. A marked loss of lignoceric and nervonic acid also noted [38] cannot be considered specific since this occurs also in other conditions [39, 40]. A lesser deficit of phospholipids and cholesterol, but not of cerebrosides, is seen in grey matter [38].

The amount of recoverable myelin in GLD is extremely low [41]. Its total lipid and cholesterol are slightly lower than in normal myelin, the PE : PC ratio is reversed, while total galactolipids and ratio of cerebrosides to phosphatides are normal. The ratio of cerebrosides to sulphatides is increased [42]. Conspicuous is the presence of gangliosides in the myelin[42]. Galactose is the only carbohydrate present in the glycolipids. Fatty acid distribution in myelin is normal with the exception of a reversed ratio of lignoceric to nervonic acid in the cerebrosides [41].

These findings suggest that a small number of oligodendrocytes are capable of producing sulphatide and a chemically normal myelin sheath [41]. The finding of more normal myelin at an earlier stage [27] suggests that there is also breakdown of myelin later in the disease, in addition to failure of myelination.

Two enzymatic defects have been discovered in GLD, and additional ones have to be postulated to explain all the observations. The imbalance between cerebrosides and sulphatides is explicable by a defect of the cerebroside-sulphotransferase [43, 44, 45], an enzyme first demonstrated in animals [46] where adenosine-3$'$-phosphate 5$'$-sulphato-phosphate serves as sulphate donor. This enzymatic deficiency is noted also in the kidneys of these patients [43]. Other enzymes such as acid phosphatase, sulphatase and other sphingolipid hydrolases, including ceramidase [45], however, show normal activity [25].

More recently, a profound deficiency of cerebroside-β-galactosidase in brain, liver and spleen of three patients with GLD has been reported [47] and corroborated on a larger series of cases [45]. This, by failure to catabolize cerebrosides normally, would lead to their accumulation and ingestion by macrophages eliciting formation of globoid cells. The latter, by their large numbers, would impair or cause death of oligodendrocytes and, thus, absence of myelin formation.

Alterations of peripheral nerves, interpreted by light microscopy as segmental demyelination [48] and degeneration of myelin [49], and ultrastructurally [50] of marked dilatation of the endoplasmic reticulum of Schwann cells and histiocytes, non-membrane bound needle or prismatic-shaped masses, and scarcity of organelles. The abnormal material in the histiocytes extrudes into the extracellular spaces.

3.II.3 METACHROMATIC LEUCODYSTROPHY

Three reports appearing in short succession indicated recognition of the metachromatic material accumulating in this disease as sulphated cerebrosides [51, 52, 53]. Birefringence of this material [54] corresponds to a pseudocrystalline structure as demonstrated by EM [55]. In addition, a variety of other inclusions, many lamellar or tubular in type, are seen within the oligodendroglia and macroglia, interpreted as lipid-protein layers of an abnormal molecular pattern [56]. The membranes surrounding the non-crystalline material with their strong acid phosphatase activity suggest lysosomal structures. Lamellar structures isolated by differential centrifugation [57] show an increased amount of sulphatides and proteins and decreased amounts of phospholipids. Myelin isolated from such cases [58, 59] reveal abnormalities both in ultrastructure [59] and chemical composition [60]. The proportion of sphingomyelin is decreased to about 40% and that of cerebrosides to less than 10% of normal, but sulphatides are increased five-fold, resulting in a cerebroside : sulphatide ratio of 1 : 20 as compared to one of 4 : 1 in controls.

The metabolic defect causing deposits of sulphatides involves also other organs, especially the kidney and leucocytes [61, 62, 63, 64, 65]. These abnormalities facilitate diagnosis by laboratory tests, such as determination of sulphatides in the urinary sediment.

The storage of sulphatides in white matter leads to reciprocal depletion of other lipids of white matter; cholesterol and phospholipids being diminished to about 50% of normal. There is no increase in cholesterol esters [66].

The disease occurs in both children and adults, the difference being that the increase of sulphatides is only 1.2- to 2.5-fold of normal in the adult in contrast to the infantile type, with an increase of 4-8 times normal. Also, depletion of white matter lipids in the adult is greater; the phrenosine type of sulphatides (hydroxy fatty acids) is more abundant, while the kerasine type sulphatides are diminished [67]. Hexosamines in the white matter ary increased [68].

Soon after identification of the accumulated material as sulphatides it was surmised that diminished sulphatase activity was the primary enzymatic defect [69]. This was supported by the demonstration of a sphingolipid sulphatase deficiency [70, 71, 72]. The defective enzyme was identified as aryl-sulphatase A [73, 74]. This, however, is the only enzymatic defect found so far in MLD; all other lysosomal enzymes in the brain being at normal levels [75]. The same defect has been demonstrated in renal tubules, peripheral leucocytes [76] and in fibroblasts cultured from skin of these patients [75], and was further corroborated by the very slow breakdown of sulphatides in human subjects with MLD [77]. Metachromatic inclusions are also present in the cytoplasm of the sural nerve [78].

Attempts to retard the synthesis of sulphatides by elimination of Vitamin A from the diet, or by intravenous and intrathecal administration of aryl-sulphatase A [79], did not succeed [76, 80].

3.II.4 SUDANOPHILIC LEUCODYSTROPHY

The problem of distinguishing SLD, Schilder's and Pelizaeus-Merzbacher disease has been discussed from the point of both morphology and chemical alterations [40, 81, 82, 83]. Although SLD and Schilder's disease appear to differ to a certain extent by chemical criteria [40], these two are combined and compared here.

White matter in SLD reveals marked depletion of lipids [40, 81, 85] with disproportionally greater loss of cerebrosides [40, 81, 84, 85, 86, 87] and deficit of long chain fatty acids, particularly lignoceric acid. Esterification of cholesterol ranges from 6% in one [40], to 70% in another case [84]. Increase of water content would correspond to formation of large extracellular spaces as seen in an ultrastructural study [88].

Lipid and non-lipid hexosamines [86, 89] are augmented. The loss of insoluble proteins and lipids [40] corresponds to the extensive loss of stainable myelin [81, 86, 88].

In the grey matter there is also decrease of phospholipids, of lignoceric acid, and presence of cholesterol esters [40]. The amount of cerebrosides, however, is comparable to that in controls.

A feature not reported so far for several demyelinating conditions including MS but found in SLD is the formation of a light myelin floating fraction showing preservation of the lamellar configuration but almost complete absence of periodicity [40]. This morphological feature, together with its chemical composition, suggests that entire segments of myelin are sequestrated. About one-half of the total cholesterol esters are present in this floating fraction. A similar fraction has been reported in a case of subacute sclerosing leucoencephalitis [90] and in one of gangliosidosis [91]. The chemistry of the low density fractions in these three conditions is fairly similar [92].

Histochemically [88], increased LDH, TPNH and TPNH-diaphorase activity is seen in astroyctes. Among the phagocytosed material are laminated structures probably representing remnants of myelin which would correspond to the data suggesting sequestration of entire myelin fragments.

An aspect of SLD awaiting elucidation is the not infrequent association with Addison's disease [93, 94, 95]. This concomitance gave rise to speculation that both diseases are due to autoimmunization. The symptoms, however, of hypo-adrenalism precede those of the cerebral disease [96, 97], and search for antibodies directed against adrenal tissue have failed to demonstrate any [97]. Also steroid replacement therapy is of no avail as far as neurological symptoms are concerned [96, 97].

Adrenalectomy in rats is followed by a disturbance of intestinal fat absorption [98], and one could assume that in a child with myelin being still in the developmental stage this may lead to improper myelination. There is, however, no experimental evidence available to support this. Adrenalectomy, being frequently employed for palliative treatment of cancer, has not resulted in a demyelinating disorder as far as can be ascertained from the literature.

The chemical findings in cases classified as "Schilder's disease" are: increase of water content, presence of large amounts of cholesterol esters, decrease of cerebrosides and of ethanolamine plasmalogen [92, 99]. An abnormal ganglioside pattern has also been reported [92], GB 2 and GB 3 being significantly increased, with a concomitant decrease of the normal major components. Qualitatively similar and quantitatively less extensive ganglioside changes have been seen in other diseases such as Jakob-Creutzfeld [100] and MLD [101]. Severe alterations of the ganglioside pattern, however, have been noted only in cases of subacute sclerosing panencephalitis [91, 102]. Since there is now evidence available that subacute sclerosing panencephalitis is of viral aetiology, the disturbed ganglioside pattern may suggest virus infection as a possible aetiology of this unusual disease.

A low density fraction has been found also in "Schilder's disease" containing a significant amount of esterified cholesterol [92], and lower proportions of protein and phospholipids than in SLD. Purified myelin in this condition [92] revealing decreased galactolipids and a moderate increase in cholesterol, however, does not differ from that in other demyelinating conditions [92].

3.II.5 PELIZAEUS-MERZBACHER DISEASE

The small number of cases classified as one of the several categories of Pelizaeus-Merzbacher disease [103, 104], and the scarcity of biochemical [105] and ultrastructural [106] data, preclude conclusions as to the sequence of events leading to the extensive absence of myelin. Three hypotheses have been advanced as to the manner in which the changes are produced, viz., through destruction or removal of myelin, similar to that in MS [107]; through faulty or incomplete formation of myelin that undergoes progressive degeneration and thus is considered to be a form of leucodystrophy [82, 108, 109]; and through arrest of myelination at an early age [23, 110].

The histopathological and electron microscopic findings infer great deficits of the lipids that are generally recognized as components of myelin. Indeed, several reports agree that, in the white matter, substantial deficits of cerebrosides [23, 105, 111] and of sulphatides [105, 106] exceeding those of cholesterol [23, 105, 106, 111] are present. In one case [104], these deficits were less in extent although there was a five-fold reduction of total lipids [112]. The proportion of unsubstituted long chain mono-unsaturated fatty acids is markedly reduced in both white and grey matter when compared with those in controls, while hydroxy fatty acids do not differ [105] in white matter. In the grey matter there is also a greater percentage of C16 : 0 and C18 : 0 acids than in controls.

If abnormal catabolism were the predominant feature of this disease one would expect cholesterol esters to be present to some degree. These, however, are minimal in amount [111]. The disproportion of lipid and fatty acid deficits would not be consonant with demyelination as the predominant or sole feature of this disease, rather improper biochemical composition due to a developmental disturbance, possibly followed by partial myelin catabolism, would best explain the data observed. The EM findings support these assumptions [106].

3.II.6 MULTIPLE SCLEROSIS

3.II.6.1 Plaques

The partial or complete absence of stainable myelin corresponds to depletion of lipids, including gangliosides [113, 114, 115] with disproportionate greater loss of plasmalogens [116, 117]. Cholesterol esters, however, varying in amount with the stage of the disease and hexosamines may be found there. The cholesterol esterifying acids are mostly made up of oleic acid while those in MS white matter consist chiefly of C16 : 0, C18 : 1 and C20 : 4 acids [118]. The increase in PUFA [115, 117] in plaques may be due to presence of cellular elements. Oligodendroglia cells, according to EM studies [119] are absent.

The proteins obtained from the centre of the plaques show absence, and those from the margin decrease, of the encephalitogenic basic protein [120]. A protein however, containing a high proportion of acidic amino acids and differing from the S-100 acidic protein [121] by amino acid composition and electrophoretic mobility comprises about 50% of the total proteins [122]. This protein is similar in amino acid composition and electrophoretic characteristics to one found in leucotomy scars and periventricular white matter.

In the centre of the plaques ATP-ase acid phosphatase [123], LDH and TPN-diaphorase [124, 125] are demonstrable, particularly in the lipid-laden macrophages. The acid phosphatase activity, on electrophorograms of protein extracts is located in a zone different from that from normal brains [125]. Oxidative enzyme activity is enhanced in early lesions and has been ascribed to cells interpreted as oligodendrocytes [126]. Active plaques as characterized by increased cell population and NADH activity show, on histochemical [126, 127] and chemical investigation [128] increased proteolytic activity in their border zones while inactive plaques reveal decreased or no proteinase activity by either method [128]. Acid phosphatase activity considered a marker for lysosomes is confined to lipid-laden microglia round plaques. Oligodendroglia cells in uninvolved white matter are devoid of these two enzyme activities [127] which corresponds to findings obtained by chemical determinations on extracts of white matter [128].

3.II.6.2 White matter

Lipids: The first report of lipid deficits in normal-appearing white matter of MS brains representing possibly a pre-demyelinating biochemical lesion was that of Cumings (1953) [129]. This has been supplemented by reports of depletion of phospholipids with disproportionately greater loss of plasmalogens [117, 130, 131], corresponding deficits of carboxyl esters and long chain mono-unsaturated long chain fatty acids [132]. More recently, deficits of eicosamonoenoic acid in the PE fraction have been reported by two groups of investigators [133, 134] associated with a higher ratio of $C22:6$ and lower ones of $C22:5$, as well as a deficiency of nervonic acid in cerebrosides [134]. Concomitant with these are reductions of cerebrosides or PE fraction in the white matter in the presence of nearly normal amounts of other lipids and of total proteins [120, 134], and a shift of cerebroside-sulphatide ratio [131]. In samples where thinning of myelin is observed in Luxol blue stained sections, proportional decrease of all lipid components is found [134]. The slight to moderate deficiency of plasmalogens in normal-appearing MS white matter is of interest in view of Cumings and Goodwin's report (1968) [131] that in brain oedema due to haemorrhage or tumour, in spite of a deficit of total phospholipids, plasmalogens are present in normal proportions. Gangliosides are present in normal amounts [115].

Lysolecithin, because of its cyto- and possibly myelinolytic effect, has been searched for and found in small quantities in normal white matter and MS plaques [135, 136]. It may represent an intermediary in the synthesis of lecithin [137]. It could be, however, a product of autolysis [138] since it accumulates in rat brain slices on incubation *in vitro* [139]. It was not, however, found in MS white matter in other investigations [134].

Proteins: The soluble proteins, easily prepared, have been most widely investigated (Cumings, 1961) [2]. On starch electrophoresis there are usually present two to four bands migrating cathodically similar to the gamma globulins of blood serum, seven to ten bands migrating anodically, and two to three prealbumin bands. One of the latter, a highly acidic prealbumin [121] is not changed quantitatively in MS white matter or CSF [140].

The amount of total soluble proteins after removal of microsomes by high speed centrifugation does not show any difference between MS and control brains [141]. Albumin is present in the soluble proteins in amounts from 25 to 29 mg/100 g wet wt in normal white matter, and no difference between MS white matter and controls is found [142].

Immunoglobulins measured by immuno-precipitation [142] or radial-immunodiffusion [141] show a wide range of the amount of IgG in both the controls and MS specimens, and a statistically significant increase in MS brains [141, 142]. This is also found in brains of individuals with multiple myeloma without any recognizable CNS lesion. The quantity of IgA does not differ in MS and controls. IgM is not present in any of the

BAND-4*

control or MS brains [141]. The immunoglobulins in MS brains may, however, be of significance as suggested by the *in vitro* myelinolytic effect of soluble proteins from MS white matter or plaques [143].

Glycoproteins [144, 145] in MS white matter have not been investigated. In the CSF, their quantity is not different in MS and controls [146]. Of the many enzymes reported to be present in white matter [147, 148, 149] only a few have been investigated in cases of MS. Acid proteinases [150] and plasmalogenase [151, 152] are increased but not peptidase or neutral proteinase. These may be implicated in the demyelinating process [151, 152].

3.II.6.3 Myelin

The advent of procedures furnishing myelin almost pure by EM criteria [153, 154] facilitates comparison between myelin prepared from the brains of MS and controls.

The amount of myelin recoverable from MS white matter is significantly less than in controls. Recovery does not apparently depend on autopsy-death interval [134]. Its PS and PI, in one series [155], and PE in another [156] were reported lower, while the former two lipids, in another investigation [131], were slightly higher than in controls. Sphingomyelin and cerebrosides, in per cent of total lipids were less in MS myelin than in the controls [157], while sulphatides were not. This resulted in a cerebroside : sulphatide ratio lower than in the controls [131]. PE and plasmalogens were also slightly but significantly reduced [157] but this was not found in another experiment [155]. The difference between the two groups of experiments may stem from different procedures for separation of the myelin.

A lower concentration of eicosamonoenoic acid and increase of polyenes noted in the PE fraction of whole white matter were also found in some MS myelin preparations [134, 155, 156]. If these findings are considered in conjunction with that of plasmalogens being reduced in amount [157] in MS myelin, then it has to be assumed that there is a shift of the PUFA from the plasmalogens to the diacyl-PE. In one series [134] the proportion of nervonic, in another [156] that of lignoceric acid in the cerebrosides was smaller than in the controls. MS myelin is free of cholesterol esters [158] which is remarkable in view of the frequent presence of increased amounts of cholesterol esters in white matter of MS.

The amount of total protein is similar to that reported for controls as found in two studies [159, 156], but increased in another [155]. The amino acid distribution [156, 160], number of —SH groups [159], and the proportions of the three classes of proteins (Folch-Lees) basic and acidic (Wolfgram) are similar in both groups [160]. Thus, there is no selective loss of any protein component from MS myelin nor could there be any significant binding of extraneous proteins, such as antibody, to the MS myelin [156].

3.II.6.4 Cerebrospinal fluid (CSF)

Proteins: The reports of Kabat and his colleagues [161, 162] on increased globulins in CSF of MS patients elicited many studies, which have clarified the following points:

    (a) Identification of the increased globulins.
    (b) Specificity of the increase of gamma globulins for MS.
    (c) Relation of increased globulins to course of disease.
    (d) Immunological aspects of CSF proteins.
    (e) Enzymatic activity of CSF proteins.
    (f) Other constituents of proteinaceous character.

(a) The increased gamma globulins consist of IgG [163].

(b) Although the increased gamma globulin level is now well established as an important diagnostic criterion in MS [164], and reports from various parts of the world have confirmed this, the elevated gamma G level is not specific for MS [165, 166]. Increased gamma globulin levels are observed in about 75% of MS cases. Close correlation between the results obtained by chemical and electrophoretic determination has been found in both MS and controls [167, 168, 169]. The gamma globulin elevation is the only significant change in the CSF of MS [167, 170]. There is no increase of alpha globulins [116, 171].

(c) Sequential studies correlating gamma globulin levels with the clinical course [172] revealed that there is no increase of gamma globulins before the time of the first attack of MS, and that elevated levels occur about six weeks after a relapse, indicating that the clinical symptoms antecede the increase of gamma globulins. Vice versa, clinical remission precedes decrease of the globulins. Likewise, there is poor correlation between clinical symptoms and the incidence of elevated gamma globulins in CSF [173, 174, 175]. The quantity of the gamma globulins depends to a certain extent on the location of the disease, being highest in cases with cerebral lesions. An abnormal ratio of kappa or lambda determinants found in the gamma globulins of the CSF but not in the autologous serum suggests their production within the CNS [176, 177].

(d) Anti-measles antibodies have been found in 12 of 20 CSF's of MS patients as against none in 10 controls [178]. For the purpose of testing for the presence of cellular hypersensitivity directed against CNS antigens, the technique of *in vitro* transformation of blood lymphocytes has been employed using cells from MS patients and autologous or homologous MS-CSF [179, 180, 181, 182]. The results differ; some of the authors [181, 182] obtain *in vitro* transformation, others not. Strandgaard [183] using the leucocyte migration technique found that autologous spinal fluid from MS patients had no inhibitory effect on the *in vitro* migration, and that no difference could be demonstrated between CSF of MS and control cases. Highly concentrated CSF of MS patients has an *in vitro* myelinolytic effect similar to that of soluble proteins of white matter of MS brains [143]. These data allow only the interpretation that CSF in MS patients does not contain a specific Ag although fragments of myelin have been found in it by EM [184], but that the gamma globulins present there, as those in white matter, may be related to the destruction of myelin.

(e) Activity of esterase, peptidase, neutral and acid proteinase in CSF of MS patients in the acute stage is markedly increased [185]. These activities with the exception of esterase activity are also enhanced in the chronic stage though less so, but are lower than those in white matter when compared on the basis of unit per mg protein. Creatine phosphokinase has been found increased in a small number of MS patients [186].

(f) Complement C^1 is lower in CSF of MS patients than in controls [187].

Lipids: Earlier studies (for reference see 188) revealed the presence of phospholipids, cholesterol and cholesterol esters, free fatty acids and beta lipoproteins in CSF. Two recent extensive studies have established that in patients not treated with steroids the total phospholipids are decreased while PE, PS, sphingomyelins and, particularly, cerebrosides, are increased, and PC and total cholesterol are present at normal or slightly lower levels [188, 189]. Free cholesterol is relatively increased [190]. There is, however, no correlation between the levels of cerebrosides and that of IgG [188, 189]. Total lipids are significantly elevated only in patients with a disease of more than eight years duration and in those with increased total proteins.

3.II.6.5 Serum lipids

Early investigations of serum lipids [191, 192] could not establish any difference between MS and controls. More recently a low level of linoleate in the fatty acids of triglycerides and cholesterol esters [193, 194] as well as in the phospholipids of platelets and RBC, have been reported. The C18 : 2 deficit in triglycerides and cholesterol esters increases with progression of the disease; while the proportion of C18 : 2 in phospholipids of platelets and RBC parallels that in the serum and increases after intake of sunflower seed oil [195]. The proportion of arachidonic acid in these three blood components, however, is similar in MS and control samples. An interrelation between these findings and increased *in vitro* adhesiveness of blood platelets [196, 197] could not be established [195, 198].

The serum lipid data corroborated by other authors [199] also contradict the assumption of insufficient absorption of lipids from the gastro-intestinal canal.

Relatively large amounts of sphingomyelin are present in both plasma and red cells. The study of their component fatty acids would be of interest since long chain monoenoic acids are present there [200, 201].

3.II.6.6 Discussion

The observation of deficits of C = 24 fatty acids in conditions as diverse as SLD, MLD, GLD, PM disease and MS white matter

points to different mechanisms producing the same biological
effect. In MLD and GLD the mechanism may be encroachment
by the accumulated abnormal metabolism products upon the
highly ordered microsomal fatty acid synthetase [202]; in
MLD, intra-oligodendroglial inclusions [54, 55, 56]; in GLD
pressure by the large globoid cells upon the oligodendroglia. In
MS, disturbance or inhibition of several enzyme systems has to
be postulated to explain all the findings: deviation from optimal
proportions of malonyl-CoA versus acetyl-CoA could account
for diminished synthesis of long chain fatty acids [202];
unavailability of the proper array of fatty acids may relate to
the deficit of cerebrosides and sphingomyelin.

A deficiency of essential fatty acids or, vice versa, a relative
oversupply of saturated fatty acids [203, 204] has been
suggested as an aetiologic factor. Indeed it has been shown that
the fatty acid composition of brain [105, 206] or its
mitochondria [207] can be altered by varying the levels of
unsaturated fatty acids in the diet. However, in the PE fraction
of MS white matter which harbours the greatest concentration
of PUFA, their proportion is increased [134, 208]. Only the PC
fraction containing a small proportion of dienes and a minimal
one of arachidonic acid showed values of dienes lower than in
the controls in three of seven of MS fractions [134] and in
another series [208] a reduction of arachidonic acid. Yet in MS
myelin [134] the ratio of essential fatty acids was similar to that
in the controls. The deficit of oleic acid reported for the serum
cholesterol esters and triglycerides correlates to the status of the
patient and increases with the progress of the disease. It is not
reflected in the fatty acids of the phospholipids [193]. Thus,
the data available do not appear to support the assumption of
an essential fatty acid deficiency.

For many years it has been hypothesized that MS may be the
result of a viral infection. The marked inflammatory response in
some cases of acute MS lent support to this.

The transmissibility of Kuru, Scrapie and Jakob-Creutzfeldt
disease demonstrated by long-term experiments, has given new
impetus to this. The failure to discover virus particles in several
EM studies [209, 210, 211, 119] would not militate against
this. In scrapie, virus-like particles have been demonstrated only
recently [212], while several previous studies had been

unsuccessful. Virus infection may alter the lipid metabolism of infected cells; for example murine and polio virus infected cells show a marked increase of turnover rate of phospholipids [213, 214] and myxovirus causes changes in the fatty acid metabolism of the host cell [215].

To shed light on this problem, numerous studies on viral antibodies in the serum as well as CSF have been undertaken. They revealed titres against measles and herpes simplex virus to be higher than in controls [216, 217, 218, 219]. The results of a recent reinvestigation [220] however, suggest that, in the United States, virus antibodies vary in type with region and ethnic group, thus weakening the concept of a viral aetiology. An additional argument against MS being due to a "slow virus" is the remitting character of the disease, all other "slow virus infections" being progressive conditions [221].

The possibility of formation of antibodies to myelin or other CNS components secondary to phagocytosis of degenerating or improperly composed CNS tissue and resulting in auto-immunizations has been suggested [222, 223, 224]. The varied deficiencies present in apparently normal MS white matter would be best explained by inadequate synthesis of sphingolipids as well as plasmalogens.

The synthesis of the latter is slower than that of fatty acids of medium chain length and similar in rate to that of long chain fatty acids [225]. Thus the extent of the deficit of these two categories being often similar would agree with this assumption [134]. Ceramides may serve as precursors of both cerebrosides and sphingomyelin [226, 227], and thus, inadequate formation of the former would explain the qualitative and quantitative deficiency of both of these compounds.

On the basis of the data presented in the preceding chapters, the following sequence of events appears to have some probability: There is qualitatively and quantitatively inadequate synthesis of cerebrosides, sphingomyelin and PE in scattered areas of white matter. If repair is not forthcoming, the PE needed for orientation of proteins [228] is insufficient, and stability of myelin reaches borderline due to the sphingolipid deficiencies. This finds its structural expression in the changes of oligodendroglia and in the separation of individual lamina, loop formation [210] and bulging of myelin layers [211]. Breakdown and phagocytosis by mononuclear cells ensues [119] followed by autosensitization. The latter, however, is not an unconditional sequelae. If the encephalitogenic basic protein in the human disease is the part of myelin that is responsible for the postulated autoimmunization, as it is in experimental animals, its antigenicity is markedly reduced by contact with serum proteins [229] If the basic protein, however, is incorporated into the macrophages without this prior contact, sensitization ensues as in experimental animals. The observation that IgG in the CSF is not elevated at the time of the first attack [172] would be concordant with this concept. Both the extent of the lipid deficits and the degree of sensitization then would determine the future course of the disease.

REFERENCES

1. I. Klatzo, *J. Neuropath. exp. Neurol.*, 26, 1 (1967)
2. J. N. Cumings, *J. clin. Path.*, 14, 289 (1961)
3. H. M. Hauser, H. J. Svien, B. F. McKenzie, W. F. McGuckin and N. P. Golstein, *Neurology (Minneap.)*, 13, 945 (1963)
4. S. Nakazawa, *Neurology (Minneap.)*, 19, 269 (1969)
5. S. Ishii, H. Tsuji, K. Ozawa, Y. Kondo and J. P. Evans, *In* Brain Edema (I. Klatzo and F. Seitelberger, eds), p. 32. Springer-Verlag, New York (1967)
6. T. Yanagihara and J. N. Cumings, *Arch. Neurol.*, 19, 241 (1968)
7. H. Jacob, *Ztschr. ges. Neurol.*, 168, 382 (1940)
8. T. Yanagihara and J. N. Cumings, *Brain*, 92, 59 (1969)
9. K. Sato, M. Yamaguchi, S. Mullan, J. P. Evans and S. Ishii, *Arch. Neurol.*, 21, 413 (1969)
10. T. Yanagihara, N. P. Goldstein, H. J. Svien and R. C. Bahn, *Neurol.*, 17, 669 (1967)
11. I. Feigin, *In* Brain Edema (I. Klatzo and F. Seitelberger, eds), p. 128. Springer-Verlag, New York (1967)
12. J. E. Kalsbeck and J. N. Cumings, *J. Neuropath. exp. Neurol.*, 22, 237 (1963)
13. R. Torack, J. Gordon and J. Prokop, *Int. Rev. Neurobiol.*, 12, 45 (1970)
14. A. Hirano, H. M. Zimmerman and S. Levine, *J. Cell Biol.*, 31, 397 (1966)
15. A. Hirano, H. M. Zimmerman and S. Levine, *J. Neuropath. exp. Neurol.*, 27, 571 (1968)

16. N. K. Gonatas, H. M. Zimmerman and S. Levine, *Amer. J. Path.*, **42**, 455 (1963)
17. J. L. Osterholm and J. Pyenson, *J. Neurosurg.*, **31**, 417 (1969)
18. E. Pausescu, R. Lugojan and M. Pausescu, *Brain*, **93**, 31 (1970)
19. K. L. Terplan, *Amer. J. Path.*, **13**, 664 (1937)
20. H. G. Knauff, D. Marx and G. Mayer, *Hoppe Seyler Z. Physiol. Chem.*, **326**, 227 (1961)
21. W. W. Wells, T. A. Pittman, H. J. Wells and T. J. Egan, *J. biol. Chem.*, **240**, 1002 (1965)
22. P. R. Huttenlocher, R. E. Hillman and Y. E. Hsia, *J. Pediat.*, **76**, 902 (1970)
23. W. Blackwood and J. N. Cumings, *J. Neurol. Neurosurg. Psychiat.*, **17**, 33 (1954)
24. R. M. Norman, O. R. Oppenheimer and A. H. Tingey, *J. Neurol. Neurosurg. Psychiat.*, **24**, 223 (1961)
25. J. Austin, *Arch. Neurol.*, **9**, 207 (1963)
26. J. H. Austin, *J. Neurochem.*, **10**, 921 (1963)
27. A. N. D'Agostino, G. P. Sayre and A. B. Hayles, *Arch. Neurol.*, **8**, 82 (1963)
28. J. H. Austin and D. Lehfeldt, *J. Neuropath. exp. Neurol.*, **24**, 265 (1965)
29. E. J. Yunis and R. E. Lee, *Science*, **169**, 64 (1970)
30. K. Suzuki and W. D. Grover, *Arch. Neurol.*, **22**, 385 (1970)
31. S. S. Schochet, J. M. Hardman, P. W. Lampert and K. M. Earle, *Arch. Path.*, **88**, 305 (1969)
32. J. M. Andrews and P. A. Cancilla, *Arch. Path.*, **89**, 53 (1970)
33. C.-M. Shaw and C. B. Carlson, *J. Neuropath. exp. Neurol.*, **29**, 306 (1970)
34. H. Mei Liu, *J. Neuropath. exp. Neurol.*, **29**, 441 (1970)
35. J. N. Cumings and B. Rozdilsky, *Neurology (Minneap.)*, **15**, 177 (1965)
36. J. Peiffer, *Arch. Psychiat. Nervenkr.*, **195**, 446 (1957)
37. H. Pilz, *Acta neuropath. (Berlin)*, **4**, 16 (1964)
38. J. H. Menkes, C. Duncan and J. Moossy, *Neurology (Minneap.)*, **16**, 581 (1966)
39. H. Jatzkewitz and E. Mehl, *Hoppe Seyler Z. Physiol. Chem.*, **329**, 264 (1962)
40. B. Gerstl, L. J. Rubinstein, L. F. Eng and M. Tavaststjerna, *Arch. Neurol.*, **15**, 603 (1966)
41. Y. Eto, K. Suzuki and K. Suzuki, *J. Lipid Res.*, **11**, 473 (1970)
42. J. N. Cumings, E. J. Thompson and H. Goodwin, *J. Neurochem.*, **15**, 243 (1968)
43. B. K. Bachhawat, J. Austin and D. Armstrong, *Biochem. J.*, **104**, 15c (1967)
44. J. Austin, B. Bachhawat, D. Armstrong, D. Stumpf, L. Kretschmer, C. Mitchell and B. Van Zee, *J. Neuropath. exp. Neurol.*, **27**, 141 (1968)

45. J. Austin, K. Suzuki, D. Armstrong, R. Brady, B. K. Bachhawat, J. Schlenker and D. Stumpf, *Arch. Neurol.*, 23, 502 (1970)
46. G. M. McKhann, R. Levy and W. Ho, *Biochem. Biophys. Res. Commun.*, 20, 109 (1965)
47. K. Suzuki and Y. Suzuki, *Proc. Nat. Acad. Sci., U.S.*, 66, 302 (1970)
48. B. D. Lake, *Nature (Lond.)*, 217, 171 (1968)
49. P. Sourander and Y. Olsson, *Acta neuropath.*, 11, 69 (1968)
50. A. Bischoff and J. Ulrich, *Brain*, 92, 861 (1969)
51. J. H. Austin, *Trans. Amer. Neurol. Ass.*, 83, 149 (1958)
52. H. Jatzkewitz, *Hoppe Seyler Z. Physiol. Chem.*, 311, 279 (1958)
53. B. Hagberg, P. Sourander, L. Svennerholm and H. Voss, *Acta Paediat.*, 48, 200 (1959)
54. G. Aurebeck, K. Osterberg, M. Blaw, S. Chou and E. Nelson, *Arch. Neurol.*, 11, 273 (1964)
55. A. Resibois, *Acta neuropath. (Berlin)*, 13, 149 (1969)
56. A. Gregoire, O. Perier and P. Dustin, Jr., *J. Neuropath. exp. Neurol.*, 25, 617 (1966)
57. K. Suzuki, K. Suzuki and G. Chen, *J. Neuropath. exp. Neurol.*, 26, 154 (1967)
58. W. T. Norton and S. E. Podulso, *In* Variation in the Chemical Composition of the Nervous System (G. B. Ansell, ed.), p. 82. Pergamon, Oxford (1966)
59. J. N. Cumings, E. J. Thompson and H. Goodwin, *J. Neurochem.*, 15, 243 (1968)
60. J. N. Cumings, *Neuropat. Pol.*, 7, 255 (1969)
61. J. H. Austin, *Neurology (Minneap.)*, 7, 415 (1957)
62. B. Hagberg and L. Svennerholm, *Acta Paediat.*, 48, 632 (1959)
63. B. Hagberg and L. Svennerholm, *Acta Paediat.*, 49, 690 (1960)
64. B. Hagberg, P. Sourander and L. Svennerholm, *Cereb. Palsy Bull.*, 3, 438 (1961)
65. A. K. Percy and R. O. Brady, *Science*, 161, 594 (1968)
66. B. Hagberg, P. Sourander and L. Svennerholm, *Am. J. Dis. Child.*, 104, 94, (1962)
67. H. Pilz and D. Müller, *J. Neurol. Sci.*, 9, 585 (1969)
68. G. W. F. Edgar, *Psychiat. Neurol. Neurochir.*, 64, 28 (1961)
69. H. Jatzkewitz, Neurochemistry Symposium, VIIth International Congress of Neurology, Rome (1961) p. 13
70. E. Mehl and H. Jatzkewitz, *Hoppe Seyler Z. Physiol. Chem.*, 331, 292 (1963)
71. J. Austin, D. McAfee, D. Armstrong, M. O'Rourke, L. Shearer and R. Bachhawat, *Biochem. J.*, 93, 15C (1964)
72. J. Austin, D. McAfee and L. Shearer, *Arch. Neurol.*, 12, 447 (1965)
73. E. Mehl and H. Jatzkewitz, *Biochim. Biophys. Acta*, 151, 619 (1968)
74. H. Jatzkewitz and E. Mehl, *J. Neurochem.*, 16, 19 (1969)
75. M. T. Porter, A. L. Fluharty and H. Kihara, *Proc. natn. Acad. Sci. U.S.A.*, 62, 887 (1969)
76. R. Julius, B. Buehler, A. Aylsworth, L. St. Petery, O. Rennert and M. Greer, *Neurology (Minneap.)*, 21, 15 (1971)

77. H. W. Moser, A. B. Moser and G. M. McKhann, *Arch. Neurol.*, 17, 494 (1967)
78. M. Ohta and T. Iwayama, *Brain Nerve (Tokyo)*, 22, 557 (1970)
79. H. L. Greene, G. Hug and W. K. Schubert, *Arch. Neurol.*, 20, 147 (1969)
80. J. C. Melchior and J. Clausen, *Acta Paediat.*, 57, 2 (1968)
81. R. M. Norman and A. H. Tingey, *In* Brain Lipids and Lipoproteins and the Leucodystrophies (J. Folch-Pi and H. J. Bauer, eds), p. 169. Elsevier, Amsterdam (1963)
82. F. Seitelberger, *In* Brain Lipids and lipoproteins and the Leucodystrophies (J. Folch-Pi and H. J. Bauer, eds), p. 187. Elsevier, Amsterdam (1963)
83. L. Crome and M. Zapella, *J. Neurol. Neurosurg. Psychiat.*, 26, 413 (1963)
84. F. Lindlar, K. Nagai and A. Vogel, *Hoppe Seyler Z. Physiol. Chem.*, 347, 1 (1966)
85. J. N. Cumings, *Brain*, 78, 554 (1955)
86. E. Bargeton-Farkas and G. W. F. Edgar, *Acta neuropath. (Berlin)*, 3, 578 (1964)
87. Y. Tsuchiya, T. Numabe and S. Yokoi, *Acta neuropath. (Berlin)*, 16, 353 (1970)
88. E. Nelson, K. Osterberg, M. Blaw, J. Story and P. Kozak, *Neurology (Minneap.)*, 12, 896 (1962)
89. P. J. Dyck, J. N. Cumings and J. Olszewski, *Neurology (Minneap.)*, 10, 765 (1960)
90. W. T. Norton, S. E. Poduslo and K. Suzuki, *J. Neuropath. exp. Neurol.*, 25, 582 (1966)
91. K. Suzuki, K. Suzuki and S. Kamoshita, *J. Neuropath. exp. Neurol.*, 28, 25 (1969)
92. Y. Suzuki, S. H. Tucker, L. B. Rorke and K. Suzuki, *J. Neuropath. exp. Neurol.*, 29, 405 (1970)
93. M. J. Eadie, *Proc. Aust. Assn. Neurol.*, 4, 63 (1966)
94. M. E. Blaw, K. Osterberg, P. Kozak and E. Nelson, *Arch. Neurol.*, 11, 626 (1964)
95. D. Hoefnagel, S. Van Den Noort and S. H. Ingbar, *Brain*, 85, 553 (1962)
96. R. W. Turkington and R. S. Stempfel, Jr., *J. Pediat.*, 69, 406 (1966)
97. A. Fanconi, A. Prader, W. Isler, F. Luthy and R. Siebenmann, *Helv. Paediat. Acta*, 18, 480 (1963)
98. W. C. Watson and E. Murray, *J. Lipid Res.*, 7, 236 (1966)
99. J. K. Smith, B. Gerstl, M. G. Tavaststjerna and W. R. Porter, *Neurol.*, 11, 395 (1961)
100. K. Suzuki and G. C. Chen, *J. Neuropath. exp. Neurol.*, 25, 396 (1966)
101. K. Suzuki, *In* Inborn Disorders of Sphingolipid Metabolism (S. M. Aronson and B. W. Volk, eds), p. 215. Pergamon Press, Oxford (1967)
102. R. Ledeen, K. Salsman and M. Cabrera, *J. Lipid Res.*, 9, 129 (1968)

103. J. Peiffer and E. Zerbin-Rüdin, *Acta neuropath. (Berlin)*, 3, 87 (1963)
104. K. Jellinger and F. Seitelberger, *Acta neuropath. (Berlin)*, 14, 108 (1969)
105. B. Gerstl, N. Malamud, R. B. Hayman and P. R. Bond, *J. Neurol. Neurosurg. Psychiat.*, 28, 540 (1965)
106. I. Watanabe, R. McCaman, P. Dyken and W. Zeman, *J. Neuropath. exp. Neurol.*, 28, 243 (1969)
107. W. Spielmeyer, *Z. ges. Neurol. Psychiat.*, 32, 203 (1923)
108. M. Bielschowsky and R. Henneberg, *J. Psychol. Neurol. (Lpz.)*, 36, 131 (1928)
109. C. M. Poser and L. van Bogaert, *Acta psychiat. scand.*, 31, 285 (1956)
110. W. Zeman, W. Demyer and H. F. Falls, *J. Neuropath. exp. Neurol.*, 23, 334 (1964)
111. A. Allegranza, P. M. Alleva, I. Cescon and G. P. Strada, *Acta Neurol. Napoli*, 23, 895 (1968)
112. H. Bernheimer (personal communication)
113. G. Brante, *Acta physiol. scand.*, 18, Suppl. 63 (1949)
114. C. M. Plum and S. E. Hansen, *Acta psychiat. neurol. scand.*, Suppl. 141, 84 (1960)
115. Y. Kishimoto, N. S. Radin, W. W. Tourtellotte, J. H. Parker and H. H. Itaboshi, *Arch. Neurol.*, 16, 44 (1967)
116. H. Bauer and R. Heitmann, *Dtsch. Z. Nervenheilk.*, 178, 47 (1958)
117. B. Gerstl, M. J. Kahnke, J. K. Smith, M. G. Tavaststjerna and R. B. Hayman, *Brain*, 84, 310 (1961)
118. P. F. Borri, R. P. Bertinelli, V. Toso, M. Taramelli, M. Paci and A. Pacini, *Acta neurol., Napoli*, 24, 593 (1969)
119. E. Sluga, *Wien. Z. Nervenheilk.*, Suppl. 2, 59 (1969)
120. E. R. Einstein, K. B. Dalal and J. Csejtey, *J. Neurol. Sci.*, 11, 109 (1970)
121. B. W. Moore, *Biochem. Biophys. Res. Comm.*, 19, 739 (1965)
122. L. F. Eng, B. Gerstl and J. J. Vanderhaeghen, *Transactions Amer. Soc. for Neurochem.*, 1, 52 (1970)
123. M. Wender and M. Kozik, *Acta neuropath.*, 13, 143 (1969)
124. R. L. Friede and M. Knoller, *Experientia*, 20, 130 (1964)
125. J. Clausen, W. Gerhardt, C. Petri *et al. Acta neurol. scand.*, 40, Suppl. 10, p. 77 (1964)
126. M. Z. M. Ibrahim and C. W. M. Adams, *J. Path. Bact.*, 90, 239 (1965)
127. J. F. Hallpike, C. W. M. Adams and O. B. Bayliss, *Histochem. J.*, 2, 199 (1970)
128. P. J. Riekkinen, J. Clausen, H. J. Frey, T. Fog and U. K. Rinne, *Acta neurol. scand.*, 46, 349 (1970)
129. J. N. Cumings, *Brain*, 76, 551 (1953)
130. A. N. Davison and M. Wajda, *J. Neurochem.*, 9, 427 (1962)
131. J. N. Cumings and H. Goodwin, *Lancet*, 2, 664 (1968)
132. B. Gerstl, M. G. Tavaststjerna, R. B. Hayman, J. K. Smith and L F. Eng, *J. Neurochem.*, 10, 889 (1963)

133. G. Arnetoli, A. Pazzagli and L. Amaducci, *J. Neurochem.*, 16, 461 (1970)
134. B. Gerstl, L. F. Eng, M. Tavaststjerna, J. K. Smith and S. L. Kruse, *J. Neurochem.*, 17, 677 (1970)
135. R. H. S. Thompson, R. Niemino and G. R. Webster, *Biochim. Biophys. Acta*, 43, 142 (1960)
136. G. R. Webster and R. H. S. Thompson, *Biochim. Biophys. Acta*, 63, 38 (1962)
137. G. R. Webster and R. J. Alpern, *Biochem. J.*, 90, 35 (1964)
138. F. Lindlar, *Naturwissenschaften*, 23, 543 (1962)
139. G. R. Webster and R. H. S. Thompson, *Nature (Lond.)*, 206, 296 (1965)
140. E. Schuller, C. Rouques, M. Loridan, *Wien. Z. Nervenheilk.*, Suppl. 2, 104 (1969)
141. B. Gerstl, C. T. Uyeda, L. F. Eng, P. Bond and J. K. Smith, *Neurology (Minneap.)*, 19, 1019 (1969)
142. W. W. Tourtellotte and J. A. Parker, *Nature (Lond.)*, 214, 683 (1967)
143. S. U. Kim, M. R. Murray, W. W. Tourtellotte and J. A. Parker, *J. Neuropath exp. Neurol.*, 29, 420 (1970)
144. K. Warecka and D. Muller, *J. Neurol. Sci.*, 8, 329 (1969)
145. K. Warecka, *J. Neurochem.*, 17, 829 (1970)
146. K. Warecka and H. J. Bauer, *Dtsch. Z. Nervenheilk.*, 194, 66 (1968)
147. C. H. Koenig, *In* Handbook of Neurochemistry (A. Lajtha, ed.), p. 235, Vol. 2. Plenum Press, New York (1969)
148. S. S. Oja and H. Oja, *J. Neurochem.*, 17, 901 (1970)
149. T. Semba and M. Civen, *J. Neurochem.*, 17, 795 (1970)
150. P. J. Riekkinen and U. K. Rinne, VI Congres International de Neuropathologie, Paris, p. 490 (1970)
151. G. B. Ansell and S. Spanner, *Biochem. J.*, 94, 252 (1965)
152. G. B. Ansell and S. Spanner, *Biochem. J.*, 106, 19-20 (1968)
153. R. H. Laatsch, M. W. Kies, S. Gordon and E. C. Alvord, Jr., *J. exp. Med.*, 115, 777 (1962)
154. L. A. Autilio, W. T. Norton and R. D. Terry, *J. Neurochem.*, 11, 17 (1964)
155. J. Clausen and I. Berg Hansen, *Acta neurol. scand.*, 46, 1 (1970)
156. F. Wolfgram, M. E. Fewster, J. F. Mead, personal communication (1970)
157. J. N. Cumings, *Neuropat. Pol.*, 7, 255 (1969)
158. M. E. Fewster, J. F. Mead, F. J. Wolfgram, W. W. Tourtellotte, *Proc. Soc. exp. Biol. Med.*, 133, 795-800 (1970)
159. B. Gerstl, L. F. Eng, R. B. Hayman, M. G. Tavaststjerna and P. R. Bond, *J. Neurochem.*, 14, 661 (1967)
160. L. F. Eng, F. C. Chao, B. Gerstl, D. Pratt and M. G. Tavaststjerna, *Biochem.*, 7, 4455 (1968)
161. E. A. Kabat, D. H. Moore and H. Landow, *J. Clin. Invest.*, 21, 571 (1942)
162. E. A. Kabat, M. Glusman and V. Knaub, *Amer. J. Med.*, 4, (1948)

163. E. R. Einstein and P. Cerutti, *Int. Arch. Allergy*, **36**, 355 (1969)
164. J. Clausen, T. Fog and E. R. Einstein, *Acta neurol. scand.*, **45**, 513 (1969)
165. S. Takase and M. Yoshida, *Tohoku J. exp. Med.*, **98**, 189 (1969)
166. S. A. Schneck and H. N. Claman, *Arch. Neurol.*, **20**, 132 (1969)
167. E. Schuller, C. Rouques and M. Loridan, *Wien. Z. Nervenheilk.*, Suppl. 2, 104 (1969)
168. R. M. Schmidt, *Dtsch. Gesundh.-Wes.*, **24**, 289 (1969)
169. J. Vymazal, *Cas Lék. ces.*, **107**, 1422 (1968)
170. R. M. Schmidt and H. Diessner, *Wien. Z. Nervenheilk.*, **27**, Suppl. 2, 138 (1969)
171. K. Arko, *Wien. Z. Nervenheilk.*, Suppl. 1, 185 (1966)
172. J. Panagiotopoulos, G. Pernhaupt and H. Tschabitscher, *Wien. Z. Nervenheilk.*, Suppl. 1, 195 (1966)
173. K. Schapira and D. C. Park, *J. Neurol. Neurosurg. Psychiat.*, **24**, 121 (1961)
174. W. W. Tourtellotte and J. A. Parker, *Trans. Amer. Neurol. Assoc.*, **90**, 107 (1965)
175. E. C. Laterre, A. Callewaert, J. F. Heremans and Z. Sfaello, *Neurology (Minneap.)*, **20**, 982 (1970)
176. H. Link and O. Zettervall, *Clin. & Exp. Immunol.*, **6**, 435 (1970)
177. H. Link and O. Zettervall, *Clin. & Exp. Immunol.*, **7**, 365 (1970)
178. G. L. Dioli, S. Mazzoni and M. Ferrucci, *Riv. Neurobiol.*, **15**, 63 (1969)
179. I. Fowler, C. E. Morris and T. Whiteley, *New Eng. J. Med.*, **275**, 1041 (1966)
180. E. Frick and H. Stickl, *Klin. Wschr.*, **46**, 1066 (1968)
181. J. A. Brody, M. M. Harlem, J. F. Kurtzke and L. R. White, *New Eng. J. Med.*, **279**, 202 (1968)
182. L. Koulischer and J. Stenuit, *Acta neurol. belg.*, **68**, 571 (1968)
183. S. Strandgaard, *Acta neurol. scand.*, **46**, 252 (1970)
184. R. M. Herndon and M. J. Johnson, *J. Neuropath. exp. Neurol.*, **29**, 320 (1970)
185. U. Rinne and P. Riekkinen, *Acta neurol. scand.*, **44**, 156 (1968)
186. A. L. Sherwin, J. W. Norris and J. A. Bulckle, *Neurology (Minneap.)*, **19**, 993 (1969)
187. E. Kuwert, K. Noll and W. Firnhaber, *Z. Immunit. forsch., Allerg. & Klin. Immun.*, **135**, 462-480 (1968)
188. J. Clausen and T. Fog, *Int. Arch. Allergy*, **36**, 649 (1969)
189. W. W. Tourtellotte and A. F. Haerer, *Arch. Neurol.*, **20**, 605 (1969)
190. C. M. Plum, *Acta psychiat. neurol. scand.*, Suppl. 148, 35 (1960)
191. E. Roboz, W. C. Hess, F. M. Forster and D. M. Temple, *A.M.A. Arch. Neurol. Psychiat.*, **72**, 154 (1954)
192. N. K. Freeman and B. V. Siegel, *Amer. J. Med. Sci.*, **238**, 101/727 (1959)
193. R. W. R. Baker, H. Sanders, R. H. S. Thompson and K. J. Zilkha, *J. Neurol. Neurosurg. Psychiat.*, **28**, 212 (1965)

194. A. Montfoort, R. W. R. Baker, R. H. S. Thompson and K. J. Zilkha, *J. Neurol. Neurosurg. Psychiat.*, 29, 99 (1966)
195. S. Gul, A. D. Smith, R. H. S. Thompson, H. Payling Wright and K. J. Zilkha, *J. Neurol. Neurosurg. Psychiat.*, 33, 506 (1970)
196. M. Nathanson and J. P. Savitsky, *Bull. N.Y. Acad. Med.*, 28, 462 (1952)
197. T. Fog, I. Kristensen and H. F. Helweg-Larsen, *Arch. Neurol.*, 73, 267 (1955)
198. H. P. Wright, R. H. S. Thompson and K. J. Zilkha, *Lancet*, 2, 1109 (1965)
199. I. Huszak and L. Heiner, Proceedings 8th International Congress of Neurology, Vienna, p. 33 (1965)
200. E. Svennerholm, S. Stallbergstenhagen and L. Svennerholm, *Biochim. Biophys. Acta*, 125, 60 (1966)
201. E. L. Hirvisalo, *Ann. Acad. Sci. Penn.*, 11 Chem., 146, 61 (1969)
202. D. Oesterhelt, C. Riepertinger and F. Lynen, *Europ. J. Biochem.*, 10, 377 (1969)
203. R. L. Swank, *New Eng. J. Med.*, 246, 721 (1952)
204. H. M. Sinclair, *Lancet*, 1, 381 (1956)
205. L. A. Witting, C. C. Harvey, B. Century and M. K. Horwitt, *J. Lipid Res.*, 2, 412 (1961)
206. H. Mohrhauer and R. T. Holman, *J. Neurochem.*, 7, 523 (1963)
207. L. Rathbone, *Biochem. J.*, 97, 620 (1965)
208. J. Clausen and I. B. Hansen, *Acta neurol. scand.*, 46, 1-7 (1970)
209. O. Perier and A. Gregorie, *Brain*, 88, 937 (1965)
210. K. Suzuki, J. M. Andrews, J. M. Waltz and R. Terry, *Lab. Invest.*, 20, 444 (1969)
211. U. K. Rinne, *Ann. Med. Int. Fenn.*, 57, 179-183 (1968)
212. A. Bignami and H. B. Parry, *Science*, 171, 389-390 (1971)
213. K. Moldave, *J. biol. Chem.*, 210, 343 (1954)
214. G. Miroff, W. E. Cornatzer and R. G. Fischer, *J. biol. Chem.*, 228, 255 (1957)
215. J. M. Tiffany and H. A. Blough, *Sci.*, 163, 573 (1969)
216. J. M. Adams and D. T. Imagawa, *Proc. Soc. Exper. Biol. Med.*, 8, 562 (1962)
217. J. M. Adams, *Neurology (Minneap.)*, 17, 707 (1967)
218. C. A. C. Ross, J. A. R. Lenman and I. D. Melville, *Brit. med. J.*, 3, 512 (1969)
219. E. A. Caspary, M. E. Chambers and E. J. Field, *Neurology (Minneap.)*, 19, 1038 (1969)
220. J. L. Sever, J. F. Kurtzke, M. Alter, G. A. Schumacher, M. R. Gilkerson, J. H. Ellenberg and J. A. Brody, VI Int. Congress of Neuropath, Paris, p. 958 (1970)
221. R. Johnson, Proc. VI Intern. Congr. of Neuropath., p. 761 (1970)
222. E. A. Caspary, E. J. Field and E. J. Ball, *J. Neurol. Neurosurg. Psychiat.*, 27, 25 (1964)
223. F. Seitelberger, *Nervenarzt.*, 38, 525 (1967)

224. H. J. Bauer, *Z. Neurol.*, 198, 5-32 (1970)
225. H. Debuch, H. Friedemann and J. Müller, *Hoppe Seyler Ztsch.*, 351, 613 (1970)
226. P. Morell and N. S. Radin, *Biochem.*, 8, 506 (1969)
227. P. Morell and N. S. Radin, *J. biol. Chem.*, 245, 342 (1970)
228. M. L. Das, E. D. Haak and F. L. Crane, *Biochem.*, 4, 859 (1965)
229. B. Gerstl, L. Eng, H. Hunt and C. Uyeda, unpublished data

CHAPTER 4

The Biochemistry of Copper in Man and Its Role in the Pathogenesis of Wilson's Disease (Hepatolenticular Degeneration)

J. M. WALSHE

4.1 WILSON'S DISEASE, DEFINITION

Wilson's disease is a hereditary metabolic disease. Clinically it is characterized by disturbances of movement, by subacute or chronic liver disease, by abnormalities of renal function and by visible deposits of copper in the cornea, the Kayser Fleischer rings. The biochemical lesion consists of excessive deposition of copper in most tissues but principally the brain, liver and kidneys; in the plasma the concentration of both copper and the copper protein caeruloplasmin are commonly, but not invariably, reduced but the amounts of copper excreted in the urine are increased. The disease, untreated, is invariably fatal.

4.2 INTRODUCTION

When the Dorian tribes descended from the mountains of the Eprius in to the Peloponesus they destroyed an artistic and sophisticated Minoan-Mycenean civilization. The reason for the success of the primitive Dorians was simple, they had iron weapons; the Achaens of the Peloponesus were armed with bronze. Not that the iron weapons of the Dorians were in any way superior to the bronze of the Achaens, indeed it has been suggested that these early iron weapons were so soft that after a few good hacks at the shield of his adversary the Dorian warrior would need to straighten his sword blade over his knee [1]; but iron is a relatively abundant metal whilst copper, for the Achaen, was a luxury so that only the elite of the kingdom were armed with metal whilst the militia, if such existed, would be equipped with staves and slings leaving them vulnerable to the well armed Dorian hordes. In evolution the relation of copper to iron is in some ways similar. Our primitive ancestors, swimming in the warm Cambrian seas, used copper not only as their respiratory pigment but also for oxygen transport; thus when some enterprising creature discovered that iron was at least as good as copper for oxygen transport and logistically very much more readily available it had taken a major step forward and one which was inevitably to relegate the copper-dependent phylla to an inferior place in the scale of evolution. Despite its relegation to a secondary place as an oxygen carrier copper has retained its primacy as an intracellular oxidase in the electron transfer chain bridging the final stage in the reduction of molecular oxygen to water thus:

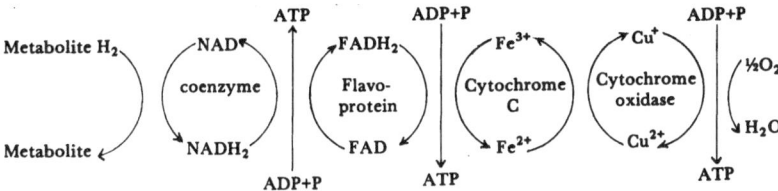

Cytochrome oxidase appears to have two components, cytochrome a and cytochrome a_3, each containing one copper atom, the unit as a whole being able to take up four electrons [2]. It is apparent that in this role as the final carrier in the electron transfer chain, the ultimate source of energy at the cellular level, copper is essential for life.

4.3 COPPER PROTEINS

Copper is present in a number of mammalian proteins and the characteristics of these have been summarized by Scheinberg and Sternlieb [3]. Amongst the copper proteins identified in man, but of unknown function, are cerebro-cuprein I, a protein extracted from normal human brain by Porter and Ainsworth [4], liver copper-protein [5], and erythrocuprein [6]. Tyrosinase, a protein of 0.25% copper content is to be found wherever melanin is present in the body, it catalyses the oxidation of tyrosine to dopa and accelerates the conversion of dopa to dopa quinone, the initial stages in the conversion of tyrosine to melanin. Lack of this enzyme is not, however, associated with deficient production of pressor amines, another pathway being present in the adrenal gland for the hydroxylation of tyrosine [7].

4.3.1 Caeruloplasmin

One of the most intensively studied copper proteins is caeruloplasmin; but despite extensive knowledge of its structure its function remains obscure. Caeruloplasmin, as its name implies, is a blue protein present in human and many animal sera; it is a glycoprotein with terminal sialic acid residues [8]. Caeruloplasmin was first isolated and characterized by

Holmberg and Laurell [9, 10, 11, 12, 13]. These authors showed it to be an alpha globulin of M.W. 151,000 each molecule containing eight atoms of copper, though recently Kasper and Deutsch [14] have reported the M.W. to be 160,000. Holmberg and Laurell further showed that caeruloplasmin was responsible for all plasma oxidase activity towards polyphenols and polyamines. These substrates include adrenaline, noradrenaline, dopa and 5 hydroxytryptamine; but all are oxidized at a pH and at a reaction rate which suggest that this is not of physiological significance [15]. Caeruloplasmin, isolated from human serum on hydroxyl apatite or DEAE cellulose, contains two components [16, 17]; no significant difference has been found in their chemical, physical or immunochemical properties nor do they appear to undergo interconversion during chromatographic separation.

The blue colour of the molecule is due to the presence of cupric copper (Cu^{2+}). The metal was originally considered to be present as cuprous-cupric pairs but recently it has been suggested that the fraction of caeruloplasmin copper present in the Cu^{2+} state depends upon the history of the preparation; possibly in the majority of samples there are only two cupric copper atoms [18]. Caeruloplasmin can be decolourized by reducing agents such as ascorbic acid and cysteine, it can also be reversibly reduced to the native protein by removal of the copper atoms. Apocaeruloplasmin has been labelled with radiocopper and this technique has been used for studying the fate of injected caeruloplasmin in the body [19, 20]. An exciting recent development has been the production of asialocaeruloplasmin with the terminal galactose exposed [21], this protein disappears from the circulation within minutes of injection and can be identified in the hepatocytes: the possible relationship of this observation to the pathogenesis of Wilson's disease will be discussed later.

Though much is known about the structure of caeruloplasmin little is known about its function. It is, as has already been stated, an oxidase for polyphenols and its ability to produce a coloured reaction compound with para-phenylenediamine or its dimethyl derivative is the basis for most assay procedures [16, 22]. Caeruloplasmin can mediate electron transfer reactions [23] but it is difficult to see of what importance this can be in the extracellular fluid compartment. Another role that has been suggested is for the mobilization of iron stores from the liver [24] and it has also been related to the formation of erythropoietin [25]. Its inability to exchange copper *in vivo* [19] makes it unlikely that caeruloplasmin is a transport protein for this metal and there is no evidence to suggest that copper derived from degraded caeruloplasmin is preferentially excreted in the bile [26]. An alternative hypothesis for the function of caeruloplasmin was put foward by Scheinberg and Morell [27] who suggested that it might control the rate of absorption of copper from the gut. Under reducing conditions, such as might occur in the intestinal wall, caeruloplasmin will release four of its eight copper atoms. If this were to occur *in vivo* it would raise the concentration of "free" copper in the plasma above that in the gut lumen and would inhibit diffusion of copper from gut to plasma. Caeruloplasmin would thus be a key factor in controlling copper balance. However later experiments with caeruloplasmin labelled with ^{67}Cu showed that such liberation of copper from caeruloplasmin did not in fact, take place *in vivo* [19].

Caeruloplasmin has also been proposed as the link between copper and iron in metabolism. Certainly in animals copper deficiency is associated with, amongst other symptoms "anaemia and alterations in iron metabolism" [28]. Frieden [29] believes that caeruloplasmin is directly involved in iron mobilization and in the rate of formation of Fe^{3+} transferrin and hence haemoglobin synthesis. Finally Broman [30] has suggested that caeruloplasmin may act by transporting a complicated copper containing prosthetic group to the cells for incorporation as an oxygen-activating unit for cytochrome oxidase.*

However, the fact not taken into consideration by any of these hypotheses is that patients with Wilson's disease, provided they are adequately treated with penicillamine, can live apparently normal lives for many years with zero levels of caeruloplasmin in the plasma. The sheer multiplicity of theories concerning the function of caeruloplasmin together with the

* This hypothesis has recently been "rediscovered" [134] and is published together with some evidence to suggest that the cytochrome oxidase activity in the leucocytes may be reduced in a patient with Wilson's disease.

failure of agreement of the various groups working in this field speak much for our inability to determine the true physiological role of this elegant but enigmatic protein.

4.4 NORMAL COPPER TRANSPORT

The normal diet contains from 2 to 4 mg of copper, more than enough to meet the body's requirements for there is little extraneous loss of the metal. It is probable that most of the dietary copper is protein or aminoacid bound but some ionic copper must be present in drinking water, particularly if this is delivered via copper pipes. Indeed outdated gas water heaters are occasionally a source of acute copper poisoning [31], an illness characterized by acute gastro-enteritis. Much of the dietary copper may well be converted to Cu^{2+} by the gastric acid, in which form it can certainly be readily absorbed from the stomach or upper small intestine; orally administered radiocopper can be detected in the liver and plasma within minutes of administration (see Figure 4.1). Once absorbed into the blood stream copper is bound to the serum albumin [32] though a small amount probably remains complexed to amino acids [33], certainly up to 5% of intravenously injected radiocopper remains available for filtration through a semipermeable membrane for some hours after injection [34].

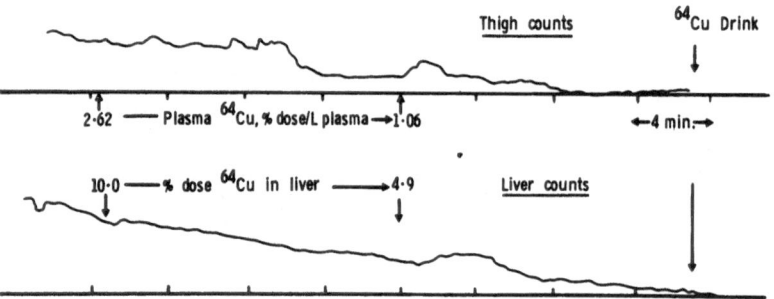

Figure 4.1. Graphical recordings showing the rise in radioactivity over the liver and thigh of a normal individual during the half hour period immediately after a drink of ^{64}CuCl (arrowed, right). Time intervals in 4 min. The liver counter was placed anteriorly over the area of maximum liver dullness and angled slightly upwards and to the right so as to avoid seeing radioactivity in the stomach.

Studies with radiocopper have also shown that the metal becomes rapidly bound to the red cells reaching a plateau level which is maintained at least as long as the half-life of radiocopper permits study; in the case of [67]Cu this may be as long as 12 days [35]. Plasma radiocopper, on the other hand, reaches a peak at 1-2 h, after ingestion [32, 36] and then disappears from the circulation as it is cleared by the liver [37]. It is returned to the plasma later incorporated into caeruloplasmin [32]. In a normal individual from 60 to 80% of an injected dose of radiocopper is concentrated in the liver at 24 h (see Figure 4.2). Thereafter the amount declines, some

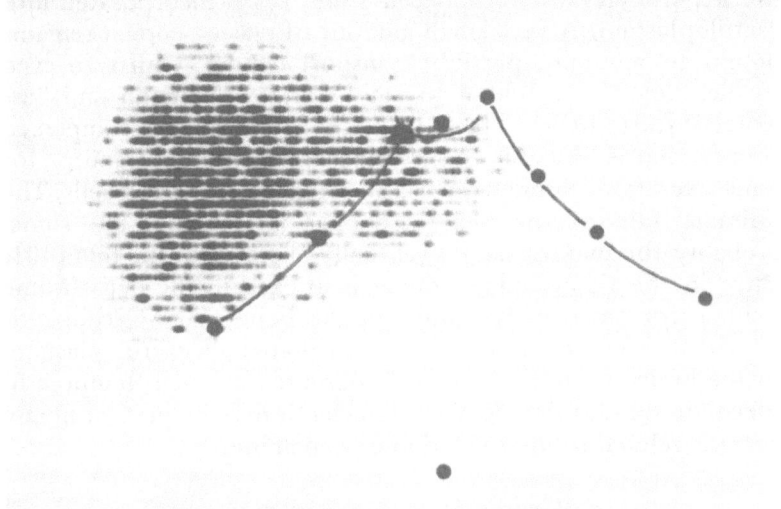

Figure 4.2. Abdominal scintiscan of a normal individual (G. B.) 3½ h after the intravenous injection of [64]Cu (as CuCl$_2$ in saline). Note normal liver outline, no extrahepatic radioactivity. Dose 186 μCi.

copper being returned to the plasma in caeruloplasmin and some excreted in the bile; Osborn and Walshe [35] have estimated that the copper so excreted may amount to 10% of the dose per 24 h. Copper isolated from bile is protein bound and is not available for reabsorption [38]. In normal individuals little copper is excreted in the urine so that balance is maintained partly by control of copper absorption and partly by biliary excretion. In man the total body copper is of the order of 100-150 mg [3]. Copper being part of the cytochrome molecule is necessarily present in all tissues but is found at the highest concentrations in the pigmented nuclei of the brain [39]: relatively high concentrations are also found in the cerebral cortex. The liver and the brain may each contain as much as 15 mg of the metal [3].

The fate of ingested copper, under normal conditions, may be summarized as follows; copper is probably freed from its organic binding by the gastric HCl; as Cu^{2+} it is rapidly absorbed in the stomach or upper small gut. It is transported to the liver as albumin bound copper, it is rapidly concentrated in the hepatocytes where between 1 and 2% is incorporated into caeruloplasmin. A very small amount of plasma copper remains bound to albumin, possibly transport copper, whilst an even smaller amount is bound to amino acids; Neumann and Sass Kortsak [33] believe that it is the amino acid complexed copper that is available for crossing cell membranes and/or for renal excretion. Some copper also remains in the red cells. The ultimate fate of the hepatic copper is doubtful but some, probably the major part, is eventually excreted in the bile [40]. Once in the tissues some copper is utilized in the cytochrome oxidase for electron transport, in the bone marrow copper is related to erythropoiesis, possibly mediated via caeruloplasmin. In the brain the role of copper is obscure but one is tempted to speculate that, in the pigmented nuclei, it may be present in any enzyme related to the oxidation of dopamine.

4.5 DISTURBANCES OF COPPER TRANSPORT

This review, as its title implies, is not interested in the wide spectrum of abnormal blood levels of copper which may be found in many conditions: these aspects of disturbed copper transport have been reviewed by Scheinberg and Sternlieb [3]. The concentration of caeruloplasmin is low at birth and remains low for about the first three months of life, representing one more facet of the functional immaturity of the foetal and neonatal liver [12, 41]. This low concentration of caeruloplasmin in the serum at birth is associated with a high concentration of copper in the liver; this excess copper is stored in the form of a unique copper protein, hepatic mitochondrocuprein [42]. As the serum caeruloplasmin concentration rises in the infant towards the normal so the liver concentration of copper falls. The mechanism of this adjustment remains unknown, unfortunately the human neonate does not lend itself to any type of balance study. Similarly the reason for the large hepatic stores of copper at birth is unknown but is, presumably related to the high blood copper levels found in late pregnancy. Perhaps it acts as a reserve for early growth needs when the main food source is milk, a product of very low copper content. Supporting this hypothesis is the fact that deliberate attempts which have been made to induce copper deficiency in premature babies have proved (happily) unsuccessful [43].

Acquired chronic copper toxicity, particularly as an industrial risk, appears to be unknown in man. In animals chronic copper poisoning occurs both naturally and under experimental conditions [3] when it is frequently associated with haemolytic anaemia and liver damage.

4.5.1 The relationship of copper to Wilson's disease, historical background

In man, to all intents and purposes, disturbances of copper transport and storage are synonymous with the genetically determined metabolic disease, hepatolenticular degeneration (Wilson's disease). The first clue to the association of abnormal copper storage and Wilson's disease came in 1913, only a year after the publication of Wilson's [44] original description of the disease which now bears his name. Rumpel [45] was the first to report finding excess copper in the liver of a patient dying of this disease. The next important clue to inculpate copper came when Siemerling and Oloff [46] noted the similarity between a sunflower cataract produced by an intraocular copper-containing foreign body and that occurring spontaneously in a patient with Wilson's disease. Other reports suggesting the involvement of copper in the pathogenesis of the disease appeared in the 1920's and 1930's but it was Cumings [47] who finally proved that excess copper was to be found in brain and liver of all fatal cases. Earlier Peters, Stocken and

Thompson [48] had reported that dimercaptopropanol (BAL), as a result of its ability to form a stable ring compound with tervalent arsenic, could be used for the management of arsenical war gas poisoning and McCance and Widdowson [49] had shown that this compound was also capable of mobilizing copper from the tissues. These observations led Cumings [47] to suggest that BAL deserved a trial as a cupruretic agent in the treatment of Wilson's disease. At about the same time it was observed that patients with Wilson's disease excreted excess copper in the urine and this could be further augmented by the administration of BAL [50].

These were indeed the halcyon days of Wilson's disease for 1947 saw the first of Holmberg and Laurell's classical series of papers on the isolation and description of caeruloplasmin [9, 13]. Three years later the harvest so well sowed began to ripen, papers appeared from Cumings [51] and Denny Brown and Porter [52] describing improvement in patients following treatment with BAL. The following year Scheinberg and Gitlin [53] and Bearn and Kunkel [54] reported that the serum copper-protein caeruloplasmin was deficient or absent from the serum of patients with Wilson's disease though subsequently it has become apparent that this is not an invariable finding [55]. In 1956 came a further advance with the introduction of penicillamine as an orally active chelating agent with a high affinity for copper [56]. This compound made it possible for the first time not only to induce complete and apparently permanent remission of the disease but also to deplete the abnormal body stores of copper and hence to demonstrate changes in the handling of radiocopper which followed.

4.5.2 Studies with radiocopper

Perhaps the major weapon which has been used in the slow process of unravelling the problem of disordered copper transport in Wilson's disease, and relating this to the pathogenesis of the illness, has been radioactive copper. Two radioisotopes have been used in clinical investigation, ^{64}Cu, H.L. 12.8 h and ^{67}Cu, H.L. 61.0 h. The longer half life of the latter confers obvious advantages but unfortunately it is difficult to produce as well as being expensive. First reports of studies with

[64]Cu appeared in 1954; Bearn and Kunkel [57] were able to show that although radiocopper was readily incorporated into caeruloplasmin by normal subjects this reaction did not take place in patients with Wilson's disease. It also became apparent from these early studies that the patients excreted copper more readily in the urine than did the controls [36, 58] but, whether the radioisotope was administered orally or intravenously, their faecal excretion was very much reduced [32, 59]. It is tempting to attribute the increased body stores of copper in Wilson's disease to impaired biliary excretion but there are too few estimations of biliary copper from such patients to draw any conclusions [52, 60, 61]. Alternatively the decreased faecal excretion of radiocopper observed after oral administration might have resulted from excess intestinal absorption [59] but this does not account for the reduced faecal excretion observed after the radiocopper has been given intravenously. Possibly the labelled copper is diluted in a greatly expanded liver pool [59] of the metal and never reaches the site of biliary excretion or possibly there is diminished excretion directly through the intestinal wall. These points are all difficult to settle experimentally in man, particularly with such a short half-life radioisotope as ^{64}Cu though in some studies with [67]Cu more than 40% of intravenously administered copper was excreted in the stool of a normal individual after 48 h [35], a finding which may well have been missed if ^{64}Cu had been used. The point therefore remains *sub judice* as to whether the positive copper balance, which must be present in patients with Wilson's disease, is due to increased intestinal absorption or decreased biliary excretion. Certain unpublished observations which bear on this topic will be discussed later.

These early studies on the concentration of radiocopper in blood, urine and stools have been followed by investigations of the distribution of the radioisotope in the body after both oral and intravenous administration. Cartwright's group [59] studied four patients with Wilson's disease and found that three had low count rates over the liver compared with their control subjects. They offered no explanation as to why the fourth patient had a normal liver uptake but the published evidence suggests that this particular patient (Dar H) was, at the time of study, in the presymptomatic stage of the illness whilst the other patients all had neurological involvement. If this explanation is correct it fully accounts for the apparent discrepancy [62]. The first attempt to estimate quantitatively the copper trapped by the liver after intravenous injection was reported by Osborn and Walshe [63]. In their control subject 90% of the radioactivity was present in the liver at 10 h and thereafter there was a steady fall to 50% at 70 h. By contrast a patient who had advanced Wilson's disease was able to concentrate only 25% of the radiocopper in the liver at 10 h but showed a steady rise to 37% at 50 h. No other localized concentrations of copper were detected in either subject. A more detailed study [37] confirmed the earlier observations that normal subjects rapidly concentrated copper in their livers and thereafter slowly released it whilst patients with Wilson's disease had a low initial uptake and little tendency for this to vary, the range of liver uptake in these patients being from 16 to 50%. However some of these patients had been receiving treatment with penicillamine though the significance of this was not at that time realized. Six patients with other forms of liver disease were also studied and the results suggested that liver damage alone did not account for the finding of impaired liver uptake of copper in Wilson's disease. As a result of this and later work Osborn and Walshe [64] concluded, wrongly as was to be shown later, that the primary genetic defect in Wilson's disease was not a failure of caeruloplasmin synthesis but an enzyme defect which resulted in an inability of the liver to concentrate copper, so that the metal never reached the site of caeruloplasmin synthesis. Evidence available at that time suggested that treatment with penicillamine did not significantly alter the handling of radiocopper by patients with Wilson's disease [65] although it appeared from other studies that the excess body stores of copper were being depleted [66]. It was because of this that Osborn and Walshe [64] concluded that "the impaired ability of the liver to concentrate copper ... is not a result of prior saturation of the binding sites with the metal". However as more cases became available for study so it became possible to build up a coherent picture of the way copper transport changed as the disease evolved. In presymptomatic patients copper uptake by the liver was found to be high, as hepatic damage became clinically apparent the liver uptake of copper fell off so that by the time the advanced neurological stage of the illness was reached there was virtually no hepatic concentrating power left (see Figure 4.3) [62, 67, 68, 69]. Following treatment with penicillamine this state of affairs was slowly reversed though it took many more years than had originally been envisaged before the hepatic concentrating power returned [62, 67].

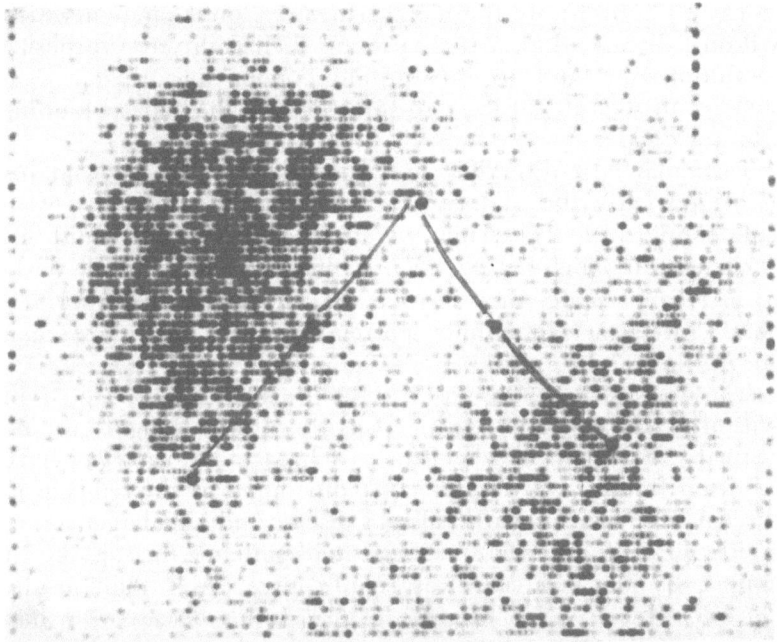

Figure 4.3. Abdominal scintiscan of a patient (R. P.) with neurological Wilson's disease, 5 h after intravenous injection of ^{64}Cu. Note poor hepatic concentration and much extrahepatic radioactivity. Dose 150 μCi.

In the light of their hypothesis that the handling of radiocopper depends upon the stage of the illness and the amount of treatment given Osborn and Walshe [69] reinvestigated the effect of liver damage on the liver uptake of copper both by patients with Wilson's disease and by patients with other forms of hepatic disease; particular attention was paid both to histological changes in the liver and to biochemical evidence of liver damage at the time of study. These results confirmed the earlier findings that liver damage, by itself, did not account for the progressive loss in efficiency of the liver trap for copper seen in Wilson's disease, but that this was accounted for by progressive saturation of the hepatic binding sites for copper and the slow reversal of this by treatment with penicillamine. More recently Gibbs and Walshe [70] have found that in patients with primary biliary cirrhosis, a condition with very large hepatic stores of copper, the liver largely retains its ability to concentrate the metal. However, unlike patients with Wilson's disease, these patients retain their ability to synthesize caeruloplasmin and to incorporate copper into this protein thereby protecting, at least to some extent, the hepatic binding sites for copper.

Particular attention has been paid by Scheinberg and his associates to the fate of caeruloplasmin labelled with radiocopper [19, 27]. They were able to show that it did not exchange the label *in vivo,* even though it could be made to do so *in vitro*. Further they showed that the copper incorporated daily into caeruloplasmin correlated well with intestinal absorption.

The handling of copper by red cells is little affected in Wilson's disease and until recently was thought to be normal [59, 64]. However, Terao, Ogihara and Mozal [71] have reported finding a low uptake of radiocopper by the red cells in three of five patients with Wilson's disease and, in a larger series, Walshe [72] found that in untreated patients the uptake of copper by the red cells was significantly lower than in the control subjects or in patients with Wilson's disease who had been treated with penicillamine. That the changes should be so small is perhaps surprising when it is realized that about 10% of patients suffer from haemolytic crises which are commonly attributed to copper toxicity.

The rate of absorption of copper from the stomach (as $^{64}CuCl_2$) has been studied by Osborn and Walshe [35] in a small series of patients with Wilson's disease and control subjects. Their findings, summarized in Table 4.1 show no difference between the concentration of radiocopper in either the plasma or the liver of the two groups during the immediate post-absorptive phase. This suggests that the rate of absorption of ionic copper is not markedly abnormal in Wilson's disease

TABLE 4.1

Uptake of Radiocopper into Liver and Plasma During
the First 30 min After Oral Administration

Subjects	No.	Plasma radioactivity % dose/litre					Liver radioactivity % dose present in liver				
		5	10	15	30	min	5	10	15	30	min
Wilson' disease	11	0.6	0.9	1.9	2.9		2.5	3.2	2.7	4.8	
Controls	5				2.8		2.6	2.9	4.0	4.4	

during the first half-hour after ingestion but it is of course possible that this state of affairs alters further down the alimentary tract. The point remains *sub judice* but the balance of evidence does not support the hypothesis that excess of absorption is the primary defect in Wilson's disease.

4.5.3 Copper proteins in Wilson's disease

The evidence at present available suggests that the formation of no copper-protein other than caeruloplasmin is disturbed in Wilson's disease. An abnormality of cytochrome oxidase itself would surely be incompatible with life, tyrosinase also does not appear to be abnormal since widespread disturbances of pigmentation are rare indeed [73]. I have seen abnormal skin pigmentation only once in over 70 cases, this was clearly melanin deposited at the site of purpuric haemorrhages on the dorsum of the feet and ankles. Neither have there been any reports of abnormal pigmentary deposits in the brain. The copper content of hair and nails is also normal [74, 75, 76].

The question of tissue proteins was once a matter of some controversy; Uzman, Iber, Chalmers and Knowlton [77] reported finding a protein in the liver of a patient with Wilson's disease which had an abnormally high affinity for copper but Walshe [78] could find no evidence to support this observation and a study of isolated copper-proteins from brain and liver led Porter [79] to state that he could find no evidence to suggest that the biochemical lesion in Wilson's disease resulted from "the accumulation of increasingly large amounts of a noxious copper-protein".

4.5.4 Biliary copper

Finally mention must be made of the biliary excretion of copper although, unfortunately, little is known of this in patients with Wilson's disease. A wide variation for values of copper in normal bile have been reported; van Ravestyn [81] found a range for copper varying from 35 to 205 μg per 100 ml but figures in excess of 1 mg per 100 ml have been reported [61, 80, 81]. In Wilson's disease it is notable that all concentrations reported, and including my own experience, are at the lower end of the normal range, the highest being 264 μg per 100 ml [61]. The data are not sufficient to draw conclusions but suggest that biliary excretion of copper may be impaired in Wilson's disease. Recently it has been reported that the affinity of bile for copper is the same in patients with Wilson's disease and in normal subjects [82], thus an abnormal enterohepatic circulation of the metal probably does not occur in these patients.

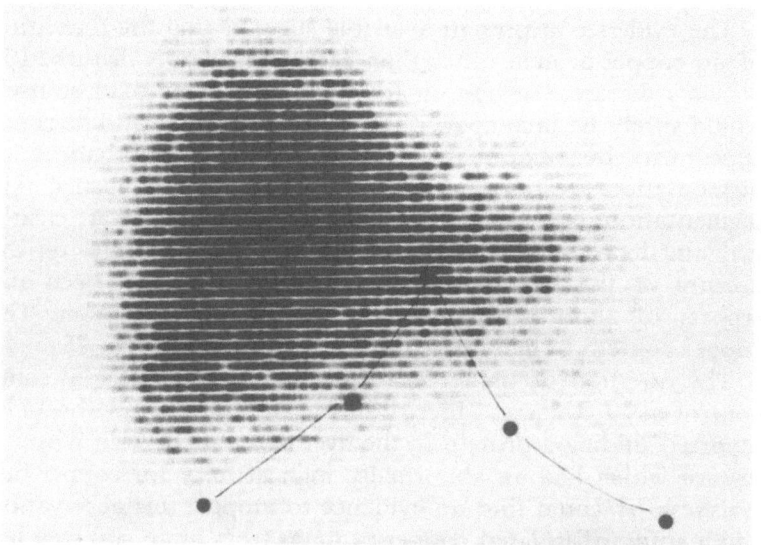

Figure 4.4. Abdominal scintiscan of a patient with presymptomatic Wilson's disease (C. D.) 5 h after intravenous injection of ^{64}Cu. Note good liver outline, little extrahepatic radioactivity. Dose 1,000 μCi.

4.5.5 Copper transport in Wilson's disease: summary

The fate of ingested copper in patients with Wilson's disease may be summed up briefly as follows. Copper is absorbed from the gut and passes up the portal vein to the liver, in the early or presymptomatic stage of the illness much of the copper is trapped (see Figure 4.4). It is not used at a normal rate in the synthesis of caeruloplasmin and it is probably not excreted at a normal rate either via the bile or the intestinal wall. As the liver proteins become saturated the excess copper is only slowly cleared from the plasma compared with various control groups (see Table 4.2). The high plasma levels of non-caeruloplasmin copper permit deposition of copper at extrahepatic sites, one of which is in the kidneys (see Figure 4.5). As the illness progresses the liver looses its ability to trap copper as also do the kidneys

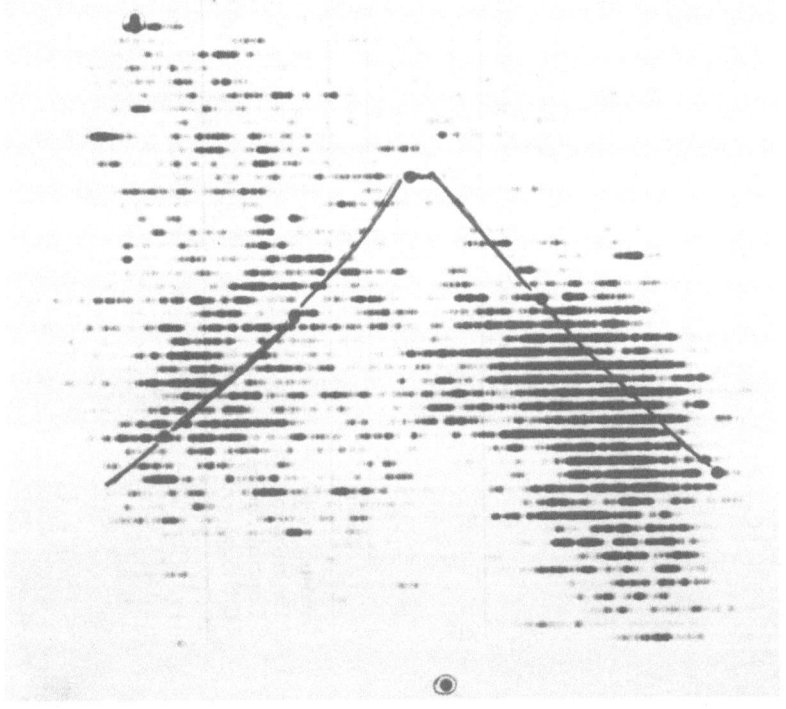

Figure 4.5. Abdominal scintiscan, early neurological Wilson's disease (Wm. McC.) 2 h after intravenous injection of ^{64}Cu. Note poor hepatic concentration and radioactivity in the renal area. Dose 300 μCi.

TABLE 4.2

Plasma Radiocopper Levels and Statistical Significance

Cases	Plasma, % dose per litre (mean ± 2 S.E.M.)				Significance differences between group		
	No	10 min	No	2 h	group	10 min	2 h
1 Wilson's disease	13	16.47 (± 3.96)	29	2.69 (± 0.60)	1 vs 3	N.S.	0.01 P
2 Heterozygote W.D	4	11.98 —	13	0.98 (± 0.08)	2 vs 3	N.S.	0.01 P
3 Controls, hepatic C.N.S. and normal	14	12.65 (± 2.36)	41	1.70 (± 0.26)			

W.D. = Wilson's disease   N.S. = not significant

so that the excess metal is deposited in the brain and corneae. This failure of the liver to remove copper from the plasma with a consequent high blood level of the metal results in high count rates being found in various areas, including the head, after radiocopper injection. This has led some workers to believe that they had detected brain uptake of radiocopper [71, 83]. In practice all that has been observed is a high ratio of tissue to liver activity consequent upon a reduced liver uptake; convincing evidence for localization of copper in the brain has not been reported. Thus as the disease progresses there is a steady rise in the plasma non-caeruloplasmin copper and an increased rate of excretion of copper in the urine. This in turn leads to the renal lesions seen in patients with advanced Wilson's disease, renal glycosuria, aminoaciduria, uricosuria, phosphaturia, hypercalcuria and inability to produce an acid urine.

Once patients with this degree of tissue saturation are treated with penicillamine the progress of events is reversed, the liver regains its ability to trap copper (see Figure 4.6), the plasma is cleared more rapidly, the blood and urine copper levels fall and the kidneys regain their ability to acidify the urine [85]. Copper deposited in the cornea as the Kayser Fleischer rings can be seen to disappear.

4.6 COPPER TOXICITY

It has already been demonstrated that copper is an essential trace element for life, it is now necessary to show that, under abnormal conditions or when present in excess, it can be toxic. In normal man copper balance is maintained throughout life so that delicate homeostatic processes must exist for providing enough copper for normal metabolic processes but no more. The big reserves of the neonate are rapidly dispersed and are not found even in young children. Unfortunately no animal model which mimics the metabolic disturbance of Wilson's disease is available for study so that experiments in which excess copper is fed to animals will not necessarily give rise to the same syndrome. Nevertheless there is experimental evidence that copper is toxic to animals when administered in quantities sufficient to produce a positive balance.

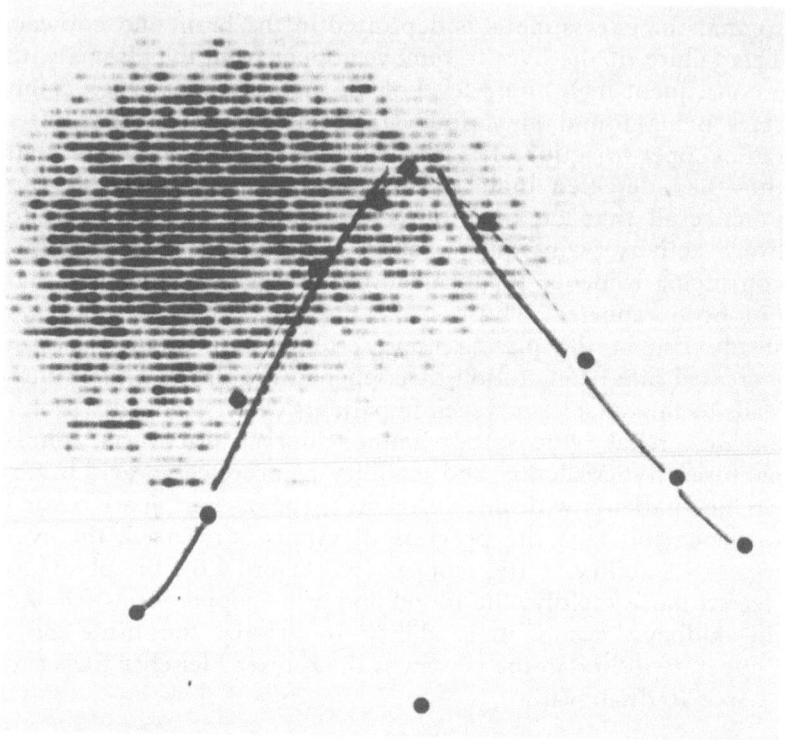

Figure 4.6. Abdominal scintiscan of a patient with Wilson's disease (G. V.) 4 h after intravenous injection of ^{64}Cu. The patient had been on treatment with penicillamine for nine years and was symptom free. Note the good liver outline and absence of extrahepatic radioactivity. Dose 400 μCi.

For instance Mallory [86] added 200 mg powdered metallic copper to the diet of rabbits and found that this led to pigment deposition in the liver and early necrosis of hepatocytes. In a later paper [87] he showed that a suspension of metallic copper given parenterally was the most reliable method of inducing copper toxicity: when given over long periods this treatment resulted in the development of "a form of pigment cirrhosis". If copper administration was discontinued the changes and the copper deposits disappeared in about five months. The central nervous system was not involved.

It has long been known that copper toxicity leads to haemolytic jaundice in sheep [88]. The pathogenesis has been thought to be a sudden massive release of copper from the liver leading to a sharp rise in the plasma copper concentration and consequent red cell lysis. Some authors believe that this same mechanism operates in the haemolytic crises sometimes seen in Wilson's disease [89]. Cartwright's group [90] studied copper induced anaemia in chickens, an animal chosen because of its low level of caeruloplasmin. Although about one-third of the birds became anaemic they found no evidence of intravascular haemolysis of the type reported in enzootic jaundice of sheep, nor was there any rise in the serum bilirubin. Further they observed that the serum copper of the birds, although it rose considerably (maximum in an anaemic chicken 393 μg per 100 ml) never approached the level of 5000 μg per 100 ml tested in an unsuccessful attempt to induce haemolysis in whole blood. Furthermore the red cells from copper treated birds showed no increase in fragility to hypotonic saline. However all birds affected by anaemia died and histological examination of their livers revealed erythrophagocytosis. This was presumed to be the method of blood destruction and anaemia production. Haemolysis associated with copper sulphate poisoning has also been described in man following the use of copper sulphate for the débridement of burns [91], and also after accidental ingestion [92].

The toxic action of copper on the red cell was investigated by Fairbanks [92] who showed that it inhibited glucose-6-phosphate dehydrogenase and accelerated the oxidation of NADPH *in vitro*, that it was able to penetrate the intact erythrocyte and inhibit glycolysis, denature haemoglobin and oxidize glutathione. He suggested that persons deficient in the enzyme glucose-6-phosphate dehydrogenase would be unusually vulnerable to copper-induced haemolysis. However deficiency of this enzyme does not appear to be necessary for haemolysis to occur in Wilson's disease for one patient has been seen who was found to have the enzyme present in normal concentration*.

In those experiments in which copper is added to the diet the central nervous system always appears to escape, an observation which led Peters and Walshe [93] to investigate the effect of copper on the brain by injecting Cu^{2+} directly into the

---

* I am grateful to Professor H. Lehmann for carrying out this determination.

subarachnoid space of pigeons. They found that as little as 20 μg of the metal rapidly led to convulsions and death. *In vitro* studies showed that Cu^{2+} inhibited oxygen uptake and pyruvate oxidation by brain slices but that this inhibition was not sufficiently rapid to account for the effect of copper on the intact animal. Further studies [94] suggested that the toxic action of copper was mediated through inhibition of the membrane ATPase; in this respect copper was the most active of the metals investigated. Copper is, in addition, an active inhibitor of a number of enzyme systems [95] particularly those dependent on an —SH group at the active catalytic centre [96, 97]. Copper has also been shown to diminish the content of phosphocreatine, ATP and potassium of guinea pig and pigeon cerebral hemisphere, an effect thought to be related to diminished ATPase activity [98].

4.7 THE PATHOGENESIS OF WILSON'S DISEASE

Two points are now established beyond reasonable doubt. *The first* that copper transport and storage are disturbed in patients with Wilson's disease; this leads to positive copper balance with the accumulation of a great excess of copper in the body, most markedly the liver, brain and kidneys. *The second* that copper is toxic to a number of enzyme systems particularly those mediated through an —SH group at the active catalytic centre. However *in vivo* studies with animals have failed to reproduce the clinical syndrome of Wilson's disease and acquired copper toxicity in man bears no striking resemblance to the genetically determined illness. Perhaps the most significant biochemical difference between individuals suffering from genetic and acquired copper intoxication is the deficiency of caeruloplasmin found in the former. However this may be no more than a coincidence, for the association does not prove a cause and effect relationship. Indeed Uzman never did believe that caeruloplasmin deficiency was related to the pathogenesis of Wilson's disease. According to his theory copper was deposited in tissue previously damaged by an underlying abnormality of protein and peptide metabolism [77]. But despite the lack of proof that a direct relationship exists between copper overload and Wilson's disease the balance of probability is much in favour of it. The slow development of the clinical syndrome, seldom manifesting itself before seven or eight years of age and often very much later, is in keeping with the slow accumulation of a toxic compound in the body. The dramatic reversal of signs and symptoms which often follows treatment with copper-binding agents greatly strengthens the hypothesis that the relationship is indeed one of cause and effect. Against this it might be argued that the two effective chelating agents used for copper removal, BAL (2,3 dimercaptopropanol) and penicillamine (β, β dimethyl cysteine), are both sulphydryl compounds and so are able to supply $-SH$ groups to the tissues; thus the removal of copper might be an interesting but unimportant side effect. Indeed it has been shown that in some patients with Wilson's disease disturbed pyruvate metabolism may be corrected by the administration of penicillamine [99]. Certainly the use of the chelating agent EDTA, which has no $-SH$ group, has proved disappointing in therapy [61]. However compared with penicillamine it is a poor chelator for copper and it requires parenteral, preferably intravenous administration, a fact which severely limits its usefulness. Recently Walshe [100] has introduced a new chelating agent, triethylene tetramine 2 HCl, for the management of Wilson's disease. This compound has no sulphydryl group so that if the initial successful reports [100, 101] are confirmed it must be taken as further evidence that ability to mobilize copper is the keystone to therapy in Wilson's disease.

It therefore appears reasonable to state that there is an incontrovertible relationship between the deposition of excess copper stores and the development of structural and functional defects in certain tissues. This sequence of events can be reversed by the establishment of a negative copper balance with chelating agents. As copper is an enzyme poison there seems little doubt that the metal must be implicated in the pathological changes observed. Now since it has been demonstrated that, in Wilson's disease, copper accumulates in the brain and liver in concentrations sufficient to inhibit essential enzymes, then it must be asked how and why this accumulation takes place. In other words what homeostatic mechanism is disturbed to permit the development of a positive copper balance?

In discussing the evidence for copper toxicity mention has been made of Uzman's hypothesis that, in Wilson's disease, tissue proteins are present which have an abnormal affinity for copper, that copper normally absorbed is bound by these proteins so firmly that it is not available for caeruloplasmin synthesis. This abnormality of protein metabolism in turn leads to the formation of an abnormal "oligopeptide" which is itself a copper carrier. This "oligopeptide" is filtered at the glomerulus and then enters into competition with amino acids for reabsorption by the renal tubules. The consequent renal amino-aciduria which is, apparently, also found in asymptomatic relatives, gives rise in turn to hepatic cirrhosis and brain damage [77, 102, 103, 104]. Copper plays no part in this scheme except as a consecutive phenomenon; "no one seriously attributes" the development of hepatic cirrhosis or brain damage "to copper intoxication *per se*" [105]. This theory has never been widely accepted because amino-aciduria is not an invariable accompaniment of the disease [61, 106], because it has not been possible to detect a specific oligopeptide in the urine [106] and because it has not been possible to repeat the finding of a particular protein in liver with a high affinity for copper [78]. Finally, as has been shown already, the association between size of the copper stores and severity of the symptoms is too close to be dismissed as mere coincidence.

In 1952 Scheinberg and Gitlin [53] reported the concentration of caeruloplasmin to be reduced in the serum of patients with Wilson's disease. This observation became the basis of an alternate theory that Wilson's disease resulted from failure to synthesize this protein. This theory was admirably summarized by Cartwright and his associates [60] as follows: the deficiency of caeruloplasmin is congenital, this permits accumulation of copper in the liver which leads to cirrhosis, in the brain giving rise to disorders of movement, in the corneae resulting in the formation of Kayser Fleischer rings and in the kidneys causing renal tubular defects involving particularly the reabsorption of amino acids and peptides. Excess copper from the tissues is chelated by amino acids and peptides and is excreted in the urine. The high level of "direct reacting" (non-caeruloplasmin) copper in the serum is a measure of the high turnover rate of copper between the gut, the tissues and the excretory routes. In a later publication these workers claimed to have shown that the positive copper balance resulted from an increased absorption of copper from the gut rather than from impaired biliary excretion [59], but examination of the figures given in this paper hardly seems to bear out their contention, viz. radioactivity excreted in the stools after intravenous administration of ^{64}Cu, five normal individuals, range 9.1-16.3%, mean 12.4%, four patients with Wilson's disease, range 1.8-3.4%, mean 2.5%.

Eventually this theory attributing the pathogenesis of Wilson's disease to caeruloplasmin deficiency has also had to bow out to later observations. The most damaging finding has been that a small number of patients with Wilson's disease may have normal or near normal concentrations of the protein yet they develop the full clinical syndrome whilst some heterozygotes (parents of patients) may have very low concentrations of this protein and remain symptom-free. For instance Sternlieb and Scheinberg [107] reported finding three heterozygotes with caeruloplasmin values of less than 10 mg per 100 ml and I have seen two with caeruloplasmin concentrations in the same range. A modification of this hypothesis has attempted to explain the apparently normal values for serum caeruloplasmin in Wilson's disease by postulating either that the protein was not broken down at the normal rate or that it was structurally abnormal and therefore unable to subserve the normal enzymatic function. But present evidence is against an abnormal half-life for caeruloplasmin in Wilson's disease [19] or a structurally abnormal protein [108] although some recent evidence suggests that in some patients the caeruloplasmin may be abnormal [109]. Another possible explanation, though one which has received little attention, is that apocaeruloplasmin may be present in the plasma of patients with Wilson's disease and this has been shown to inhibit normal caeruloplasmin oxidase activity [110].

Yet another hypothesis linking caeruloplasmin deficiency with the synthesis of an abnormal protein is that of Morell, Irvine, Sternlieb, Scheinberg and Ashwell [21]. These workers succeeded in preparing caeruloplasmin labelled with both radiocopper and tritium, but devoid of its terminal sialic acid grouping. Unlike native caeruloplasmin this asialocaeruloplasmin disappeared from the circulation within minutes of injection. After its disappearance from the plasma the asialocaeruloplasmin could be detected in the hepatocytes but not the Kupffer cells. This rapid uptake by the hepatocytes was dependent upon the exposure of the terminal galactosyl residue following the removal of sialic acid. As a result Morell and his associates [21] suggested that deficiency of caeruloplasmin in Wilson's disease could result from the production of caeruloplasmin normal in all respects except for the terminal galactosyl grouping, the consequence being "those molecules synthesized with incomplete carbohydrate chains either would not be released from their site of synthesis, or, if secreted, would not survive in circulation".

Oestrogens will induce caeruloplasmin synthesis [111] both in normals and patients with Wilson's disease [112, 113]. This led Scheinberg and Sternlieb [114] to postulate that the raised caeruloplasmin values found occasionally in Wilson's disease were but a temporary phenomenon resulting from liver damage and failure of oestrogen catabolism. I have seen six patients with Wilson's disease with caeruloplasmin concentrations in excess of 15 mg per 100 ml. Three of these did indeed have severe liver damage, but two were presymptomatic and one had nervous system involvement only, the liver having escaped virtually unscathed. On the other hand two children have been seen both with severe liver disease but with zero caeruloplasmin concentrations. Thus severe hepatic involvement does tend to be associated with a raised serum caeruloplasmin level in Wilson's disease but the relationship does not appear to be so close that it can be the sole explanation of the anomaly.

The interpretation of results from studies with radiocopper in patients with Wilson's disease are all bedevilled with the possibility that the radiocopper has simply been diluted in a greatly expanded body pool of the metal. If this is the case the finding of a low concentration of labelled copper in tissue, urine or faeces is simply a measure of dilution [59, 115]. However, the distribution of radiocopper in both patients and control subjects does not correspond with the distribution of total body copper [116]. This certainly shows that for at least 48 hours after injection uniform dilution of the radioisotope does not take place in the body pool of the metal. More direct evidence has come recently from the work of Gibbs and Walshe [70]. They investigated copper transport in patients with primary biliary cirrhosis; these are of particular interest because of the very large stores of copper in their livers, comparable with those found in patients with Wilson's disease [117]. Their studies led them to conclude that "newly arrived radiocopper is preferentially handled in the presence of copper overload, thus dilution of radiocopper in an expanded hepatic pool of the metal cannot alone account for the delayed incorporation (of radiocopper into caeruloplasmin) found in patients with Wilson's disease". One interesting by-product of this work was the development of a technique for estimating the hepatic turnover times for radiocopper. In normal individuals this was of the order of 20-30 days, for patients with primary biliary cirrhosis the time was 600-700 days but in patients with Wilson's disease it was in excess of 1,800 days. "In all cases the turnover time for radiocopper was significantly less (than for stable copper)." Obviously injected radiocopper must eventually mix with the body pool of copper but the evidence suggests that for short term studies this is not a major source of inaccuracy. It would thus seem that the positive copper balance that is found in patients with Wilson's disease is in some way related to the inability of the liver to incorporate copper into caeruloplasmin, further supporting the hypothesis that the primary defect in this disease is more likely to be impaired excretion of copper via the bile rather than increased intestinal absorption of the metal.

4.8 MECHANISMS OF SYMPTOM PRODUCTION

Copper, as has already been discussed, is an enzyme poison and the sulphydryl-dependent enzymes are probably those most vulnerable to attack.

4.8.1 The liver

In the liver, once cell necrosis has been initiated, the mechanism of symptom production scarcely needs further discussion. As liver damage proceeds to cirrhosis so portal hypertension and splenomegaly commonly result, leading eventually to the development of oesophageal varices and haematemesis, a complication which has a particularly evil prognosis in this disease [118]. However it remains unexplained why some patients will undergo an apparent spontaneous recovery from an episode of liver damage only to present perhaps years later with central nervous system involvement. The clue may lie in the changing distribution of copper in the liver at different stages of the disease, in the youngest patients copper is found diffusely distributed in the cytoplasm of the hepatocytes where its presence is associated with cytopathological changes, whilst in older patients and in normal neonates copper is concentrated in the lysosomes [119] and here it appeared to be non-toxic.

4.8.2 Haemolysis

Nor is the situation with regard to understanding the mechanism of haemolysis any easier. It must be related to copper toxicity, the clinical and experimental evidence for this is overwhelming. Nevertheless the commonly accepted hypothesis of massive copper liberation from the liver being the precipitating cause is not entirely above criticism. First, the haemolysis seen in Wilson's disease is not, like that in sheep, intravascular with haemoglobinaemia and haemoglobinuria; second the concentrations of plasma copper that have been reported during haemolysis, 103-163 μg per 100 ml [89] are not even of the same order of magnitude as that needed to cause haemolysis in plasma [90]. This modest rise in plasma copper recorded during haemolysis could, at least in part, result from the liberation of the metal from lysed red cells; 70% of a normal red cell mass contains between 1,000 and 2,000 μg of copper. It would seem that haemolysis must take place in the reticuloendothelial system, cells which have a peculiar freedom from copper overload. Goldberg and his associates [90] suggested that the haemolysis observed in copper intoxicated chicks took place in the hepatic sinusoids. Like these workers Gibbs and Walshe [120] found no increase in osmotic fragility of normal red cells after exposure to copper or of the red cells of a patient who had recently undergone a series of haemolytic crises. On the other hand it is tempting to postulate that the red cell membrane ATPase is inhibited by copper, that this is followed by breakdown of the sodium pump with consequent swelling and destruction of the cells. If this is the case the final act of haemolysis must be sudden for spherocytosis has not been reported in Wilson's disease.

4.8.3 The brain

If the sequence of events in the liver is often enigmatic and the mechanism of haemolysis remains unexplained it must be admitted that the distribution of lesions in the brain is mysterious indeed. It has been suggested [56] that the reason why the brain and particularly the basal ganglia are so severely affected is because of their dependence on carbohydrate oxidation via the tricarboxylic acid cycle for their energy supply, the cycle operating via a number of sulphydryl enzymes.

Assuming that normal functioning of the neurone is particularly sensitive to copper why, one must ask, does the sensory nervous system always escape completely? Published information suggests that copper concentrations are increased uniformly throughout the brain in Wilson's disease [60, 61, 73] but the sensory cortex seems to have escaped specific mention. Recently it has been possible to repair this omission with copper determinations from the brain of a patient who died with a severe neurological lesion. This patient belonged to a religious sect which discouraged orthodox medical treatment. He was therefore virtually without medication for several years before his final admission to hospital.

Sensory cortex	48.4µg/g wet weight
Motor cortex	53.7µg/g wet weight
Mid brain	66.5µg/g wet weight
Basal ganglia	55.0µg/g wet weight
Loci caerulei	58.3µg/g wet weight

Why indeed do the sensory neurones escape functional damage? One is left to wonder at the wide variation in the clinical picture if the basic biochemical defect is uniform. For instance some patients present with wild tremor or spontaneous movements, some with dystonia, some with choreiform movements, whilst others are akinetic. Transient lapses of consciousness are occasionally seen as are epileptic seizures and a few patients may suffer severe psychiatric disturbances which, on occasion, precede the onset of other signs of nervous system disease. In fact it is probably true to say that no two patients with neurological Wilson's disease are ever alike.

It is useless to pretend that the answer to these questions lies just around the corner but it is interesting, and perhaps not entirely unhelpful to speculate on some mechanisms which may be involved. To do so may lay the writer open to criticism but if it provokes others to seek clues on those happily rare occasions when the brain from a patient with Wilson's disease becomes available for study the exercise will have been worth while.

In the Parkinsonian syndrome there is degeneration of the pigmented nuclei of the brain, those areas with the highest copper content [39], many patients with Wilson's disease have Parkinsonian symptoms. Dopamine is found at the highest concentration in the substantia nigra, probably in the melanin containing cells. The pigment may well be derived from dopamine or its precursor dopa [121]. The concentration of dopamine is low in patients dying with Parkinsonism suggesting a reduced ability of the brain to form this amine which appears essential for mediating the motor functions of the basal ganglia. It does not seem unreasonable to suggest that a disturbance in the metabolism of this transmitter system occurs in Wilson's disease under the influence of excess copper. In the early stages copper may potentiate dopamine synthesis leading to abnormal movements; later, when the concentration of copper exceeds a critical level, synthesis is inhibited and a more typically Parkinsonian syndrome, leading finally to akinesia, develops. One patient has been seen, who in addition to severe tremor, had marked exophthalmos and hyperidrosis suggesting sympathetic over-activity. These symptoms all responded to decoppering treatment with penicillamine.

4.8.4 The kidneys

Finally brief mention must be made of the renal lesion. Heavy metals are known to affect renal tubular function and there is no reason why copper should be an exception. Radiocopper studies have shown that, after the liver, the kidney is the next site of copper deposition [122] (Figure 4.5) so that the finding of functional renal defects [123] is hardly surprising. However, Reynolds, Tannen and Tyler [124] were unable to find a good correlation between the functional defect and the histological changes on the one hand and copper deposition on the other. By contrast Wolff [125] demonstrated a relationship between the presence of copper and the functional lesion, a finding which has since been confirmed [126]. The renal tubular acidosis which develops in Wilson's disease [127] can be reversed by treatment with penicillamine [85]. Possibly as Walshe [85] suggested, the failure of Reynolds and his associates to demonstrate copper in association with other histological changes in the kidney [124] was a further demonstration of the unreliability of histochemical techniques for the metal.

4.9 THE INFLUENCE OF PENICILLAMINE ON COPPER TRANSPORT AND STORAGE

Brief mention has been made earlier of the ability of penicillamine to deplete the excess copper deposits in patients with Wilson's disease. There are four main lines of evidence to support this contention (1) Visible copper deposits in the corneae, the Kayser Fleischer rings, can be seen to regress and finally disappear under the influence of treatment, only to reappear if this is interrupted or reduced to an inadequate level [78, 128]. (2) The concentration of copper in the plasma falls once treatment is established, in some cases it may fall to virtually undetectable levels [66, 129, 130]. (3) The concentration of serum caeruloplasmin falls, not only in patients with Wilson's disease [130], but also in patients with other diseases treated with penicillamine [131] (see Figure 4.7). (4) There is a fall in the basal excretion of copper in the urine

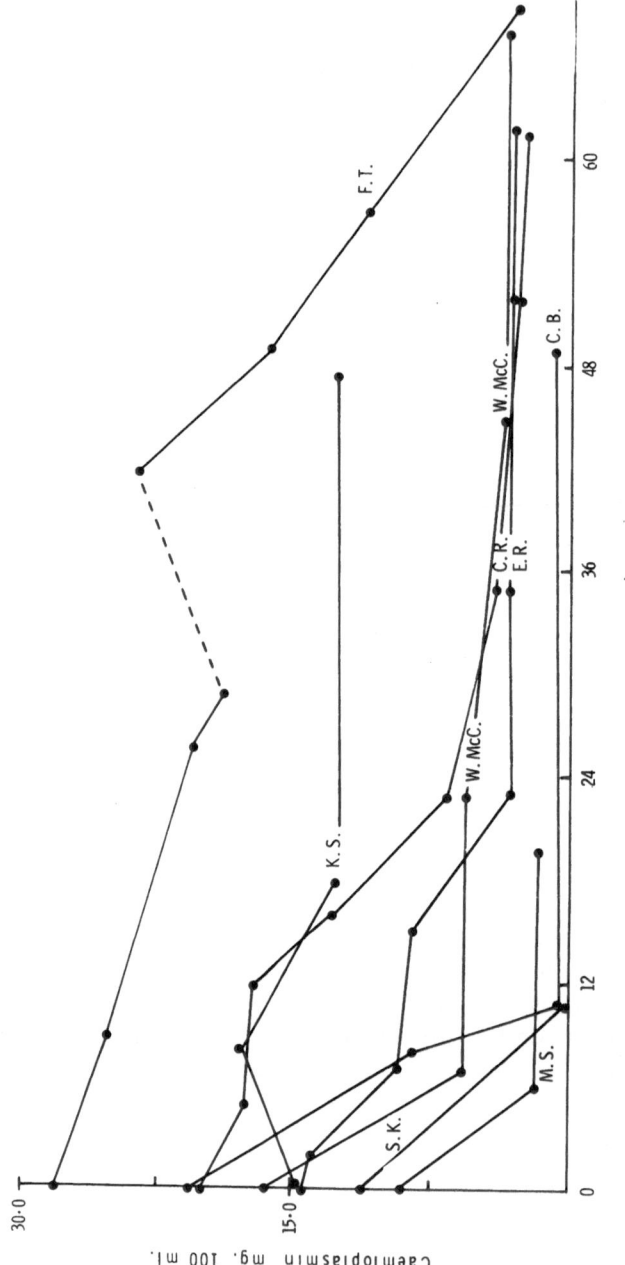

Figure 4.7. Graph showing the decline in concentration of serum caeruloplasmin in patients with Wilson's disease after the start of treatment with penicillamine. Note in the case of F.T. the rise in caeruloplasmin concentration between 30 and 45 months, during which time treatment was temporarily discontinued.

and a corresponding fall in the amount of copper excreted in response to a test dose of penicillamine [66, 132]. These four points all strongly support the hypothesis that penicillamine depletes body stores of copper.

The time of administration of penicillamine relative to the time of administration of radiocopper is crucial. Most published reports concerning the excretion of radiocopper, under basal conditions, have shown that patients with Wilson's disease excreted of the order of 5% or less of the dose in 24 hours [58, 59] and by this time radiocopper excretion has reached very low levels. From this base line it can be increased by the administration of penicillamine to a figure of between 2 and 6% in the next 6 h, the exact amount depending on the previous therapeutic history of the patient and hence the size of the copper load [133]. If however the penicillamine is given before the radiocopper, so that the drug is present in the plasma before protein binding of the copper has taken place, then the amount of the radioisotope excreted is enormously increased, for six patients so studied the average was 50% in 24 h (see Table 4.3). The therapeutic implications of this are obvious, penicillamine is a much more active copper chelator if given before exposure to copper rather than afterwards*. Predictably this massive excretion of radiocopper, under conditions of priming with penicillamine, has resulted in a low hepatic uptake of the metal and a low liver thigh ratio not only in patients with Wilson's disease but also in the single control subject so studied [67].

Theoretically perhaps the most important observation which has resulted from the study of the effect of penicillamine on copper transport is the fall in caeruloplasmin concentration. In a few patients the protein has become undetectable in the serum and has remained so for many years. This iatrogenic acaeruloplasminaemia has given rise to the development of no symptoms which might be attributed to deficiency of the protein. Certainly none of the functions which have been attributed to caeruloplasmin have been affected. If the protein carried the prosthetic group of cytochrome oxidase to the cells

---

* For workers at hazard from radioactive spill it is clearly of great advantage to have an adequate blood level of penicillamine, or the preferable chelating agent, before entering the area of risk.

TABLE 4.3

% Dose Radiocopper (Given I.V.) Present in Urine of Patients With Wilson's Disease
Under Basal Conditions and after 500 mg D-penicillamine Base
(Mean ± 2 S.E.M.)

Cases	No.	0 – 24 h	24 – 30 h
W.D. (no previous therapy)	7	3.4 ± 1.7 (basal)	6.3 ± 3.4 (after penicillamine)
W.D. (maintenance penicillamine)	22	1.2 ± 0.2 (basal)	2.4 ± 0.3 (after penicillamine)
W.D. Penicillamine before ^{64}Cu	6	50.2 ± 5.1	

or was essential in iron mobilization and haemoglobin synthesis its deficiency would rapidly become apparent. The fact that acaeruloplasminaemia, when accompanied by penicillamine administration, is so well tolerated would seem to point to a key role in maintaining copper balance, but the mechanism involved remains quite obscure.

4.10 SUMMARY

Normal handling of copper in man has been reviewed and compared with the abnormal handling in Wilson's disease. The excess copper stores in this disease must be due either to increased absorption or decreased biliary excretion; there is no direct evidence to settle this point but the latter hypothesis, at present, appears the more likely.

Experimental demonstration of copper toxicity has been discussed with particular reference to Wilson's disease. The balance of evidence leaves no reasonable room for doubt that copper is directly related to the development of the pathological changes in this disease. The role of caeruloplasmin, its structure and function have been reviewed but its relation to Wilson's disease remains obscure.

The ability of penicillamine to deplete the body stores of copper has been recorded and the significance of its ability to produce acaeruloplasminaemia without apparent disturbances of intermediary metabolism noted. The importance of attaining a therapeutic blood level of penicillamine before, rather than after, exposure to copper has been reported; this procedure ensures the maximum cupruresis. While throwing little extra light on the pathogenesis of Wilson's disease the therapeutic advantages of this procedure are self evident.

ACKNOWLEDGEMENTS

I am greatly indebted to my collaborators Miss K. Gibbs and Dr. S. B. Osborn who have allowed me to draw so freely on the results of observations hitherto unpublished, to Dista Products Limited for generous gifts of penicillamine and to the many physicians who have referred to me their patients with Wilson's disease. Without the help of any of these the writing of this chapter would not have been possible.

REFERENCES

1. J. Alsop, *In* From the Silent Earth, p. 129. Secker and Warburg, London, (1965)
2. H. Beinert, *In* The Biochemistry of Copper (J. Peisach, P. Aisen and W. E. Blumberg, eds), pp. 213-234. Academic Press, New York and London, (1966)
3. I. H. Scheinberg and I. Sternlieb, *Pharmacol. Revs.*, 12, 235 (1960)
4. H. Porter and S. Ainsworth, *J. Neurochem*, 5, 91 (1959)
5. A. G. Morell, J. R. Shapiro, and I. H. Scheinberg, *In* Wilson's disease: some Current Concepts (J. M. Walshe and J. N. Cumings, eds), p. 36. Blackwell's Scientific Publications, Oxford, (1961)
6. T. Mann and D. Keilin, *Proc. roy. Soc. B.* 126, 303 (1938-9)
7. T. B. Fitzpatrick and W. C. Quevedo, *In* Metabolic basis of inherited disease, 2nd Edition, (J. B. Stanbury, J. B. Wyngaarden and D. S. Fredrickson eds), p. 324. McGraw-Hill, New York, (1966)
8. C-B. Laurell, *In* The Plasma Proteins, (F. W. Putnam ed.), Vol. 1, p. 349. Academic Press, New York, (1960)
9. G. C. Holmberg and C-B. Laurell, *Acta Chem. Scand.*, 1, 944 (1947)
10. G. C. Holmberg and C-B. Laurell, *Acta Chem. Scand.*, 2, 550 (1948)
11. G. C. Holmberg and C-B. Laurell, *Acta Chem. Scand.*, 5, 476 (1951)
12. G. C. Holmberg and C-B. Laurell, *Acta Chem. Scand.*, 5, 921 (1951)
13. G. C. Holmberg and C-B. Laurell, *Scand. J. clin. Lab. Invest.*, 3, 103, (1951)
14. C. B. Kasper and H. F. Deutsch, *J. biol. Chem.*, 238, 2325 (1963)
15. C. Curzon, *In* Wilson's disease: some Current Concepts (J. M. Walshe and J. N. Cumings, eds), p. 96. Blackwell's Scientific Publications, Oxford (1961)
16. L. Broman, *Nature, (Lond.)*, 182, 1655 (1958)
17. H. F. Deutsch and G. B. Fisher, *J. biol. Chem.*, 239, 3325 (1964)
18. W. E. Blumberg, J. Eisinger, P. Aisen, A. G. Morell and I. H. Scheinberg, *J. biol. Chem.*, 238, 1675 (1963)
19. I. Sternlieb, A. G. Morell, W. D. Tucker, M. W. Greene and I. H. Scheinberg, *J. clin.Invest.*, 40, 1834 (1961)
20. T.A. Waldman, A. G. Morell, R. D. Wochner, W. Strober and I. Sternlieb, *J. clin. Invest.*, 46, 10 (1967)
21. A. G. Morell, I. Sternlieb, I. H. Scheinberg and G. Ashwell, *J. biol. Chem.*, 243, 155 (1968)
22. H. A. Ravin, *J. lab. clin. Med.*, 58, 161 (1961)
23. O. Waalas and E. Waalas, *Arch. Biochem. Biophys.*, 95, 151 (1961)
24. S. Osaki and D. A. Johnson, *J. biol. Chem.*, 244, 5757 (1969)

25. M. Shimizu, *Birth Defects, Original Article Series* 4, no. 2, 49 (1968)
26. P. Aisen, A. G. Morell, S. Alpert and I. Sternlieb, *Nature (Lond.),* 203, 873 (1964)
27. I. H. Scheinberg and A. G. Morell, *J. clin. Invest.* 36, 1193 (1957)
28. G. E. Cartwright and M. M. Wintrobe, *Amer. J. clin. Nutrit.,* 15, 94 (1964)
29. E. Freiden, *Nutrit. Revs.,* 28, 87 (1970)
30. L. Broman, *Acta Soc. med. Upsaliensis,* 69, Suppl. 7 (1964)
31. A. B. Semple, W. H. Parry and D. E. Phillips, *Lancet* 2, 700 (1960)
32. A. G. Bearn and H. G. Kunkel, *J. lab. clin. Med.,* 45, 623 (1955)
33. P. Z. Newmann and A. Sass Kortsak, *J. clin. Invest.,* 46, 646 (1967)
34. S. B. Osborn and J. M. Walshe, *Clin. Sci.,* 26, 213 (1964)
35. S. B. Osborn and J. M. Walshe, (unpublished)
36. C. J. Earl, M. J. Moulton and B. Selverstone, *Amer. J. Med.,* 17, 205 (1954)
37. S. B. Osborn, C. N. Roberts and J. M. Walshe, *Clin. Sci.,* 24, 13 (1963)
38. P. A. Farrer and S. P. Mistilis, *Birth Defects, Original Article Series,* 4, no. 2, 14 (1968)
39. P. J. Warren, C. J. Earl and R. H. S. Thompson, *Brain,* 83, 709 (1960)
40. D. Gitlin, W. I. Hughes and C. A. Janeway, *Nature, (Lond.),* 188, 150 (1960)
41. J. Schorr, A. G. Morell and I. H. Scheinberg, *A.M.A. J. Dis. Child.,* 96, 541 (1958)
42. H. Porter, M. Sweeney and E. M. Porter, *Arch. Biochem. Biophys.* 104, 97 (1964)
43. J. F. Wilson and M. E. Lahey, *Pediatrics, Springfield,* 25, 40 (1960)
44. S. A. K. Wilson, *Brain,* 34, 295 (1911-12)
45. A. Rumpel, *Dtsch. Z. Nervenheilk,* 49, 54 (1913)
46. E. Siemerling and H. Oloff, *Klinische Wochenschrift,* 1, 1087 (1922)
47. J. N. Cumings, *Brain,* 71, 410 (1948)
48. R. A. Peters, L. A. Stocken and R. H. S. Thompson, *Nature (Lond.),* 156, 616 (1945)
49. R. A. McCance and E. M. Widdowson, *Nature (Lond.),* 157, 837 (1946)
50. B. M. Mandelbrote, M. W. Stanier, R. H. S. Thompson and M. N. Thurston, *Brain,* 71, 212 (1948)
51. J. N. Cumings, *Brain,* 74, 10 (1951)
52. D. Denny Brown and H. Porter, *New Engl. J. Med.,* 245, 917 (1951)
53. I. H. Scheinberg and D. Gitlin, *Science,* 116, 484 (1952)
54. A. G. Bearn and H. G. Kunkel, *J. clin. Invest.,* 31, 616 (1952)
55. G. E. Cartwright, H. Markowitz, G. S. Shields and M. M. Wintrobe, *Amer. J. Med.,* 28, 555 (1960)
56. J. M. Walshe, *Amer. J. Med.,* 21, 487 (1956)
57. A. G. Bearn and H. G. Kunkel, *Proc. Soc. Exp. Biol. and Med.,* 85, 44 (1954)
58. W. B. Matthews, *J. Neurol. Psychiat.,* 17, 242 (1954)

59. J. A. Bush, J. P. Mahoney, H. Markowitz, C. J. Gubler, G. E. Cartwright and M. M. Wintrobe, *J. clin. Invest.*, **34**, 1766 (1955)
60. G. E. Cartwright, R. E. Hodges, C. J. Gubler, J. P. Mahoney, K. Daum, M. M. Wintrobe and W. B. Bean, *J. clin. Invest.*, **33**, 1487 (1954)
61. H. Bickel, F. C. Neale and G. Hall, *Quart. J. Med.*, N.S.**26**, 527 (1957)
62. S. B. Osborn and J. M. Walshe, *Lancet*, **1**, 346 (1967)
63. S. B. Osborn and J. M. Walshe, *Lancet*, **1**, 70 (1958)
64. S. B. Osborn and J. M. Walshe, *Clin. Sci.*, **29**, 575 (1965)
65. A. Sass Kortsak, B. S. Glatt, M. Cherniak and I. Cederlund, *In* Wilson's disease: some Current Concepts, (J. M. Walshe and J. N. Cumings eds), p.151. Blackwell's Scientific Publications, Oxford (1961)
66. J. M. Walshe, *Clin. Sci.*, **26**, 461 (1964)
67. S. B. Osborn and J. M. Walshe, *Birth Defects, Original Article Series*, **4**, No. 2, 41 (1968)
68. W. N. Tauxe, N. P. Goldstein, J. B. Gross and R. V. Randall, *Birth Defects, Original Article Series*, **4**, No. 2, 45 (1968)
69. S. B. Osborn and J. M. Walshe, *Lancet*, **2**, 17 (1969)
70. K. Gibbs and J. M. Walshe, *Clin. Sci.*, **41**, 189 (1971)
71. T. Terao, K. Ogihara and T. Mozal, *Birth Defects, Original Article Series*, **4**, No. 2, 29 (1968)
72. J. M. Walshe, *In* S.S.I.E.M. Symposium No. 5. Some Inherited Disorders of brain and muscle. (J. D. Allan and D. N. Raine eds), p.130. Livingstone, Edinburgh (1969)
73. J. N. Cumings, *In* Heavy Metals and the Brain, p.27. Blackwell's Scientific Publications, Oxford (1959)
74. G. M. Martin, *Nature, (Lond.)*, **202**, 903 (1964)
75. E. W. Rice and N. Goldstein, *Metabolism*, **10**, 1085 (1961)
76. K. Gibbs and J. M. Walshe, *J. med. Genet.*, **2**, 181 (1965)
77. L. L. Uzman, F. L. Iber, T. C. Chalmers and M. Knowlton, *Amer. J. med. Sci.*, **231**, 511 (1956)
78. J. M. Walshe, *Brain*, **90**, 149 (1967)
79. H. Porter, *Birth Defects, Original Article Series* **4**, No. 2, 23 (1968)
80. C. J. Gubler, H. Brown, H. Markowitz, C. E. Cartwright and M. M. Wintrobe, *J. clin. Invest.*, **36**, 1208 (1957)
81. H. A. van Ravestyn, *Acta Med. Scand.*, **118**, 163 (1944)
82. K. W. Buchwald and L. Hudson, *Cancer Res.*, **4**, 645 (1944)
83. D. J. Fromer, *Clin. Sci.*, in press (1971)
84. W. H. Oldendorf and M. Kitamo, *Arch. Neurol.*, **13**, 5333 (1965)
85. J. M. Walshe, *Lancet*, **1**, 775 (1968)
86. F. B. Mallory, *Amer. J. Path.*, **1**, 117 (1925)
87. F. B. Mallory and F. Parker, *Amer. J. Path.*, **7**, 351 (1931)
88. H. E. Albiston, L. B. Ball, A. T. Dick and J. C. Keast, *Australian Vet. J.*, **16**, 233 (1940)
89. N. McIntyre, H. M. Clink, A. J. Levi, J. N. Cumings and S. Sherlock, *New Engl. J. Med.*, **276**, 439 (1967)

90. A. Goldberg, C. B. Williams, R. S. Jones, M. Yanagita, G. E. Cartwright and M. M. Wintrobe, *J. lab. clin. Med.*, **48**, 442 (1956)
91. N. A. Holtzman, D. A. Elliott and R. H. Heller, *New Engl. J. Med.*, **275**, 347 (1966)
92. V. F. Fairbanks, *Arch. Int. Med.*, **120**, 428 (1967)
93. R. A. Peters and J. M. Walshe, *Proc. roy. Soc. B.*, **116**, 273 (1966)
94. R. A. Peters, M. Shorthouse and J. M. Walshe, *Proc. roy. Soc. B.*, **116**, 285 (1966)
95. K. R. Rees, *In* Wilson's disease: some Current Concepts (J. M. Walshe and J. N. Cumings eds), p.49. Blackwell's Scientific Publications, Oxford (1961)
96. C. Veeger and M. Massey, *Biochim. Biophys. Acta*, **37**, 181 (1960)
97. M. Massey and C. Veeger, *Biochim. Biophys. Acta*, **48**, 33 (1961)
98. P. S. Epstein and H. McIlwain, *Proc. roy. Soc. B.*, **116**, 295 (1966)
99. J. M. Walshe, *Clin. Sci.*, **20**, 197 (1961)
100. J. M. Walshe, *Lancet*, **2**, 1401 (1969)
101. R. S. Dubois, D. O. Rodgerson, T. L. Slovis, K. M. Hambidge and T. A. Bianchi, *Lancet*, **2**, 775 (1970)
102. L. L. Uzman and D. Denny Brown, *Amer. J. med. Sci.*, **215**, 509 (1948)
103. L. L. Uzman and B. Hood. *Amer. J. med. Sci.*, **223**, 392 (1952)
104. L.L. Uzman *Amer. J. med. Sci.*, **226**, 645 (1953)
105. L. L. Uzman, *Arch. Neurol. Psychiat.*, **77**, 164 (1957)
106. W. H. Stein, A. G. Bearn and S. Moore, *J. clin. Invest.*, **33**, 0 (1954)
107. I. Sternlieb and I. H. Scheinberg, *J. Amer. Med. Assoc.*, **183**, 747 (1963)
108. N. A. Holtzman, M. A. Naughton, F. L. Iber and B. M. Gaumnitz, *J. clin. Invest.*, **46**, 993 (1967)
109. S. B. Needleman, V. Shagal and B. Boshes, *Separatim Experentia*, **26**, 495 (1970)
110. J. M. Walshe, *J. clin. Invest.*, **42**, 1048 (1963)
111. E. M. Russ and J. Raymunt, *Proc. Soc. exp. Biol. (N.Y.)*, **92**, 465 (1956)
112. E. M. Russ, J. Raymunt and S. Pillar, *J. clin. Endocr.*, **17**, 908 (1957)
113. J. L. German and A. G. Bearn, *J. clin. Invest.*, **40**, 445 (1961)
114. I. H. Scheinberg and I. Sternlieb, *Lancet*, **1**, 1420 (1963)
115. A. Sass Kortsak, M. Cherniak, D. W. Geiger and R. J. Slater, *J. clin. Invest.*, **38**, 1672 (1959)
116. J. M. Walshe, *In*Wilson's disease: some Current Concepts (J. M. Walshe and J. N. Cumings, eds), p.148. Blackwell's Scientific Publications, Oxford, (1961)
117. A. H. Hunt, R. M. Parr, D. M. Taylor and N. G. Trott, *Brit. med. J.*, **2**, 1498 (1963)
118. I. Sternlieb, I. H. Scheinberg and J. M. Walshe, *Lancet*, **1**, 638 (1970)
119. S. Goldfischer and I. Sternlieb, *Amer. J. Path.*, **53**, 883 (1968)
120. K. Gibbs and J. M. Walshe, (unpublished)
121. O. Hornykiewicz, *Pharmacol. Revs.*, **18**, 925 (1966)

122. S. B. Osborn, K. Szaz and J. M. Walshe, *Quart. J. Med., N.S.*, 38, 467 (1969)

123. A. G. Bearn, *Amer. J. Med.*, 22, 747 (1957)

124. E. S. Reynolds, R. L. Tannen and H. R. Tyler, *Amer. J. Med.*, 40, 518 (1966)

125. S. M. Wolff, *Lancet*, 1, 843 (1964)

126. Y.Yoshitoshi, T. Oda, Y. Yamane, N. Nagase, K. Mori and T. Shikata, *Birth Defects, Original Article Series*, 4, No. 2, 104 (1968)

127. M. Fulop, I. Sternlieb and I. H. Scheinberg, *Ann. Int. Med.*, 68, 770 (1968)

128. W. Sussman and I. H. Scheinberg, *Arch. Ophthal.*, 82, 738 (1969)

129. J. M. Walshe and V. Clarke, *Arch. Dis. Child.*, 40, 651 (1965)

130. J. M. Walshe, *Birth Defects, Original Article Series*, 4, No. 2, 126 (1968)

131. R. I. Henkin, H. R. Keiser, I. A. Jaffe, I. Sternlieb and I. H. Scheinberg, *Lancet*,2, 1268 (1969)

132. J. M. Walshe, *Brit. J. Hosp. Med.*, 4, 91 (1970)

133. J. M. Walshe, (unpublished)

134. M. H. K. Shokier and D. C. Shreffler, *Proc. nat. Acad. Sci.*, 62, 867 (1969).

CHAPTER 5

Brain Amine Metabolism in Some Neurological and Psychiatric Disorders

G. CURZON

Abbreviations

A, adrenaline; COMT, catechol-0-methyl transferase; CSF, cerebrospinal fluid; DA, 3,4-dihydroxyphenylethylamine (dopamine); Dopa, 3,4-dihydroxyphenylalanine; 5HIAA, 5-hydroxyindoleacetic acid; 5HT, 5-hydroxytryptamine (serotonin); 5HTP, 5-hydroxytryptophan; HVA, 3-methoxy-4-hydroxyphenylacetic acid (homovanillic acid); MAO, monoamine oxidase; MAOI, monoamine oxidase inhibitor; MHPG, 3-methoxy-4-hydroxyphenylglycol; NA, noradrenaline; VMA, 3-methoxy-4-hydroxymandelic acid (vanillomandelic acid).

5.1 Introduction

The principal amines which will be considered here in relation to neurological and psychiatric disease are the catecholamines, dopamine (DA) and noradrenaline (NA), and the indolealkylamine, 5-hydroxytryptamine (5HT) or serotonin.

The initial indications that the amines might be important for the functioning of the nervous system were probably the almost simultaneous reports of the isolation of adrenaline (A) from the adrenal gland [1] and of the similar effects of administering adrenal extracts and stimulating sympathetic nerves [2]. Eventually it was demonstrated [3] that the material secreted by the sympathetic nerves was NA and that this had a characteristic distribution in the brain [4] suggesting a relationship with specific brain functions.

While the biological importance of DA·as a precursor of NA was first suggested [5] in 1939 it was only thought of as a possible neurohormone many years later. This was mainly because, unlike A and NA, its activity in standard pharmacological assay systems is slight. Not until the development of the modern spectrophotofluorometer was it possible to, determine readily the low concentrations of the catecholamines present in brain and show that almost all the brain DA was localized in the basal ganglia [6]. This immediately suggested a special importance of DA in the control of movement.

Recognition of the importance of 5HT in the nervous system stems from the finding in 1953 that the hallucinogen LSD powerfully inhibited its action on smooth muscle [7] and therefore perhaps also on brain and from the demonstration in 1954 of a specific distribution of 5HT in the brain [8].

More recently the use of the histofluorescence method for the localization of brain amines led to the finding that DA, NA and 5HT are present in the brain not merely in a characteristic distribution by region but in DA, NA and 5HT neuronal tracts [9], each one containing a specific amine. Furthermore, it has been shown that electrical stimulation of the cell bodies of the NA [10], DA [10] or 5HT [11] neurones results in depletion of the corresponding amine at the nerve terminals. Also, experiments using microelectrophoretic application of amines [12, 13] provided evidence that each activates or inhibits particular neuronal populations. These observations point very strongly to transmitter functions for the amines. The various tracts may thus be termed DA-ergic, NA-ergic and 5HT-ergic respectively.

That disturbed amine metabolism or action may have a role in psychiatric illness was indicated by the structural relationships between many hallucinogens and either the catecholamines or 5HT. Another key finding was the association between the mood elevating effects of iproniazid and its inhibitory action upon monoamine oxidase [14] (MAO), an enzyme which is involved in amine destruction. Conversely, the tranquillizer reserpine was found to deplete brain 5HT [15] and NA [16]. A host of drugs have subsequently been recognized or developed which modify mood or behaviour and influence the metabolism, disposition or action of brain amines (see Ref. 17 for review). These relationships strongly suggest that psychiatric illness involves brain amine disturbance. The most striking indication that abnormal brain metabolism has a role not only in psychiatric but also in neurological disease was the finding at autopsy of very low concentrations of DA in the basal ganglia of patients with Parkinson's disease [18] and also the effectiveness of L-dopa, the DA precursor, in the treatment of parkinsonian symptoms [19].

5.2 Amine Metabolism in the Brain

This topic will be dealt with relatively briefly. Detailed accounts of amine metabolism can be found elsewhere [20, 21].

The amines under consideration are all aromatic substances, containing benzene or indole rings and are synthesized *in vivo* from the two aromatic L-amino acids, L-tyrosine and L-tryptophan. The latter is an essential amino acid in so far as man cannot synthesize it and thus depends on dietary sources. Tyrosine is not essential, being formed by p-hydroxylation of the benzene ring of phenylalanine. Tyrosine and tryptophan have many routes of metabolism, the pathways leading to amine formation only accounting for a small fraction of their total metabolism. The amines derived from tyrosine are the catecholamines DA, NA and A, while from tryptophan are derived the indolealkylamines of which most attention has been paid to 5HT.

There are many similarities between the pathways of synthesis and degradation of the catecholamines and those of 5HT. Thus, in both cases the first step in synthesis (Figure 5.1) is ring hydroxylation by tyrosine hydroxylase [22] and tryptophan hydroxylase [23] respectively to give L-3,4-dihydroxy-phenylalanine (L-dopa) and L-5-hydroxytryptophan (5HTP). These substances are α-amino acids but are not among the 17 α-amino acids from which protein molecules are synthesized. Dopa and 5HTP are decarboxylated by aromatic amino acid decarboxylase to DA and 5HT respectively. A method by which this enzyme can be satisfactorily measured in human brain has only recently been described [24]. Indeed failure to detect appreciable decarboxylase activity in human brain [25, 26, 27] has led to the speculation that although the rate limiting step in brain amine synthesis in animals is ring hydroxylation, the subsequent decarboxylation step may also be rate limiting in man. This question has not been resolved and is important in relation both to hypotheses concerning pathological brain amine disturbances and also to the rationale of their chemo-therapy.

After decarboxylation, the two pathways become less similar, the enzyme dopamine-β-oxidase [28, 29] converting DA to NA, but a similar pathway of 5HT metabolism is not known. Adrenaline is formed through N methylation of NA by phenylethanolamine N-methyl transferase [30]. The adrenal medulla is rich in this enzyme but only slight activity is present in brain. Whether A occurs in brain is doubtful although its formation therein from labelled injected NA has been reported [31]. Therefore the characteristic catecholamines of the brain are DA and NA.

Recently an indolethylamine N-methyl transferase has been detected in the brain of various animals including man [32, 33]. However, the products of its action, the singly and doubly N-methylated 5HT derivatives N-methyl 5HT and N-dimethyl

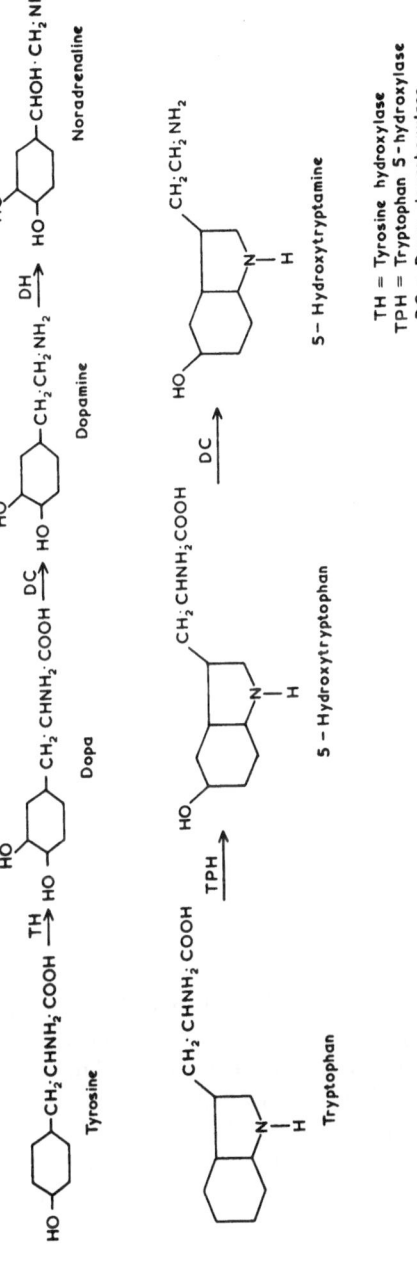

Figure 5.1. Synthesis of dopamine, noradrenaline and 5-hydroxytryptamine in the brain.

5HT (bufotenine) have not been reliably detected in the brain under physiological conditons. They may possibly be formed when tryptophan is given together with a monoamine oxidase inhibitor (MAOI).

Inside the neurones the amine is synthesized and largely contained in storage vesicles within which it is not available to destructive enzymes. This stored material is in equilibrium with free amine in the neuronal cytoplasm where it is susceptible to destruction by mitochondrial MAO (Figure 5.2). The latter plays a part in the breakdown of both the catecholamines and 5HT, the initial products being various aldehydes [34]. Normally these are not detectable being largely oxidized further to acids. A pathway of reduction of the aldehydes to the corresponding alcohols also exists [35, 36] but this is in general (although not in all cases—vide infra) quantitively much less important. Through the action of MAO followed by the oxidation of the aldehyde products, DA is converted to 3,4-dihydroxyphenylacetic acid (dopacetic acid), NA to 3,4-dihydroxymandelic acid and 5HT to 5-hydroxyindoleacetic acid (5HIAA). Only in the latter case however is the acid the major metabolite of the amine as another enzyme catechol-0-methyl transferase (COMT) [37, 38, 39] is also involved in the metabolism of DA and NA converting them to the corresponding 0-methylated derivatives, 3-methoxytyramine and nor-metanephrine. The two enzymes MAO and COMT are localized differently. MAO occurs in mitochondria contained within the neuronal cytoplasm but COMT apparently occurs in the synaptic cleft [40, 41]. Thus DA may be converted to 3,4-dihydroxyphenylacetic acid by MAO inside the neurone which can be methylated extraneuronally by COMT to 3-methoxy 4-hydroxy phenylacetic acid (homovanillic acid, HVA). Alternatively DA molecules released into the synaptic cleft may be methylated by COMT to 3-methoxytyramine which on re-entering neurones or in other cells can be oxidized by MAO to the same final product, HVA. This substance is normally the principal DA metabolite and by determining it a measure of DA metabolism can be obtained.

Outside the brain the main pathway of NA and A metabolism is exactly analogous to that of DA, COMT and MAO acting on either NA or A to give, in each case, 3-methoxy 4-hydroxy mandelic acid (vanillomandelic acid, VMA). However, VMA is not detectable in the brain, the aldehydes formed by immediate action of MAO on NA or its 0-methylated derivative being not oxidized to acids therein but largely reduced to the corresponding alcohols [36, 42]. Thus the characteristic metabolite of NA in the brain is 3-methoxy 4-hydroxy phenylglycol (MHPG).

An important difference between the metabolism in the brain of the catecholamines and of 5HT is that there is no known enzyme destroying 5HT in the synaptic cleft and it is presumably mainly destroyed after re-uptake by neurones.

The brain contains all the enzymes necessary for the synthesis of the amines from their precursors tyrosine and tryptophan and for their destruction. The immediate precursors, dopa [43] and 5HTP [44] and also the more distant precursors L-tyrosine and L-tryptophan can penetrate to the brain when given systemically and therefore can increase brain amine concentrations. However, catecholamines or 5HT synthesized or introduced peripherally are generally found to penetrate the blood-brain barrier only slightly [45, 46] although one group reports uptake and very rapid metabolism in the brain of 5HT given peripherally to rats [47].

Various other amines are present or have been suggested to be present in the brain or nervous system, although there are as yet no related pathological findings and (except for melatonin) evidence of hormonal or transmitter properties is negligible. In one study [48] ethanolamine, piperidine, putrescine, spermidine, spermine, histamine and methyl-histamine were found in the human brain. Spermidine and spermine were present in relatively high concentrations. Very recently [49], an unknown substance with characteristics suggesting an indolethylamine was found in rat spinal cord apparently intraneuronally localized. Tryptamine has not yet been detected in normal brain except after giving large doses of its precursor tryptophan plus MAO1 to guinea-pigs [50]. Intravenous infusion of ^{14}C-tryptophan in the rat did not lead to detectable ^{14}C in a brain extract which would have contained any tryptamine present [51]. Tyramine is detectable, being particularly concentrated in the

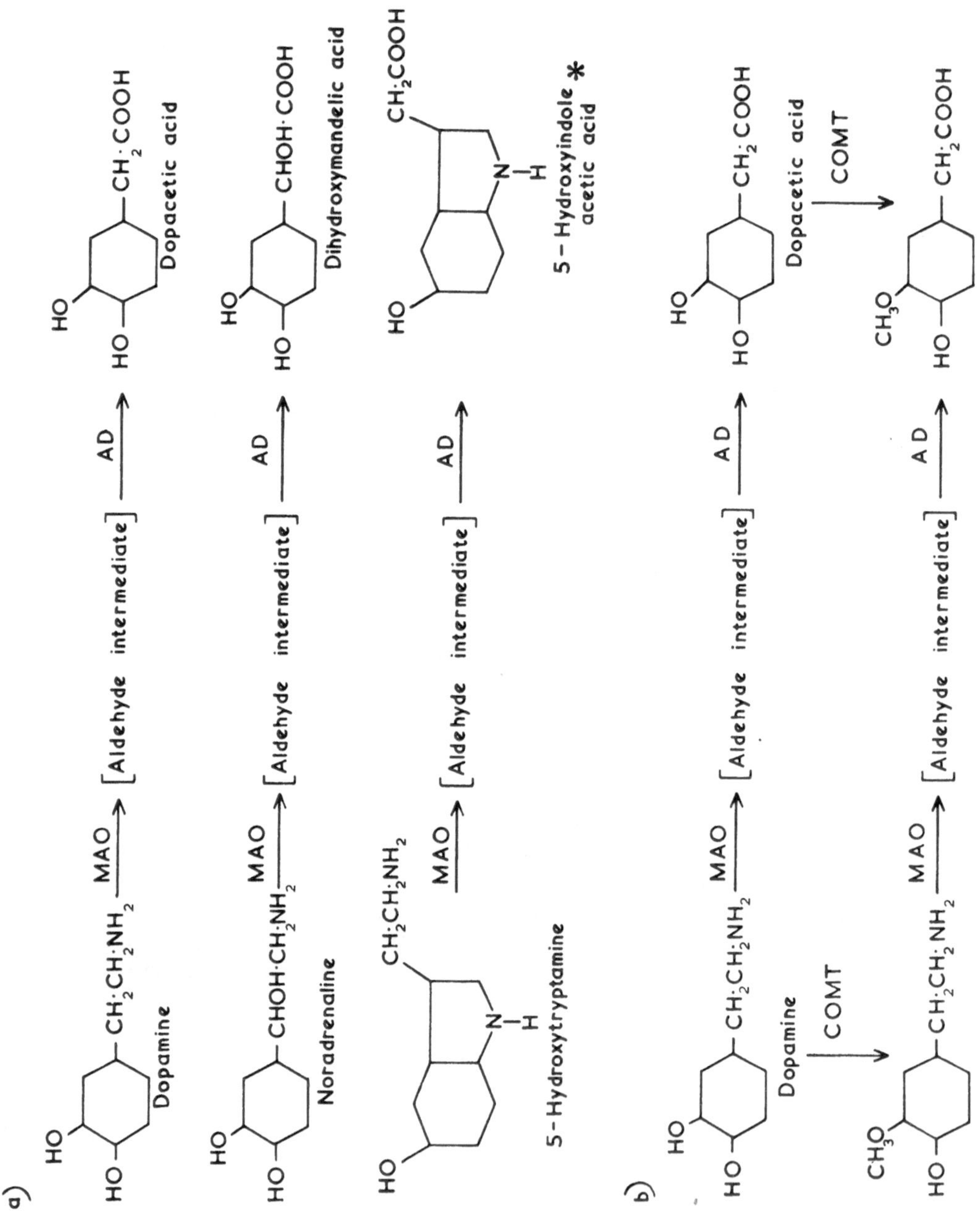
a)
Dopamine
MAO
Aldehyde intermediate
AD
Dopacetic acid
Noradrenaline
Dihydroxymandelic acid
5-Hydroxytryptamine
5-Hydroxyindole acetic acid *
b)
COMT

c)

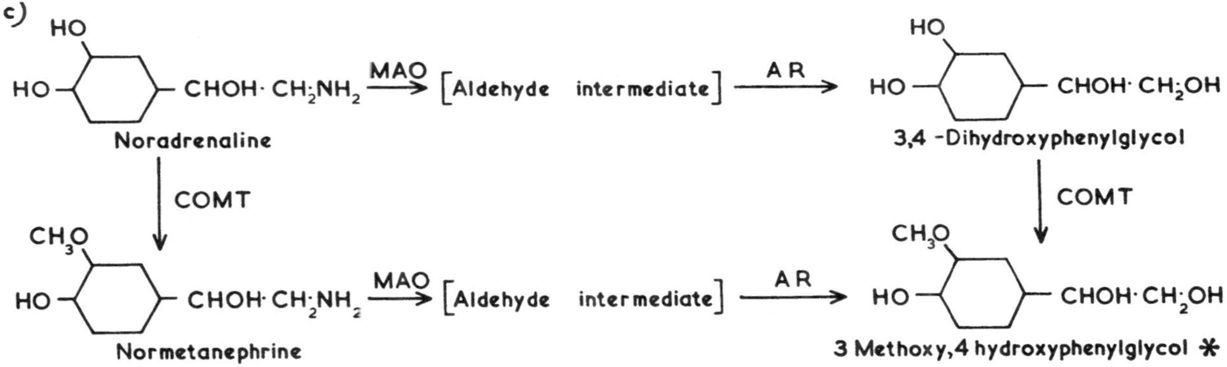

MAO = Monoamine oxidase
AD = Aldehyde dehydrogenase
AR = Aldehyde reductase
COMT = Catechol O-methyl transferase

Figure 5.2. Destruction of amines in the brain.

(a) Monoamine oxidase pathway with oxidation of aldehyde intermediate-major pathway of 5-hydroxytryptamine destruction
(b) Combined monoamine oxidase and catechol-0-methyl transferase pathway with oxidation of aldehyde intermediate-major pathway of dopamine destruction
(c) As (b) but with reduction of aldehyde intermediate-major pathway of noradrenaline destruction.

* = Principal terminal amine metabolite in brain.

hypothalamus [52]. Finally, while the pineal is not strictly part of the brain it should be mentioned that 5HT has a special route of metabolism therein leading to N-acetyl-5-methoxytryptamine (melatonin) (see ref. 53 for review).

5.3 METHODS OF STUDY OF AMINES IN MAN WITH SPECIAL REFERENCE TO DETECTION OF METABOLIC ABNORMALITIES IN THE BRAIN

5.3.1 Urine and blood

The availability of urine and blood samples has led to many investigations on brain disorders in which these fluids have been utilized. In particular, urinary 5HIAA and VMA have been determined to give measures of whole body 5HT and NA + A turnover. The main disadvantage of this approach is that extracerebral metabolism of amines accounts for all but a very small fraction of the total amine metabolite content of the urine. Therefore, detection of abnormal amounts of the metabolites in urine, while suggestive by no means proves abnormal brain metabolism. Conversely, failure to detect a urinary abnormality does not prove normal brain metabolism, as a gross abnormality of the latter which was not paralleled in the general metabolism would hardly be detectable in the urine. A borderline exception to this generalization may be the determination of urinary MHPG (see 5.2) as about 25% of this was found in the dog [54] to be derived from the metabolism of brain NA. Also, for example in phenylketonuria (where there is disturbed brain function associated with defective conversion of phenylalanine to tyrosine in the liver) investigation of urinary metabolites can be relevant.

5.3.2 Cerebrospinal fluid

The difficulties of interpretation of urine findings do not apply to cerebrospinal fluid (CSF) and thus determination of HVA and 5HIAA in human lumbar CSF is becoming an important tool in the study of the metabolism in the brain of their respective precursors DA and 5HT and in the interpretation of the effects of drug treatment upon their metabolism. The assumption is made that the concentrations of

HVA and 5HIAA in the lumbar CSF give a measure of the amount of turnover of the parent amines in the brain. This is supported by a number of findings. (1) Amine metabolite concentrations in the lateral ventricular CSF of the dog correlate with their concentrations in adjacent brain regions [55]. (2) Peripherally administered HVA only penetrates slightly or not at all to lateral ventricular CSF in the cat [56] or dog [57], similar results being also obtained for 5HIAA in the dog [58]. (3) Drugs which alter brain amine turnover in laboratory animals alter the concentrations of the acidic metabolites in dog [57], rabbit [59] and human [60] CSF appropriately. (4) In parkinsonism and in senile and pre-senile dementia, conditions in which there is evidence of defective turnover of amines in the brain, low concentrations of HVA and 5HIAA in the CSF are also found [61].

The first determinations of human CSF HVA were reported in 1963 [62] and the first determinations of 5HIAA in 1960 [63]. Most subsequent papers in which this approach was used were published relatively recently, i.e. 1966 [56, 64-67], 1967 [68, 69], 1968 [70-73], 1969 [61, 74-79], 1970 [59, 60, 80-91]. This is probably because evidence for the relationship between the CSF amine metabolite levels and brain amine metabolism accumulated only recently [55-61] and also because of the recent improvements in methodology enabling determination of both HVA and 5HIAA in 5 to 8 ml of lumbar CSF. In general, methods available for the determination of MHPG, the brain NA metabolite, are not sufficiently sensitive although one method [92] which has been used for urine is suggested by its authors to be suitable for application to CSF and some values obtained by another method have been reported [93].

While the determination of lumbar CSF amine metabolites has considerable advantages over urine or blood determinations in the study of human brain amine metabolism, abnormal values do not necessarily indicate abnormal metabolism of the precursors in the brain. Abnormality of transport of the acidic metabolites from brain to CSF, from CSF to blood or from the ventricles to the lumbar sac could also be responsible. Ventricular levels are much higher than lumbar levels [71, 82, 88] as an active process of transport of the acids from the CSF to the blood occurs together with the movement of CSF down the spinal canal. Therefore, abnormally low lumbar concentrations are found in some but not all patients with probable meningeal damage [94] or in patients with myelographic evidence of restricted flow of CSF to the lumbar sac due to tumours or cord lesions [95]. This relationship between low levels and restricted flow incidentally provides direct evidence that lumbar CSF HVA originates above the area of restriction and almost certainly from the brain. In these subjects, the decrease of HVA was more marked than that of 5HIAA suggesting that some of the latter may be of local spinal origin. This correlates with animal work as while nerve terminals containing 5HT are found at high concentrations in the lumbar part of rat and mouse spinal cord, DA terminals are not detectable in the spinal cord [96].

Defective transport of the acidic metabolites from CSF to blood may result in high lumbar concentrations. Thus a patient has been reported with high CSF 5HIAA and HVA but in whom treatment with probenecid (which blocks transport of these substances from CSF to the blood) indicated that the abnormality was due to defective transport [74]. After probenecid the CSF concentrations of the subject did not change but those of other patients rose markedly.

Determination of CSF HVA and 5HIAA after probenecid is of great value as their concentrations are then more closely related to brain amine turnover. However, in most probenecid studies only moderate increases of HVA and 5HIAA were found [72, 74, 77, 87]. Recently it has been given in much larger and more prolonged dosage [90] and much larger increases found. This suggests that in the earlier work the transport block was only partial or intermittent and therefore some doubt must be cast upon its interpretation.

Even in the absence of the above extracerebral mechanisms by which abnormal CSF HVA and 5HIAA may arise, CSF levels of these substances, while reflecting brain metabolism of their parent amines, do not allow a full balance sheet to be drawn up for any brain amine. This is clear from Figure 5.2. For example, estimation of the ratio of intraneuronal to extraneuronal metabolism of a catecholamine requires determination of the ratio of its deaminated to its 0-methylated metabolites [40, 41]. Only one brief report [97] has appeared on the determination in CSF of 3,4-dihydroxyphenylacetic acid, the deaminated but not 0-methylated metabolite of DA. Determination of other relevant metabolites in CSF has not yet been described. Another possibility is the oxidation of DA or 5HT by MAO to aldehydes followed by an abnormal diversion to the alcoholic metabolites 3-methoxy-4-hydroxyphenylethanol (dopaminol) or 5-hydroxytryptophol [35, 36]. This would probably be confused with low net amine turnover as HVA and 5HIAA concentrations would tend to be low.

However, notwithstanding these limitations the determination of amine metabolites in the lumbar CSF is at present the most practical and fruitful method for the study of human brain amine metabolism.

5.3.3 Brain

It is obvious that indications of abnormal brain amine metabolism obtained using CSF are greatly strengthened if supplemented by direct study of brain material. Relatively little relevant work has yet been done, firstly because of the limited availability of material, as the usual methods used for fixation of brain render amine determinations impossible. Secondly, there are considerable gaps in our knowledge of the effects on brain amines of changes during terminal processes, between death and autopsy and during subsequent storage. Also, these changes may differ in different brain regions.

Work on human post-mortem brain 5HT has been stimulated by investigations [98] suggesting that its concentration in brain areas probably does not alter markedly during routine storage of bodies before autopsy. Subsequently, human brain stem 5HT was found not to vary significantly with time between death and autopsy [99] although there was a tendency for it to decrease as time increased from 12 to 92 h while storage in a deep freeze after autopsy resulted in an exponential fall of brain stem 5HT and 5HIAA to about two-thirds of initial concentration in 25 days but little further change up to 50 days further storage [100]. These findings for 5HT are consistent with the lack of significant relationship between hind-brain 5HT concentration and times of storage in the deep freeze between 39 and 300 days [101]. However, there is some indication that 5HIAA increases during these prolonged periods of storage (see 5.6.2).

Much less information is available on post-mortem changes of DA and NA. Rat and mouse brain DA and NA [102, 103] fell to half or less of initial concentrations within a few hours of death under conditions roughly comparable with those of humans before autopsy. However DA and NA concentrations were similar in human brains taken at autopsies performed either at 3 or 20 h after death [18]. The distribution of DA, NA and 5HT between human brain regions [6, 104] is generally comparable to that found in animals while human brain HVA distribution [105] approximately follows that of its precursor DA.

While relatively little work has been done on amines and their metabolites in autopsy material still less is known about the activities of the enzymes involved. This field might be usefully explored further especially as activities in the rat brain remain unchanged [26] after storage of the dead animals for 16 h at 4° and 20°. Tyrosine hydroxylase, aromatic amino acid decarboxylase, dopamine β-oxidase, MAO and COMT were studied and activities of these enzymes in various regions of some human brains were also obtained [26]. Recently the histofluorimetric method for localization of NA has been successfully applied to cryostat sections of human non-brain material obtained during surgery [106]. Results suggest that the method might be applied to human brain material if the time between death and autopsy was short.

5.4 PARKINSON'S DISEASE

5.4.1 Introduction

Parkinson's disease is the brain disease in which clearest evidence has been obtained that a disturbance of brain amine metabolism plays a major role in the development of symptoms. It is also a striking example of a common brain disease of which a knowledge of the biochemical disturbance has led to the prediction of a successful rational therapy. Some useful general accounts of developments in this area have recently appeared [107, 108, 109].

5.4.2 The disturbance of amine metabolism

The basal ganglia (the caudate nucleus, putamen and globus pallidus) and the related substantia nigra have long been known to have a role in the control of movement (see ref. 110 for review). Therefore, as soon as these regions (especially the two striatal regions, the caudate nucleus and putamen) were found to contain most of the DA of the brain it became apparent that this substance might be a neurohormone with a special function related to movement [111]. The distribution of DA in human brain [6, 9, 112] is strikingly different to that of NA. Almost concurrently with these findings it was reported [18] that both DA and NA concentrations were very low in the basal ganglia of a small group of subjects with Parkinson's disease or postencephalitic parkinsonism. The DA content of the substantia nigra was also very low [113] and furthermore 5HT concentration was low in various parts of the brain [114]. DA levels were particularly low in postencephalitic parkinsonism which may be related to the particularly severe brain lesions found in this condition. In more recent work, in which an improved method was used, the earlier findings in the striatal regions were confirmed but normal DA was found in the globus pallidus [115].

Findings on brain amine concentrations in Parkinson's disease are shown in Table 5.1 which summarizes the data of the Vienna group [115, 116].

If the low DA values were due to a particularly rapid breakdown of DA which was formed at normal rate then concentrations of HVA the main DA metabolite would be high. However, abnormally low HVA concentrations have been found in the caudate nucleus and putamen of patients with Parkinson's disease [105, 115] and therefore defective DA formation is indicated. The high HVA/DA ratio reported suggests that DA in surviving DA-ergic neurones is turned over abnormally rapidly.

The above work was published in 1960-1965 and subsequently there has been a lack of further reports on amine biochemistry in post-mortem brain material from parkinsonian subjects. However, the findings have been strengthened by studies on amine metabolites in the CSF. Thus low lumbar CSF

TABLE 5.1

Brain Amines in Normal Human Subjects and in Patients with Parkinson's Disease[a]

Brain Region	Dopamine (μg/g)		Noradrenaline (μg/g)		5-Hydroxytryptamine (μg/g)	
	Normal[b]	Parkinson[b]	Normal[b]	Parkinson[b]	Normal[b]	Parkinson[b]
Caudate nucleus	3.50(12)	0.32(12)	0.07(8)	0.03(12)	0.33(6)	0.12(5)
Putamen	3.57(15)	0.23(12)	0.11(10)	0.03(12)	0.32(6)	0.14(5)
Globus pallidus	0.15(4)	0.15(6)	0.09(6)	0.11(7)	0.23(6)	0.13(5)
Thalamus	0.01(2)	0.01(2)	0.09(4)	0.05(2)	0.26(4)	0.13(4)
Hypothalamus	0.02(7)	0.00(5)	1.29(7)	0.67(9)	0.29(6)	0.12(5)
Substantia nigra	0.46(13)	0.07(10)	0.04(11)	0.02(10)	0.55(6)	0.26(5)

[a] Data from refs. 115, 116.
[b] Numbers in parentheses indicate the number of brains for which the value given represents a mean.

HVA has been reported many times [61, 65, 69, 72, 75, 82, 83, 94]. HVA concentration was also found to be lower than that of a control group after probenecid was given to impede its transport from CSF to blood [72]. While the mean lumbar HVA concentration of parkinsonian groups is consistently found to be significantly less than that of controls a wide scatter of values and some overlap is often reported. Furthermore, low CSF HVA may also occur in other disorders involving proven or possible basal ganglia disturbance (vide infra) and in disturbances of HVA transport (see 5.3.2). Therefore low HVA concentration in lumbar CSF is hardly a pathognomic test for Parkinson's disease. Also, no correlation has been found between lumbar HVA and the severity of parkinsonian symptoms [65]. However, analysis of data is limited somewhat by the low accuracy of lumbar HVA determination at lower concentrations. In work using ventricular CSF, in which HVA concentrations are much higher the most akinetic patients were found to have a mean level significantly lower than that of the others [88].

Lumbar CSF 5HIAA concentrations are lower than those of controls but much less marked differences have been found by some workers [82, 84, 117] than by others [61, 69, 72]. This discrepancy may partly stem from the different kinds of control groups used, as while the Scandinavian workers [61, 69, 72] used healthy volunteers others used patients with miscellaneous neurological conditions. Also heterogeneity of the Parkinson group may be involved (see Table 5.2). Furthermore, while lumbar CSF HVA is almost all derived from the striatum most of the 5HIAA comes from other regions. Therefore a deficiency in striatal or basal ganglia 5HT metabolism would not necessarily be clearly reflected in the lumbar CSF. The 5HIAA content of lateral ventricular CSF, which more closely reflects striatal 5HT metabolism, is however strikingly low in patients with parkinsonism [118].

While work on post-mortem brain material and CSF indicates that not only low DA but also low NA and 5HT are present in the brain in Parkinson's disease and that these latter abnormalities are not restricted to the basal ganglia most attention has been given to the low striatal DA. This is because of the special significance of the striatum in movement

TABLE 5.2

CSF Amine Metabolites Before and After L-Dopa Treatment of Patients with Parkinsonism

Subjects	Amine metabolites in CSF before L-dopa treatment		Regression equation relating increase of CSF HVA (y) to L-dopa/day (x)	Improvement on L-dopa
	HVA µg/ml	*5HIAA µg/ml*		
Patients with parkinsonism and large increase of CSF HVA/g L-dopa	0.032 ± 0.027(5)	0.029 ± 0.015(5)	$y = 0.187x + 0.004$ (5) Correlation = 1.000 (significant at better than 1% level)	Negligible
	} $P < 0.05$	} N.S.		
Other patients with parkinsonism	0.009 ± 0.007(11)	0.018 ± 0.007 (13)	$y = 0.0342x + 0.030$(10) Correlation = 0.668 (significant at better than 5% level)	Definite in subjects whose CSF HVA increased to > 0.100 µg/ml
	} $P < 0.001$	} $P < 0.02$		
Neurological patients without parkinsonism	0.045 ± 0.016 (9)	0.027 ± 0.010 (9)		

Numbers of subjects are indicated in brackets. Data from ref. 117. Values are given ± one S.D. The above data is discussed on pages 174-175.

disorders, the high DA concentration there and the proportionally greater decrease of DA than of the other substances. That low DA is more specifically related to symptoms than is 5HT is perhaps suggested by work on the brain of a senile patient with unilateral parkinsonian tremor as while the DA concentration of the caudate nucleus and putamen on the side contralateral to the tremor was much lower than on the other side the 5HT concentration was similar on both sides [119]. Also, patients with Parkinson's disease treated with MAOI drugs had markedly higher striatal NA and 5HT, but not DA, than those who had not received the drug [120]. While these important observations should not encourage neglect of the significance of the other amines they do indicate the importance of low striatal DA synthesis in Parkinson's disease.

Work on enzymes required for DA metabolism has shown normal MAO activity of the caudate nucleus and other parts of the brain [121]. This topic might however be worth further study as there is evidence suggesting an MAO with a particular affinity for DA in the basal ganglia [122]. There is no evidence of a defect in dopa decarboxylase [123], although this topic requires re-investigation using the recently improved method for determining human brain decarboxylase [24]. Tyrosine hydroxylase, the probable rate determinant enzyme for catecholamine synthesis [22] does not seem to have been determined in Parkinson's disease.

Work in which experimental brain lesions were made in animals has led to important clues on the origin of the low striatal DA and its relationship to the classical neuropathology of Parkinson's disease. As loss of pigmented cells in the substantia nigra has long been recognized as the most definite brain lesion in the disease [124, 125] it is most suggestive that stereotactic lesions in the rat substantia nigra deplete DA in the caudate nucleus [126]. Depletion only occurred when the substantia nigra lesions were made in the melanin-containing part of the substantia nigra, the pars compacta [127]. Lesions of nerve fibres between the substantia nigra and the striatum resulted in depletion specifically where the particular fibres damaged entered the striatum. If part of the striatum was removed then the catecholamine content of the substantia nigra increased and also that of the nerve fibres between it and the internal capsule [128]. These results showed that nigro-striatal DA tracts exist and explain how lesions in the substantia nigra can lead to low striatal DA. As electrical stimulation of the cell bodies in the substantia nigra depletes DA from the striatal nerve endings [10, 129] the fibres may reasonably be termed DA-ergic.

A relationship between substantia nigra lesions, striatal DA and movement disturbance was demonstrated by making unilateral lesions in the ventromedial tegmentum of the upper brain stem. This caused loss of cells in the substantia nigra, decrease of striatal DA and NA but not 5HT and contralateral hypokinesis [130, 131]. If lesions were made in dorsomedial fibres of the cerebral peduncle then striatal 5HT decreased [132]. Lesions of the above types cause not only depletion of the amines but also of the enzymes necessary for their synthesis, tyrosine hydroxylase, tryptophan hydroxylase and aromatic amino acid decarboxylase [133, 134].

Striatal DA can also be depleted by stereotactic injection of 6-hydroxy DA (which causes degeneration of catecholaminergic terminals) into the pars compacta of the substantia nigra [135]. The DA cell bodies immediately start to degenerate and the whole nigrostriatal DA system degenerates in 48 h. Unilateral injection causes unilateral degeneration and asymmetric posture, the body being turned towards the side with the lesion [136]. Various drugs which affect DA metabolism or DA receptors cause the animal to rotate. The possibility that a deviation of DA metabolism to 6-hydroxy DA occurs in Parkinson's disease is intriguing especially as it is conceivable that 6-hydroxy DA is formed during melanin synthesis in the substantia nigra.

The above methods for producing degeneration of the substantia nigra provide interesting models for Parkinson's disease and for other movement disorders. A number of questions concerning the role of melanin, the pigmented material of the substantia nigra, remain unanswered. Its synthesis, nature and relationship to nigrostriatal function and degeneration all require more study. The term "melanin" does not necessarily indicate a specific chemical substance and there are reports of differences between brain melanin and the more intensively studied skin melanin [137, 138, 139]. However, evidence that the substantia nigra can form melanin from tyrosine [140] points to a pathway of synthesis which is at least similar to that of skin melanin and which may be related to catecholamine metabolism. Indeed it has been suggested that brain melanin is derived from catecholamines themselves [141] perhaps from DA which is present at considerable concentration in the melanin containing pars compacta of the substantia nigra [113]. Also rat brain has been claimed to contain an enzyme able to convert DA but not dopa or NA to a melanin like pigment [142, 143]. There is a general parallelism between the distribution of the melanin containing cells of the substantia nigra, associated nuclei and other parts of the brain stem and the distribution of catecholamine containing cell bodies [144]. Furthermore, synthetic melanin made from catecholamines but not from dopa resembles nigral pigment spectroscopically [145] and also NA binds particularly strongly in the pericellular area of brain melanin cells suggesting the presence there of many impinging catecholamine containing synaptic endings [146]. Thus, defective melanin formation in Parkinson's disease may itself conceivably reflect disturbed amine metabolism. Study of the brain melanin forming enzyme system and its substrate specificity using recent methods of assay [147] would be worth while.

Whether demelanization of the substantia nigra in Parkinson's disease is simply a consequence of overall degeneration of the nigrostriatal DA-ergic tracts or whether it has a causative role in the degeneration is unknown. However, it has been suggested that the semiconductor properties of melanin granules [148] might be required for normal basal ganglia function [149] and that the properties of melanin as a sink for free radicals [150] could also be involved [143].

There have been many studies of urinary amine metabolites in Parkinson's disease. Early work (reviewed in ref. 151) showed low DA concentration and is contradicted by one recent study [152] but confirmed by another [153] in which excretion of free but not of conjugated DA by a group of subjects with parkinsonism of various origins was significantly lower than that of a control group on the same diet. Excretion of the DA metabolite 3,4-dihydroxyphenylacetic acid was also lower [153]. The authors suggest that low urinary DA may result from chronic drug treatment of the parkinsonian patients whose current drugs were not withdrawn during the study and refer to the finding [154] of low free urinary DA in schizophrenics—another group subjected to chronic drug treatment. The low excretion might also be related to reduced physical activity especially as DA is low in urine formed during sleep [155]. A third possibility is that it results from reduced activity of the enzyme tyrosine hydroxylase required for DA synthesis. Evidence consistent with this hypothesis has been obtained using phenylalanine and tyrosine oral load tests, although other interpretations of these findings are as likely [156]. Tyrosine utilization via transamination to p-hydroxyphenylpyruvic acid may be enhanced in parkinsonism as elevated excretion of the latter substance is found [157], perhaps due to increased tyrosine transaminase activity, which is a likely non-specific result of severe illness.

The finding of low 5HIAA excretion in Parkinson's disease [158] has not been confirmed [159, 160]. The protean "pink spot" has been reported [161], refuted [162], suggested to be due to 3,4-dimethoxyphenylethylamine [161] (dimethyl DA), or tyramine [163] and has recently been correlated with tea drinking [164]. Urinary tyramine was also found to be significantly increased in severely but not in mildly affected subjects with Parkinson's disease [165]. Finally, elevated tryptamine excretion has been claimed [165, 166] but even if confirmed is unlikely, for quantitative reasons, to result from or cause defective hydroxylation of tryptophan to 5HT as originally suggested [166].

Thus, while brain amine disturbance in Parkinson's disease is well authenticated, evidence for urinary abnormalities is not striking and is unlikely to reflect metabolic disturbances of primary importance.

5.4.3 Drug treatment of Parkinson's disease in relation to the disturbance of brain amine metabolism

As soon as the striatal DA deficiency in Parkinson's disease was recognized, DA replacement became a rational therapeutic goal. As DA does not pass readily into the brain its precursor dopa was used. Slow intravenous injection to patients with Parkinson's disease or postencephalitic parkinsonism was followed by improved movement and speech but little change of tremor or rigidity [167]. The effect was transient but MAOI treatment enhanced and prolonged it. In a confirmatory study by other workers [168] a rapid but very transient alleviation of tremor and rigidity was shown electromyographically to precede the above effects. Although a number of other reports of benefit from dopa appeared [169, 170, 171] the results of two controlled trials were largely negative [172, 173]. However, when DL-dopa was given at larger dosage than previously (3-16 g/day orally for up to 350 days) then 8 out of 16 patients showed marked improvement [19]. As dosage was gradually increased, decreased rigidity appeared and at higher levels tremor in some patients decreased or disappeared. Transient granulocytopenia which occurred in four patients has not been noted in subsequent work in which not DL-dopa but L-dopa was given. Another aromatic amino acid DL-phenyl-alanine increased both tremor and rigidity. This amino acid would be extremely inefficient as a DA precursor. Its structural similarity to tyrosine and dopa suggest its harmful effects may be due to competitive interference with residual endogenous DA synthesis.

The beneficial effects on Parkinson's disease of dopa in large oral dosage have been confirmed in a number of trials [174-177] in which the L-isomer caused marked or dramatic improvements in about half the patients. Some improvement, especially of functional disabilities was found in most subjects [176]. These, and other manifestations of hypokinesia and rigidity improved most. Tremor improved to a lesser extent and more obviously [174] when the drug was given for 12 months. "Side-effects" such as running down of a self-winding wrist-watch previously kept wound by wrist tremor [178] and fractures caused by playing football are anecdotal though striking indications of improvement. Some patients with post-encephalitic parkinsonism also bene-fited [179] though they could not tolerate as large doses of L-dopa as those with Parkinson's disease and only a minority showed useful benefit in prolonged trials as harmful side-effects were frequent [180, 181]. These disadvantages may be related to post-encephalitic patients having more extensive and long-standing brain damage than those with Parkinson's disease.

L-dopa therapy involves giving a daily dose of the drug of the order of a thousand times the amount of striatal DA normally synthesized per day. It is therefore hardly surprising that side-effects of the treatment are fairly frequent [19, 174-177, 179-185]. Hyperkinetic and behavioural side-effects are of interest in relation to Huntington's chorea and depression and are commented on in sections 5.5.1 and 5.6.3 respectively.

To what extent does L-dopa act by replacing deficient striatal DA? Direct evidence of restoration of normal DA-ergic function is not available, but in the near future post-mortem data on striatal DA metabolism in patients who have been on L-dopa should accumulate and at least contribute to the solution of the above question. Increase of CSF HVA during L-dopa treatment [75, 83, 117] points to increased synthesis of DA in the brain and there are indications of relationships between this increase and improvement (Table 5.2). For example subjects whose lumbar HVA only increased slightly (i.e. to levels comparable with those of an untreated non-parkinsonian control group) showed no more than slight improvement but a group attaining higher HVA improved more markedly [83, 117]. The low HVA levels of the first group are consistent with the low average L-dopa dose per day of 1.75 g though patients on similar dosage but attaining higher HVA showed clear benefit. Variable gastrointestinal absorption of L-dopa may be an important factor here [186]. Results however, suggest that the CSF HVA derived from exogenous L-dopa does not represent an equally effective amount of DA as does a similar concentration of HVA in untreated normals. This could indicate more rapid turnover of DA derived from exogenous L-dopa or the persistence of disability due to other biochemical abnormalities such as defective brain 5HT synthesis. Another possibility is that while DA is normally present in a restricted distribution in the brain, decarboxylase and MAO required to convert dopa successively to DA and HVA are present in many non-striatal areas including the cerebral vasculature [187]. Therefore some of the CSF HVA derived from exogenous dopa might have been synthesized via therapeutically ineffective DA.

It is superficially paradoxical that not only the subjects with particularly small increase of CSF HVA after L-dopa showed little benefit but also a group of five subjects with a particularly large increase of HVA per g L-dopa. These were significantly older than other subjects and were arteriosclerotic. As they had a significantly higher mean CSF HVA before L-dopa than the other patients results suggest that most of the DA synthesis from exogenous dopa in this particular group was at normal sites of brain DA synthesis. Also the failure of L-dopa to benefit patients in whom striatal DA synthesis was apparently unimpaired before treatment suggests that its action in subjects with low pre-dopa HVA involves increased striatal DA synthesis and that it is not merely a drug which alleviates parkinsonian symptoms and which is coincidentally a precursor of striatal DA. Another interesting point is that when the latter group of patients are excluded (Table 5.2) then both CSF HVA and 5HIAA concentrations before L-dopa treatment of the residium are more significantly below those of a control group than when they are included.

Now if Parkinson's disease is due to nigrostriatal DA containing neurones dying off and if dopa restores striatal DA then the question arises—is this DA contained in surviving neurones? That the increased DA would enable them to perform functions of their dead neighbours is uncertain but seems likely in view of the extensively branched and therefore presumably polysynaptic nature of striatal dopaminergic terminals [188] and the conceivable possibility of compensatory rearrangement of synaptic contacts. Also such a mechanism would be assisted if nigrostriatal degeneration induces supersensitivity of the corresponding deprived receptors. This is possible as unilateral nigrostriatal degeneration produced by 6-hydroxy DA causes apparent hypersensitivity of the denervated side to L-dopa [189, 190].

The proliferation of hypotheses and suggestions concerning the mechanism of therapeutic action of L-dopa illustrates the intense recent interest in this topic, e.g.

(1) Increase of DA in surviving DA-ergic terminals.

(2) Formation of DA in striatal 5HT-ergic neurones [191]. This mechanism could occur in the complete absence of surviving DA-ergic terminals. Evidence for it has been obtained *in vitro* [191]. The assumption is made that DA

released from 5HT-ergic nerve endings is available to synaptic DA receptors.

(3) Therapeutic dosage of L-dopa is enormously greater than amounts metabolized normally and some of it is metabolized on normally undetectable or negligible pathways [192, 193] including one to 3-methyldopa [193]. This substance is only slowly metabolized or excreted and is distributed almost evenly through the body [194]. Animal experiments suggest that human brain levels slowly increase during L-dopa treatment and slowly decline after withdrawal. If 3-methyldopa can be converted to DA in the body these observations might be relevant to the understanding of the frequently considerable time lag between initiation of dopa treatment and therapeutic effect.

(4) Animal experiments [105] suggest that methylation of administered L-dopa to 3-methyldopa may lead to deficiency of the methyldonor methionine. As this is also required [40, 41] for the extraneuronal COMT pathway of DA metabolism it has been pointed out [195] that the synaptic effect of DA could be enhanced by the methionine deficiency.

(5) Possible or proven minor pathways of L-dopa metabolism, e.g. formation of tetrahydropapaveroline or apomorphine-like [196, 197] or of m-hydroxylated derivatives [198] have been suggested to be therapeutically significant.

Only a very small fraction of the DA formed from administered L-dopa is synthesized in the brain. This is largely because decarboxylase in the walls of the gut and of the cerebral capillaries destroys much dopa converting it to DA which cannot enter the brain [199, 200]. Therefore if an inhibitor of the decarboxylase which inhibits the extracerebral but not the cerebral enzyme is also given then the dose of L-dopa required for therapeutic effect is decreased manifold [201]. The increase of brain DA in the rat after L-dopa administration is much enhanced by the inhibitor [202]. Degree of L-dopa penetration to different brain regions depends inversely on DA formation from it within the brain capillaries of the regions, and penetration is greatest in the striatum. This dependence is abolished by the inhibitor [203] but catecholamine still increases in the basal ganglia but not in areas containing NA-ergic neurones. However, in these circumstances there is *in vivo* evidence that DA replaces 5HT in 5HT-ergic neurones [204].

A number of other approaches to enhancing the effectiveness of L-dopa is possible. One suggestion is to replace it by a derivative which is more easily able to penetrate to the brain [205, 206]. Inhibition of dopamine-β-oxidase, the enzyme converting DA to NA does not increase L-dopa effectiveness [207] which is understandable as brain NA formation from administered L-dopa is probably quantitatively relatively unimportant [208].

Another possible therapeutic manoeuvre is to assist surviving striatal DA synthesis or effectiveness without L-dopa administration. For example, animal work [209, 210] suggests that anticholinergic drugs which have long been used in the treatment of Parkinson's disease may alleviate symptoms by inhibiting neuronal reuptake of released DA thus potentiating its synaptic action. Another drug with a related effect is L-amphetamine which (unlike D-amphetamine which inhibits catecholamine uptake in the brain as a whole) inhibits uptake strongly in the striatum but only weakly elsewhere in the brain [211]. This may explain the therapeutic effect of DL-amphetamine on parkinsonism and suggests that side-effects would be decreased by the use of the L-isomer.

Whether amantadine [212] benefits patients with Parkinson's disease by influencing DA metabolism or action is obscure. The lack of response to the drug by patients already on optimal dosage of L-dopa [213] is consistent with the two drugs having similar mechanisms of action. It is of interest that amantadine potentiates the L-dopa provoked increase of motor activity in mice [214]. Also, though effects on rat brain DA metabolism are slight [215] and amantadine treatment of patients with Parkinson's disease does not alter lumbar CSF HVA concentration [216] those with lowest pre-treatment HVA responded best.

Apomorphine, which stimulates DA receptors [217] has a transient L-dopa-like action on parkinsonian symptoms when injected [218]. Therefore, synthetic neurotransmitters related to apomorphine have been proposed as a possibly more specific way of stimulating DA receptors than by giving L-dopa [219].

Such a stimulation would be of a threshold lowering kind unless the drug was also taken up by surviving DA-ergic neurones and released in their firing.

5.5 OTHER DYSKINESIAS

5.5.1 Drug provoked dyskinesias

Movement disorders caused by drugs used therapeutically were virtually unknown before the advent of modern psychotropic drugs (in particular, reserpine, phenothiazines and butyrophenones). Relationships between the mechanisms of the behavioural and motor effects of these drugs are strongly indicated. Drug provoked disorders provide experimental animal models for human dyskinetic states and also have clinical importance as unpleasant side-effects of drugs used in medical practice.

Reserpine treatment of human subjects may lead to various reversible parkinsonian symptoms and rats given the drug also exhibit akinesia, tremor and rigidity [220, 221]. Symptoms in animals appear to be related to the brain amine depleting effect of reserpine as they were reversed by intravenous L-dopa and L-5HTP but not by DA and 5HT which do not penetrate to the brain [222]. That they are due specifically to a striatal DA decrease is consistent with the absence of reversal by MAOI + dihydroxyphenylserine [223] (a precursor of NA but not of DA) but appear to be contradicted by reversal with 5HTP. Furthermore, reserpine caused akinesia even when given to rabbits from which the caudate nuclei had been removed [224].

Phenothiazines and butyrophenones may cause various movement disturbances in man. Dystonia in children and young adults and parkinsonism or restlessness in older subjects may occur during treatment and are reversible. The facial dyskinesia which may occur in elderly subjects, especially those with evidence of brain damage, is often irreversible (see ref. 225 for review). Unlike reserpine, these substances have little effect on brain amine levels in animals. They behave as if they block amine receptors so that there is a compensatory activation of monoaminergic neurones with increased but functionally ineffective release of amines into the synaptic cleft. Thus, increased synthesis occurs of those catecholamine metabolites requiring the extraneuronal OMT for their synthesis [226], e.g. concentrations of the DA metabolites 3,4-dihydroxyphenyl-acetic acid and HVA increase in the corpus striatum [227] without alteration of DA. The lack of change of DA concentration together with increased concentrations of its metabolites implies increased DA synthesis and this together with a smaller increase of NA synthesis [228, 229] has been demonstrated in the rat brain after treatment with the phenothiazine drug chlorpromazine.

Animal experiments indicate some correlation between potency of these drugs in producing movement disturbances and the increase of brain HVA caused by them [230, 231] although correlation is only partial [231]. The full spectrum of movement disturbance seen in humans is not observed in animals which mainly exhibit tremor [231]. Species differences in effects of the drugs may be relevant here. For example, while metabolism of brain DA but not of 5HT is altered in the rabbit [227] both are affected in the dog [57] and man [60].

There is no evidence of a relationship between CSF amine metabolite changes and development of symptoms in human drug provoked movement disturbances [60, 232] though an amine disturbance is suggested by the finding of cellular degeneration in the substantia nigra of subjects with tardive drug induced dyskinesias [233]. The alleviatory action upon facial dyskinesia of α-methyl dopa [234] which particularly decreases catecholamine stores and the enhancement of symptoms by L-dopa [235] are consistent with a mechanism involving a brain amine imbalance.

Involuntary movements caused by L-dopa treatment of parkinsonism are well known [83, 175, 179] and may be due to resultant local excessive DA-ergic activity/5HT-ergic activity. A number of animal studies are relevant. Thus stereotyped hyperactive behaviour often of a bizarre kind has been produced in rats by drugs which increase levels of turnover of brain DA or act on DA-ergic receptors [236, 237].

5.5.2 Manganese dyskinesia

Manganese miners who inhale large amounts of ore dust may develop psychiatric followed by neurological disturbances. The majority of affected subjects show typical parkinsonian symptoms, while about 10% suffer from muscular dystonia [238]. Symptoms are not simply related to manganese deposition as the brain, blood and other organs do not contain high manganese concentrations [239]. Experimental manganese poisoning has been produced in monkeys [240], the movement disturbance being more severe in chimpanzees than in Rhesus monkeys [241]. This is of interest as brain melanin is much less apparent in Rhesus monkeys than in chimpanzees [242] and it has been suggested that manganese poisoning may involve brain melanin disturbance [149] and that susceptibility to experimental dyskinesia in different species correlates with melanin content of the substantia nigra [243]. A more definite indication of disturbed brain amine metabolism is that squirrel monkeys which developed rigidity, dystonia and tremor after treatment with manganese dioxide had markedly lower caudate nucleus DA and 5HT concentrations after treatment than control or unaffected animals [244]. The brain amine disturbance appears specific to the basal ganglia as 5HT and NA in the rest of the brain were normal. It is also significant that repeated i.m. manganese dioxide injection into Rhesus monkeys caused neuronal degeneration in the globus pallidus [241], as electrocoagulation of this region in the rabbit leads to a large decrease of caudate nucleus DA concentration [245].

There are no published findings on brain amine metabolism in human manganese poisoning but the above considerations provide a sufficient rationale for the therapeutic use of brain amine precursors. Five subjects showed marked improvement of rigidity and hypokinesis and improved postural reflexes when given L-dopa [246]. The symptoms of a sixth patient were exacerbated by L-dopa and by apomorphine except that the latter caused tremor to disappear [218]. This patient showed general improvement on 5HTP. Two dystonic subjects were also improved by L-dopa.

5.5.3 Huntington's chorea

To some extent Huntington's chorea represents an opposite pole to Parkinson's disease with hyperkinesis and involuntary movements as major symptoms instead of hypokinesis. As involuntary movements are a not infrequent result of L-dopa treatment of Parkinson's disease [83, 175, 179] and as these may appear strikingly Huntingtonian [247] it might be thought that over-production of DA was involved in the disease. The precipitation by L-dopa of classically Huntingtonian symptoms in subjects with the juvenile akineto-rigid form of the disease [248, 249] is also consistent with the hypothesis. However it is not supported by biochemical studies. Urinary DA metabolite concentrations are not high [250, 251, 252] and loading with L-dopa does not cause an abnormal elevation of these substances [250]. The abnormally strong red colour on iodine oxidation of urine [253] and interpreted as indicating high urine DA was shown not to be due to a catecholamine and was not confirmed when a quantitative version of the test was used [254]. More significantly DA concentrations in the basal ganglia are normal [18]. The total catecholamine content of the basal ganglia presumably tends to be low as shrinkage of this area is found at autopsy [255].

The suggestion has been made that as in Huntington's chorea, striatal cell bodies are severely degenerated, the amount of DA at striatal nerve endings available per surviving non-DA-containing cell body might be abnormally high [256]. However, the rather low lumbar CSF HVA found [65, 68] and the significant negative correlation between this and severity [257] are not obviously consistent with the above. Lumbar CSF 5HIAA concentration on the contrary was not low and unlike parkinsonian and control groups was unusual, showing negative correlation with HVA concentration. It is of interest that CSF HVA and 5HIAA concentrations of a single subject with severe akineto-rigid Huntington's chorea were markedly below those found for the rest of the group and were comparable to those of a parkinsonian group [257].

The therapeutic effects of various drugs are consistent with decreased synaptic DA concentrations or effectiveness being beneficial. Thus, phenothiazines have been used [258] which seem to block DA receptors, while tetrabenazine, an amine depletor, gives marked benefit in Huntington's chorea and other hyperkinetic states such as oral dyskinesia [259, 260, 261]. Particularly striking benefit [262] is reported with tetrabenazine together with Pimozide, the latter drug being a butyrophenone said to be an especially powerful blocker of DA receptors. Whether tetrabenazine acts entirely by DA depletion is not clear. That both brain DA and 5HT are depleted in man is indicated by both HVA and 5HIAA levels being raised in the CSF during the first few days of treatment [263] and beneficial action of 5HT depletion would be consistent with the exacerbation of symptoms by 5HTP [264]. During more prolonged tetrabenazine treatment HVA and 5HIAA levels eventually fall to or even below their initial values, although benefit persists. The CSF changes might suggest a continuing amine synthesis and increased amine store depletion together with a gradually increasing reduction of the aldehydes formed by MAO action to alcohols instead of their oxidation to HVA and 5HIAA. Another amine depleter, reserpine is known to divert amine metabolism to the alcohol pathway [265, 266]. The depression which is a common side-effect of tetrabenazine treatment [263, 267] may well be due to brain 5HT depletion (see 5.6.2) and may restrict the utility of the amine depleters in the treatment of Huntington's chorea.

A relationship between decreased brain DA and therapeutic action is also suggested by the beneficial action on Huntington's chorea of α-methyl-p-tyrosine [268] which inhibits both DA and NA synthesis [269] and the lack of effect of α-methyl dopa [270] which mainly depletes NA stores.

5.5.4 Miscellaneous dyskinesias

The relationship of brain amines to Parkinson's disease is now encouraging their study in movement disorders in general and various CSF studies are being made and the effects of drugs influencing amines are being investigated. Low CSF HVA and 5HIAA has been reported for example, in the parkinsonian dementia associated with amyotrophic lateral sclerosis which occurs in Guam [84]. Guamese subjects with amyotrophic lateral sclerosis but without parkinsonism had values intermediate between those of controls and of the group with the full symptom complex. These findings suggest that all the symptoms have a common mechanism of origin. However, patients with amyotrophic lateral sclerosis in the United States (where there is no general association between this condition

and parkinsonism) also showed HVA concentrations intermediate between those of subjects with Parkinson's disease and
of controls

Little is known about amine metabolism in Wilson's disease.
Brain amine or CSF amine metabolite concentrations have not
been reported and urine studies (previously reviewed, ref. 151)
indicate no consistent abnormalities. The high but variable DA
excretion may be a consequence of defective metabolism due to
liver damage [271]. While 5HT is an *in vitro* substrate for
caeruloplasmin [272, 273]. which is deficient in Wilson's disease
it seems unlikely that 5HT metabolism by caeruloplasmin is
quantitatively significant *in vivo* as 5HIAA excretion is
normal [271, 274]. There have been two reports of the use of
L-dopa in the treatment of Wilson's disease, respectively
describing benefit of a subject previously unresponsive to
penicillamine [275] and the lack of benefit when L-dopa was
given as a supplement to penicillamine [276].

Very low DA, NA and 5HT are reported in the basal ganglia
of a seven month-old child with familial subacute necrotizing
encephalopathy who had shown akinesia and muscular
hypotonia [277]. Very low glutamic acid decarboxylase
activity was also found suggesting a deficiency of pyridoxal
phosphate dependent decarboxylases including those involved
in amine formation. As pyridoxal metabolism appeared not
deficient but strikingly elevated a defect of its utilization is
indicated. Urinary DA concentration was very high and
tryptamine (normally not detectable in brain) was apparently
present in the basal ganglia. These amines are also formed by
decarboxylation and thus the general picture is rather complex.
Deficiency of both decarboxylase and MAO was suggested. A
somewhat more economical mechanism might involve a
substance preventing the binding of pyridoxal phosphate to
certain carboxylases but not others, thus resulting in decreased
formation of normally found brain amines. As low brain amine
synthesis causes a feed back increase of pyridoxal phosphate
synthesis [278] this could lead to saturation of previously
unsaturated decarboxylases with cofactor and perhaps result in
detectable brain tryptamine formation.

A single patient with progressive supranuclear palsy and low
CSF HVA has been reported who benefited from L-dopa

treatment [86], but most subjects with this condition do not improve on L-dopa. More CSF determinations will presumably clarify this problem. Recently lumbar CSF HVA and 5HIAA values have been reported for six patients suffering from torsion dystonia [91]. Mean concentrations were not significantly different from those of a control group though that of HVA was lower. One out of five of the subjects improved markedly when given L-dopa, while another showed increased disability on α-methyl-p-tyrosine which inhibits catecholamine formation. A third patient was unaffected by p-chlorophenylalanine, an inhibitor of 5HT synthesis. In another' study rather better results were obtained with L-dopa [279]. It may be significant that 5HTP was said to improve the hypotonia of Down's syndrome 5HTP [280, 281] but the pre-existing oral dyskinesia of one patient worsened [280]. Low blood 5HT has been found in patients suffering from this syndrome [282, 283] but CSF 5HIAA is normal both in Down's syndrome and in other myotonias [79].

It is likely that determinations of CSF amine metabolites during life, supplemented by detailed investigation of amines and relevant enzymes in brain autopsy material will lead to greatly increased understanding of movement disorders and their therapy. As well as the dyskinesias discussed above other conditions requiring study include Hallervorden-Spatz disease, Kuru disease, the so-called red nucleus tremor in some subjects with multiple sclerosis, the movement disorder in some phenylketonurics, the parkinsonism associated with hypothyroidism [284], the familial tremor occurring in Sweden and a number of obscure juvenile dyskinesias. The suggested association between alkaptonuria and parkinsonism [285], the dyskinesias often associated with traumatic and other brain lesions, Gilles de la Tourette syndrome, the "jumping Frenchmen of Maine" syndrome [286] and various other conditions would probably also repay attention.

5.6 DEPRESSION

5.6.1 Introduction

The strongest indication that amine disturbance or inadequacy may be involved in depressive illness is provided by the effects on mood of drugs which influence brain amine levels. Thus, reserpine [287] and tetrabenazine [263, 267, 288] deplete brain amines and not infrequently cause depression. Conversely, MAOI drugs alleviate depression and raise human brain DA, NA and 5HT concentrations [289, 290] on a time course approximately paralleling that of improvement [99] with therapeutically equipotent amounts of different MAOI drugs having quantitatively comparable effects on brain amines [290]. Similarly, the tricyclic anti-depressants, though they do not inhibit the destruction of catecholamines and 5HT, block their neuronal reuptake, thus tending to make amine molecules available at receptor sites for a longer time (reviewed in ref. 291). Thus, drugs which increase effective concentrations of brain amines elevate depressed mood. Conversely, lithium, which alleviates mania may have an opposite effect on the amines, inhibiting the release upon stimulation of neurones of both NA and 5HT [292], although the situation may be complex as only 5HT appears to be affected by chronic lithium treatment [293] and stimulation of the midbrain raphe results in greater brain 5HT turnover in lithium treated than in control rats [294].

As all the above drugs can influence both catecholamine and 5HT metabolism it is not obvious whether their effects on mood are due to effects on a specific amine, on more than one amine, on relative concentrations of amines or on different amines in different subjects. Also, even if the therapeutic properties of MAOI and tricyclics are due to effects on amine concentrations or disposition it does not necessarily follow that depressions alleviated by them are primarily due to brain amine deficiencies.

The claim that abnormally high and low urinary cyclic AMP excretion occurs in mania and depression respectively [295, 296] is of interest as AMP may mediate responses of target tissues to amine action at receptors. However, the finding may well reflect different motor activities of depressed and manic subjects [297]. The concentration of cyclic AMP in lumbar CSF is similar in mania, depression and various neurological disorders [298].

Much animal work has been done on the biochemical changes responsible for the action of reserpine on behaviour. This is a difficult area and its relevance to human depressive illness is unclear, although the precipitation of depression by reserpine is suggestive. One major difficulty is that the effect of reserpine is probably related not to total brain amine concentrations, but to a small mobile pool as recovery from sedation occurs when only a small fraction of the depleted amine stores are replaced [299]. Furthermore, administration to human subjects of more or less specific inhibitors of catecholamine or 5HT synthesis has not resulted in clear evidence for involvement of either in depression.

Direct evidence suggesting that disturbed indolealkylamine or catecholamine metabolism have significant roles in depressive illness is summarized below. A number of important discussions of the biochemistry of depression and of other psychotic states place amine studies within a general context [300-303].

5.6.2 The indolealkylamine hypothesis

Human CSF and brain studies and the alleviatory effect of tryptophan point to (without proving) a role for 5HT in the chemical pathology of depressive illness.

A suggestion that some depressives may have an overall defect of 5HT synthesis is provided by two studies [304, 305] in which it was found that depressed patients responding to the MAOI drug iproniazid had a lower initial urinary 5HIAA excretion than those who did not respond. This was not confirmed in a third study [306].

Low CSF 5HIAA has been reported in depression [64, 66, 307] and confirmed either by a trend [77] or significantly [87] after probenecid treatment. Low values are also usually obtained in mania [66, 78, 307] though in one study concentrations were higher than in depression [66] and in another [78] some positive correlation between 5HIAA and degree of mania was found. While the low 5HIAA findings in mania discourage the equating of a depression-mania polarity with a low 5HT-high 5HT polarity they do at least suggest that the results in depression are not simply a reflection of motor inactivity.

Low 5HT concentration is reported in the hind brains of depressive suicides [308] though values varied widely, possibly due to factors discussed in section 5.3.3 and to different modes of suicide and previous medications and also to diagnostic uncertainties and age differences [309]. In another study, low brain 5HIAA but not 5HT was found in suicides though there was . no significant difference between the depressed and apparently non-depressed suicides [101]. These low 5HIAA findings may be artefactual as hind brain 5HIAA concentrations of the control subjects (who died of a coronary thrombosis or occlusion) taken together with those of the depressed suicides correlate significantly with storage time before assay 5HIAA in ng/g = 415 (+ 5.91 x days) stored. The low results for the depressed group are at least partly explicable by this relationship. It is suggestive that in another investigation in which the time between autopsy and determination was minimal the brain stem 5HIAA concentrations of suicides though lower than controls were not significantly so [309].

The alleviation of depression by MAOI drugs is potentiated by tryptophan [310-313], a precursor not only of 5HT but also of tryptamine. While evidence is against tryptamine being present in the brain under physiological conditions [50, 51] the possibility that it may be deficient in depression or in excess in mania has been energetically proposed [314] and has been the subject of some controversy [315-318]. However, tryptamine [319] did not enhance the effects of MAOI drugs. On the other hand there is little evidence that 5HTP which is a specific precursor of 5HT directly influences mood [320, 321] though caution is necessary as the distribution in the brain of 5HT derived from exogenous 5HTP but not from exogenous tryptophan is different from that of endogenous brain 5HT [322].

While tryptophan without MAOI has been both claimed [312, 323] and denied [324] to have anti-depressive action, both the positive and negative trials are open to criticism [324, 325]. It is however remarkable that although when tryptophan is given to schizophrenic [85] or neurological [89] patients their brain 5HT metabolism is elevated (as indicated by increased CSF 5HIAA) it is consistently found that CSF 5HIAA does not increase when tryptophan is given to depressed patients [85, 89, 307]. This points strongly to defective tryptophan metabolism in depression but renders difficult the interpretation of any anti-depressive effect of tryptophan without MAOI in terms of increased brain 5HT. These findings raise again the possibility that tryptamine formed from the ingested tryptophan may be therapeutically significant. Another possibility is that the beneficial effect of tryptophan with or without MAOI is related not to amines formed from it but to some other property, e.g. its crucial role in protein synthesis [326] which could affect metabolic processes involving any class of substance.

The failure of CSF 5HIAA to increase when tryptophan is given to depressed subjects could be due to enhanced diversion of tryptophan via the pyrrolase pathway, as depressives given an oral tryptophan load excrete larger amounts of its metabolites formed through liver tryptophan pyrrolase action than do a control group [327]. This is reasonable as pyrrolase is induced by adrenocorticoids [328] and there is much evidence of elevated adrenocortical secretion in depressive illness [329, 330, 331] especially in the early morning [332-335]. Defective feedback inhibition of ACTH release may be responsible [336, 337]. Whether raised adrenocorticoid secretion is a primary or secondary manifestation of the illness is debatable [338, 339] and raised adrenocorticoid levels without depression (and vice versa) are commonplace.

It has been suggested that elevated pyrrolase activity may not only influence the fate of a tryptophan load but may decrease endogenous 5HT synthesis [340, 341]. Various animal experiments show this to be feasible. Thus in the rat, cortisol injection [342], immobilization stress [343] and injection of α-methyl tryptophan [344, 345] all increased liver pyrrolase activity and decreased brain 5HT. Furthermore the decrease of brain 5HT was prevented by injecting pyrrolase inhibitors [344]. These findings have received some support [346, 347] though the mechanism of the brain 5HT change remains obscure. The most obvious mechanism is for pyrrolase to divert tryptophan metabolism away from the 5HT pathway. However, though rat plasma tryptophan falls transiently after cortisol injection total brain tryptophan does not change significantly.

The above adrenal-cortex-brain 5HT relationship provides a model for studying possible metabolic interactions in endogenous and reactive depressions. It does not explain why CSF 5HIAA is low in endogenous depressives independently of the stage of illness or of plasma cortisol concentration [307]. Perhaps defective brain 5HT metabolism alone may be insufficient to cause depression but may result in a predisposition towards it. It is of interest that low rat brain 5HT obtained either by midbrain raphe lesions [348] or by inhibition of synthesis [349] is associated with increased sensitivity to external stimulation.

A well defined but at present unexplained finding is that the urinary excretion of tryptamine is low in depression [319, 350]. Excretion by recovered patients is higher [319].

There has been some discussion of the possibility that depression occurring as a side-effect of oral contraceptives may involve a decrease of brain 5HT. Women taking combined oestrogen-progestogen preparations excrete increased amounts of tryptophan metabolites [351] and rats given these drugs chronically are reported to show transiently increased liver pyrrolase activity and transiently decreased brain 5HT [352]. If these drugs significantly increase extracerebral tryptophan metabolism on the pyrrolase pathway, even in the absence of a tryptophan load [353], then the possibility of a functional pyridoxal deficiency arises as both 5HT synthesis and tryptophan metabolism subsequent to pyrrolase action require pyridoxal. Women on oral contraceptives and suffering from depression are said to benefit from pyridoxine treatment [354] and a controlled trial of pyridoxine seems warranted. However, the fall of brain 5HT associated with increased pyrrolase activity obtained when cortisol is given to rats is not prevented by pyridoxine [355].

5.6.3 The catecholamine hypothesis

A correlation between mood and NA and A excretion by manic depressives has been reported [356]. This relationship could possibly be secondary to changes of fluid intake, water metabolism [357] or motor activity, although in a longitudinal study of a manic-depressive patient [358] it is claimed that increased excretion of DA and of NA and its metabolites during mania correlated with mood rather than with the other variables or with drug treatment. High DA excretion in mania has been confirmed [359] and seems unlikely to be simply a consequence of increased motor activity [360]. The low urinary MHPG excretion in depression may be of importance as it could indicate defective brain NA metabolism [361] (see 5.2). The finding that after an oral tyrosine load both manic and depressed subjects had higher plasma tyrosine levels than did normal controls [362] is of interest. Recently similar findings were briefly reported after a tryptophan load [363]. Tolerance curves were normal in schizophrenics and in recovered patients.

No evidence of abnormal brain DA metabolism in affective states is provided by the limited CSF HVA studies reported [66, 77, 78]. Similarly, hind brain [101] and hypothalamic [309] NA and caudate nucleus [309] DA concentrations are comparable in brains of depressive suicides and control subjects.

The above findings do not convincingly support the hypothesis that disturbed brain catecholamine metabolism plays much part in abnormal mood states. However, the reversal by dopa of reserpine sedation in animals [364] has led to the trial of dopa as an antidepressant but until recently with little or no success [304, 365, 366, 367]. However, the successful treatment of parkinsonism with large amounts of L-dopa (5.4.3) has encouraged further investigation and some depressed patients studied benefited from treatment with L-dopa plus a peripheral decarboxylase inhibitor [368] though others became more psychotic. Depressive symptoms worsen in some parkinsonian patients given L-dopa [185].

A greater sensitivity of manic depressives than of unipolar depressives to the activating effect of L-dopa and thus presumably to catecholamines is reported [369]. The precipitation of manic episodes by drugs which would tend to increase functional brain amine concentrations [370] is consistent with the above finding especially in the absence of reports of the induction of mania by tryptophan or 5HTP.

It may well eventually be found that mood abnormalities cannot be completely correlated with defective synthesis of any single amine. Different amines could be important in different subjects in which case pharmacological manipulation of a single amine might influence symptoms only in specific sub-groups. Also relative as well as absolute levels of individual amines may be important [371, 372].

Finally, transient brain amine disturbances might well occur in normal subjects and be adequately compensated for, while in chronic depressive or other chronic states defective regulatory mechanisms might prolong abnormal amine metabolism. Relevant studies are however at an early stage [373].

5.7 SCHIZOPHRENIA

The possibility of abnormal brain amine metabolism in schizophrenia is suggested by the structural similarities and the indications of interactions between hallucinogens and brain amines although the extent to which the effects of hallucinogens can be considered as a model for schizophrenia is not clear [374]. There is some evidence that a more schizophrenia-like pattern occurs when LSD is given to subjects showing biochemical evidence of high cortisol levels or abnormal tryptophan metabolism [375]. This might indicate an interaction of LSD either with an abnormal biochemical state or with a personality under stress.

The inhibition of the action of 5HT on smooth muscle by the hallucinogen LSD led to the suggestion that an antiserotonin effect was also responsible for its effect on the brain [7, 376] and that schizophrenia or other psychotic states might be due to disturbed 5HT metabolism. An interaction between LSD and 5HT-ergic neurones in the brain was subsequently shown. Thus, LSD causes a small but definite increase of brain 5HT and a decrease of 5HIAA [377], while electrical stimulation of 5HT-ergic neurones has an opposite effect causing brain 5HT to fall and 5HIAA to rise [11]. The effect of LSD on brain 5IIT metabolism is associated with a depression of the firing rate of 5HT-ergic neurones [378]. NN-Dimethyltryptamine, another N-methylated hallucinogenic indolethylamine, has a similar effect on firing while 2 brom-LSD (a powerful peripheral anti-5HT but with little hallucinogenic potency) only has a weak effect. Hallucinogens such as mescaline which are related to the catecholamines also depress firing, but only of one group of the neurones depressed by the indolic hallucinogens.

The hallucinogenic effect of mescaline also suggested that metabolism of the catecholamines might be disturbed in

schizophrenia. A possible diversion of catecholamine metabolism by O-methylation to a psychotoxic mescaline-like
substance [379], or various diversions of catecholamine
metabolism to psychotoxic agents have been suggested to occur
in schizophrenia, e.g. in the adrenochrome [380] and
taraxein [381] hypotheses. Studies supporting these hypotheses
have been criticized and the general methodological difficulties
which face biochemical research on schizophrenia have been
pointed out in various reviews [382, 383, 384].

Further attention however has been paid more recently to
the possibility of abnormal methylation of either catecholamines or indolealkylamines in schizophrenia, not only because
many hallucinogens are O- or N-methyl derivatives of these
substances, but also because of the temporary deterioration of
schizophrenic patients when given MAOI together with the
methyl donor methionine [385, 386, 387]. Abnormal
O-methylation of catecholamines was suggested by the reported
presence of 3,4-dimethyoxyphenylethylamine (which is structurally very similar to mescaline) in schizophrenic urine [388].
The relationship between this substance, dietary factors and the
so-called "pink spot" detected on urinary chromato-
grams [389] is somewhat confused. The latter is probably a
complex mixture which may or may not contain 3,4-di-
methoxyphenylethylamine [163, 390, 391]. Furthermore clear
evidence that this substance is either a product of endogenous
metabolism or that its excretion is elevated in schizophrenia is
lacking [392].

Psychosis associated with amphetamine addiction is well
known and is similar to paranoid schizophrenia [393]. This is
relevant to the possible role of catecholamines in schizophrenia,
as the drug has multiple interactions with them inhibiting MAO
and neuronal catecholamine uptake, releasing catecholamines
from nerve endings and possibly itself forming a false
transmitter, or a hallucinogenic O-methylated catecholamine
derivative [394]. A further complication is the increased firing
of rat brain 5HT-ergic neurones caused by i.v. injection of
amphetamine [395]. In these circumstances the biochemical
mechanism of amphetamine psychosis is obscure though further
research might well lead to a valid schizophrenia model.

The O-methylation of 5HT to melatonin (5-methoxy-N-acetyl 5HT) occurs in the pineal. However, nothing specific is known about its formation in schizophrenia though it may have significant effects on behaviour [53, 396]. The possibility that N-methylation of 5HT to N-methyl 5HT and NN-dimethyl 5HT (bufotenine) can occur in the brain is of great interest as most psychotoxic indoles contain an NN-dimethyltryptamine residue [397, 398]. An N-methyl transferase able to N-methylate indolealkylamines [399] has been detected in animal and human extracerebral tissues and activity has recently been found in brain [32, 33]. Whether N-methylated indoles are formed *in vivo* is less certain, earlier claims having been based on artefacts or non-specific methods of detection [400]. More recently [401] bufotenine was detected in the urine of schizophrenic but not mentally defective subjects at very low concentration which increased about two weeks before symptoms worsened. However, other workers [402] find bufotenine is excreted equally by schizophrenic and control subjects. Studies on the effect of administration of MAOI and methyl donors appear more well defined, it being claimed that while six control subjects under this treatment excreted elevated amounts of tryptamine, two chronic schizophrenics also excreted NN-dimethyltryptamine, bufotenine and 5-methoxy-NN-dimethyltryptamine [403]. Furthermore, behavioural changes were more prominent in the schizophrenics and preceded by the biochemical changes. While these findings suggest a psychotoxic effect of methylated indoles on schizophrenics the lack of benefit resulting from reduced tryptophan and methionine intake is consistent with the methylated indole not being responsible for spontaneous schizophrenic symptoms [404]. However, rigid interpretation is impossible as withdrawal of the two amino acids could not be complete.

To summarize, there are many indications of relationships between brain amines and drugs causing states with similarities to schizophrenia and some information on the exacerbation of schizophrenia by drugs which can influence amine metabolism. However, direct evidence concerning abnormal brain amine metabolism in spontaneous schizophrenia is not yet available.

5.8 VARIOUS MENTAL DISORDERS

Inherited defects of amino acid metabolism especially those involving the aromatic acids may lead to abnormal brain amine metabolism. One possible mechanism for an amine disturbance is that the amino acid may itself be an amine precursor so that a defect in its absorption or metabolism may result in defective amine synthesis. Another possibility is that abnormally high levels of the amino acid or a derivative may inhibit the transport of an amine precursor to sites of amine synthesis in the brain or inhibit enzymes involved in amine synthesis. Thus defective 5HT metabolism occurs in phenylketonuria and is probably secondary to the high levels of phenylalanine. Both serum 5HT and urinary 5HIAA are low [405] though evidence is against a correlation between their levels and intelligence [406]. However, when a phenylketonuria-like state is produced in rats by feeding a high phenylalanine diet then learning is impaired and brain 5HT decreased [407]. Similar results are obtained on feeding leucine, while conversely a high tryptophan diet improved learning and increased brain 5HT. In these circumstances determination of 5HIAA in the CSF of phenylketonurics would be of interest.

The high incidence of psychotic illness in relatives of phenylketonurics has suggested that heterozygosity for this disease might predispose to endogenous depression [408, 409]. The indications of defective 5HT metabolism in both conditions and the similarity between the morbidity risk for endogenous depression and the frequency of heterozygozity for phenyl-ketonuria are consistent with the hypothesis. However, a phenylalanine tolerance test able to discriminate between a group of heterozygotes and controls did not discriminate between controls and depressives [410].

Decreased brain 5HT and DA in rats on a high dietary leucine intake is probably due to inhibition of amine precursor transport to the brain [411, 412]. Similar biochemical changes might be responsible for the mental retardation associated with maple syrup disease in which keto acids derived from leucine and other branched chain amino acids accumulate [413]. Decreased brain 5HT might also be involved in the mental changes which occur in the variant of pellagra associated with a high leucine diet [414]. The possibility that abnormal amine metabolism may play a part in the mental symptoms occurring in ordinary pellagra is also worth consideration especially as nicotinamide deficiency might well lead to diversion via the pyrrolase pathway [415] of the already low tryptophan intake away from 5HT synthesis. Again, decreased brain 5HT synthesis could have a role in causing the psychotic symptoms [416] shown by some patients with Hartnup disease, as intestinal absorption of tryptophan is defective [417]. The resultant enhanced bacterial tryptophan metabolism in the colon may also be important here as for example tryptamine (which penetrates readily to the brain [418]) might be produced.

A number of other rare disturbances of aromatic amino acid metabolism associated with mental defect and usually with evidence of inheritance have been reported (see ref. 419 for review) and might well also lead to disturbed brain amine metabolism, e.g. tyrosinaemia, increased urinary dopa with dwarfism, tryptophanuria, hydroxykynureninuria and hypercalcaemia with indicanuria.

A preliminary communication [420] reports low blood 5-hydroxyindoles in a group of children with behavioural disturbance and hyperactivity. The relevance of these findings to brain 5HT depends on the degree of reliability of the platelet as a model for central 5HT neurones [421]. It is worth noting however, that significant negative correlations are found between motor activity and brain 5HT in rats [349, 350, 422].

There is some suggestion of abnormal brain amine metabolism in senile and presenile dementia [61]. CSF HVA and 5HIAA decreased in the order: healthy aged volunteers, senile dementia, presenile dementia, parkinsonism. HVA concentration in the basal ganglia was lower in senile dementia than in dementia associated with vascular disease or in non-specific senile diseases though there was considerable overlap between groups [423]. However, there were significant negative correlations between degree of dementia and HVA and 5HIAA concentrations. There were no significant correlations between concentrations and degree of motor impairment [424].

5.9 MIGRAINE

As vascular changes characteristically occur in migrainous headache attacks, vasoactive substances, i.e. acetylcholine, substance P, bradykinin, histamine, 5HT and NA have been discussed [425], in relation to migraine. A role for 5HT, NA or A has seemed particularly likely. Thus: (i) they are powerfully vasoactive; (ii) N and NA secretion into the blood is increased in stressful situations—suggesting a biochemical link between migrainous symptoms and the so-called migrainous personality, (iii) reserpine liberates amines from body stores and provokes migrainous headache [426]; (iv) methysergide and other drugs used in the treatment of migraine antagonize pharmacological actions of 5HT [427]; (v) at very low concentrations 5HT induces pain—at least when applied to blisters [428].

Migrainous subjects were reported to excrete large amounts of the terminal metabolites of NA, A and 5HT—VMA and 5HIAA on days when they had attacks [429, 430]. This was confirmed in one more recent study [431] though the changes found were less striking. In another study [432] one subject was described with markedly increased 5HIAA excretion during and preceding attacks though most other subjects did not show increases and in no subject was VMA excretion related to headaches.

Increased 5HIAA excretion could be associated with increased blood hydration which occurs in the prodromal and early stages of migraine attacks [433]. Haemodilution can cause increased urinary 5HIAA [434] and alternatively might itself result from liberation of 5HT which has anti-diuretic properties [435]. Gastrointestinal symptoms which are common in migrainous attacks may also be related to 5HT changes, as not only is peristalsis increased by intra-luminal administration of 5HT, but also itself causes 5HT liberation [436], while administration of magnesium sulphate or carbachol elevates serum 5HT [437]. However, high 5HIAA excretion was found to precede the onset of nausea and vomiting in migrainous attacks [431] and attacks may occur with nausea and vomiting but without 5HIAA peaks [432].

While injection of 5HT in the area of the superficial temporal artery was found in one study [438] to induce headache in migrainous subjects this was not confirmed in another study in which 5HTP also did not cause headache [439], and migraine is not prominent in carcinoid disease in which enormous amounts of 5HT may be metabolized.

These negative findings which were followed by the observation later confirmed [440] that 5HT or MAOI treatment alleviated headache while reserpine provoked attacks [426], and also the findings of high urinary 5HIAA in headache episodes suggest some migrainous headaches may be due to depletion of 5HT from certain sites. In agreement with this hypothesis it is found that plasma 5HT falls at the onset of migraine attacks [431, 440] apparently due to a factor which depletes 5HT from platelet stores [441].

Thus, study of the migrainous attacks provoked by the amine depleter reserpine may be relevant to the understanding of spontaneous attacks. Reserpine however probably causes a more general amine disturbance than occurs in spontaneous attacks as indicated by the vasomotor changes it commonly precipitates [442]. After injecting reserpine into migrainous subjects the urinary excretion of 5HIAA and VMA is increased most in those subjects in whom headache is provoked. Similarly, when headaches are induced with glyceryl nitrate there is a large increase of urinary 5HIAA and VMA which does not occur in subjects who do not have attacks [443]. Results do not suggest that amine stores of the subjects in whom reserpine provokes headache are abnormally sensitive to the drug, while the absence or mildness of headache in non-migrainous subjects after reserpine injection [426, 440] suggests that an abnormal response to amine changes is involved. Both headache induction after reserpine and the associated changes of amine metabolism were more prominent in younger subjects [442]. Whether this indicates an age dependence of reserpine metabolism and distribution or a decreased depletability of amines in older subjects is unknown. The latter possibility is of interest as it suggests that the frequent disappearance or decreasing severity of migraine in middle age could be due to a decreasing sensitivity of amine stores to endogenous depleters.

Many migrainous subjects have attacks after eating certain foods, chocolate and cheese being the most common dietary precipitants [444]. Cheese contains the amine tyramine and it has been shown that this substance precipitates severe migraine in many subjects who suffer from dietary migraine [445] but only causes infrequent and mild headache in non-migrainous subjects [444]. It is likely that other dietary precipitants will be discovered. Tyramine is present in many foodstuffs as a product of the decarboxylation by microorganisms of the amino acid tyrosine. It probably acts indirectly on blood vessels through the release of NA and it is of interest that the drug Catapres (ST. 155) which antagonizes the action of NA on blood vessels has a prophylactic effect against migrainous headache [446].

Tyramine sensitivity may be caused by a defect in its metabolism, probably defective conjugation with sulphate [447, 448] and it is likely that tyramine sensitive subjects will also be found to exhibit defective detoxication of a variety of drugs.

Amine metabolites have not yet been determined in the CSF of migrainous patients. However, it is not found to differ from that of non-migrainous subjects in its content of 5HT and other pharmacologically active substances [449].

REFERENCES

1. J. J. Abel, *Hoppe-Seyler's Z. physiol. Chem.*, **29**, 318 (1899)
2. M. Lewandowsky, *Archs. Anat. Physiol., Lpz (Physiol. Abt.)*, 360 (1899)
3. U. S. Von Euler, *Acta physiol. scand.*, **16**, 63 (1948)
4. M. Vogt, *J. Physiol.*, **123**, 451 (1954)
5. H. Blaschko, *J. Physiol.*, **96**, 50P (1939)
6. A. Bertler, *Acta physiol. scand.*, **51**, 97 (1961)
7. J. H. Gaddum, *J. Physiol.*, **121**, 15P (1953)
8. A. H. Amin, T. B. B. Crawford and J. H. Gaddum, *J. Physiol.*, **126**, 596 (1954)
9. K. Fuxe, T. Hökfelt and U. Ungerstedt, *In* Metabolism of Amines in the Brain (G. Hooper, ed.), p. 10. Macmillan, London (1969)
10. G. W. Arbuthnot, T. J. Crow, K. Fuxe, L. Olson and U. Ungerstedt, *Brain Res.*, **24**, 471 (1970)
11. G. K. Aghajanian, J. A. Rosecrans and M. H. Sheard, *Science*, **156**, 402 (1967)
12. P. B. Bradley, *Int. Rev. Neurobiol.*, **11**, 2 (1968)
13. J. D. Connor, *Science*, **160**, 899 (1968)
14. E. A. Zeller, J. Barsky, J. R. Fouts, W. F. Kirchheimer and L. S. Van Ordern, *Experientia*, **8**, 349 (1952)
15. B. B. Brodie, J. S. Olin, R. G. Kuntzman and P. A. Shore, *Science*, **125**, 1293 (1957)
16. M. Holzbauer and M. Vogt, *J. Neurochem.*, **1**, 8 (1956)

17. I. J. Kopin, *In* Brain Chemistry and Mental Disease (B. T. Ho and W. M. McIsaac, eds), p. 73. Plenum Press, New York and London (1971)
18. H. Ehringer and O. Hornykiewicz, *Klin. Wschr.*, 38, 1236 (1960)
19. G. C. Cotzias, M. A. Van Woert and L. M. Schiffer, *New Engl. J. Med.*, 276, 374 (1967)
20. G. H. Acheson (ed.), 2nd Symposium on catecholamines. *Pharmac. Rev.*, 18 (1966)
21. E. Costa and M. Sandler (eds), *Biological Role of Indolealkylamine Derivatives in Adv. Pharmac.*, 6, Supp. p. 1 (1968)
22. T. Nagatsu, M. Levitt and S. Udenfriend, *J. biol. Chem.*, 239, 2910 (1964)
23. E. M. Gal, J. C. Armstrong and B. Ginsberg, *J. Neurochem.*, 13, 643 (1966)
24. K. Lloyd and O. Hornkiewicz, *Brain Res.*, 22, 426 (1970)
25. E. Robins, J. M. Robins, A. B. Croninger, S. G. Moses, S. J. Spencer and R. W. Hudgens, *Biochem. Med.*, 1, 240 (1967)
26. W. H. Vogel, V. Orfei and B. Century, *J. Pharmac.*, 165, 196 (1969)
27. W. H. Vogel, H. McFarland and L. N. Prince, *Biochem. Pharmac.*, 19, 618 (1970)
28. E. Y. Levin, B. Levenberg and S. Kaufman, *J. biol. Chem.*, 235, 2080 (1960)
29. S. Udenfriend and C. R. Creveling, *J. Neurochem.*, 4, 350 (1959)
30. J. Axelrod, *J. biol. Chem.*, 237, 1657 (1962)
31. P. L. McGeer and E. G. McGeer, *Biochem. biophys. Res. Commun.*, 5, 502 (1964)
32. M. Morgan and A. J. Mandell, *Science*, 165, 492 (1969)
33. A. J. Mandell and M. Morgan, *Nature (New Biol.)*, 230, 85 (1971)
34. J. Renson, H. Weissbach and S. Udenfriend, *J. Pharmac.*, 143, 326 (1964)
35. D. Eccleston, A. T. B. Moir, H. W. Reading and I. M. Ritchie, *Br. J. Pharmac.*, 28, 367 (1966)
36. G. R. Breese, T. N. Chase and I. J. Kopin, *J. Pharmac.*, 165, 9 (1969)
37. J. Axelrod, *Physiol. Rev.*, 39, 751 (1959)
38. J. Axelrod, R. W. Albers and C. D. Clemente, *J. Neurochem.*, 5, 67 (1959)
39. T. Persson, *Acta pharmac. tox.*, 27, 397 (1969)
40. I. J. Kopin and E. Gordon, *J. Pharmac.*, 138, 351 (1962)
41. I. J. Kopin, *Pharmac. Rev.*, 18, 513 (1966)
42. J. W. Maas and D. H. Landis, *Psychosom. Med.*, 28, 247 (1966)
43. G. F. Murphy and T. L. Sourkes, *Archs. Biochem.*, 93, 338 (1961)
44. S. Udenfriend, H. Weissbach and D. F. Bogdanski, *J. biol. Chem.*, 224, 803 (1957)
45. H. Weil-Malherbe, J. Axelrod and R. Tomchick, *Science*, 129, 1226 (1959)
46. L. G. Whitby, J. Axelrod and H. Weil-Malherbe, *J. Pharmac.*, 132, 193 (1961)
47. M. Bulat and Z. Supek, *J. Neurochem.*, 15, 383 (1968)

48. T. L. Perry, S. Hansen and L. Macdougall, *J. Neurochem.*, **14**, 775 (1967)
49. A. Björklund, B. Falck and U. Stenevi, *J. Pharmac.*, **175**, 525 (1970)
50. D. Eccleston, G. W. Ashcroft, T. B. B. Crawford and R. J. Loose, *J. Neurochem.*, **13**, 93 (1966)
51. R. C. Lin, E. Costa, N. H. Neff, C. T. Wang and S. H. Ngai, *J. Pharmac.*, **170**, 232 (1969)
52. A. A. Boulton and L. Quan, Abst. 2nd Internat. Meeting, Internat. Soc. for Neurochemistry, 101 (1969)
53. R. J. Wurtman, J. Axelrod and D. E. Kelly, The Pineal. Academic Press, New York (1968)
54. J. W. Maas and D. H. Landis, *J. Pharmac.*, **163**, 147 (1968)
55. H. C. Guldberg, *In* Metabolism of Amines in the Brain (G. Hooper, ed.), p. 54. Macmillan, London (1969)
56. G. Bartholini, A. Pletscher and R. Tissot, *Experientia*, **22**, 609 (1966)
57. H. C. Guldberg and C. M. Yates, *Br. J. Pharmac.*, **33**, 457 (1968)
58. G. W. Ashcroft, R. C. Dow and A. T. B. Moir, *J. Physiol. (Lond.)*, **199**, 397 (1968)
59. M. B. Bowers, *J. Neurochem.*, **17**, 827 (1970)
60. T. N. Chase, J. A. Schnur and E. K. Gordon, *Neuropharmac.*, **9**, 265 (1970)
61. C. G. Gottfries, I. Gottfries and B. E. Roos, *J. Neurochem.*, **16**, 1341 (1969)
62. N. E. Anden, B. E. Roos and B. Werdinius, *Life Sciences*, **2**, 448 (1963)
63. G. W. Ashcroft and D. F. Sharman, *Nature (Lond.)*, **186**, 1050 (1960)
64. G. W. Ashcroft, T. B. B. Crawford, D. Eccleston, D. F. Sharman, E. J. MacDougall, J. B. B. Stanton and J. K. Binns, *Lancet*, ii, 1049 (1966)
65. H. Bernheimer, W. Birkmayer and O. Hornykiewicz, *Wien. klin. Wschr.*, **78**, 417 (1966)
66. S. J. Dencker, U. Malm, B. E. Roos and B. Werdinius, *J. Neurochem.*, **13**, 1545 (1966)
67. H. Andersson and B. E. Roos, *Experientia*, **22**, 539 (1966)
68. G. S. Barolin and O. Hornykiewicz, *Wien. klin. Wschr.*, **79**, 815 (1967)
69. B. Johansson and B. E. Roos, *Life Sciences*, **6**, 1449 (1967)
70. M. B. Bowers and F. A. Gerbode, *Nature (Lond.)*, **219**, 1256 (1968)
71. F. A. Gerbode and M. B. Bowers, *J. Neurochem.*, **15**, 1053 (1968)
72. R. Olsson and B. E. Roos, *Nature (Lond.)*, **219**, 503 (1968)
73. T. Persson and B. E. Roos, *Nature (Lond.)*, **219**, 854 (1968)
74. M. B. Bowers, *Brain Res.*, **15**, 522 (1969)
75. W. Weiner, W. Harrison and H. Klawans, *Life Sciences*, **8**, 971 (1969)
76. T. Persson and B. E. Roos, *Br. J. Psychiat.*, **115**, 95 (1969)
77. B. E. Roos and R. Sjöström, *Pharmacologia Clinica*, **1**, 153 (1969)
78. M. B. Bowers, G. R. Heniger and F. Gerbode, *Int. J. Neuropharmac.*, **8**, 255 (1969)

79. V. Dubowitz and K. J. Rogers, *Dev. Med. Child Neurol.*, 11, 730 (1969)
80. K. J. Rogers and V. Dubowitz, *Dev. Med. Child Neurol.*, 12, 461 (1970)
81. C. G. Gottfries, I. Gottfries and B. E. Roos, *Acta psychiat. scand.*, 46, 99 (1970)
82. A. T. B. Moir, G. W. Ashcroft, T. B. B. Crawford, D. Eccleston and H. C. Guldberg, *Brain*, 93, 357 (1970)
83. G. Curzon, R. B. Godwin-Austen, E. B. Tomlinson and B. D. Kantamaneni, *J. Neurol. Neurosurg. Psychiat.*, 33, 1 (1970)
84. J. A. Brody, T. N. Chase and E. K. Gordon, *New Engl. J. Med.*, 282, 947 (1970)
85. M. B. Bowers, *Neuropharmacology*, 9, 599 (1970)
86. J. R. Mendell, T. N. Chase and W. K. Engel, *Lancet*, i, 593 (1970)
87. H. M. Van Praag, J. Korf and J. Puite, *Nature (Lond.)*, 225, 1260 (1970)
88. R. Papeschi, P. Molina-Negro, T. L. Sourkes, J. Hardy and C. Bertrand, *Neurology, Minneap.*, 20, 991 (1970)
89. D. Eccleston, G. W. Ashcroft, T. B. B. Crawford, J. B. Stanton, D. Wood and P. H. McTurk, *J. Neurol. Neurosurg. Psychiat.*, 33, 269 (1970)
90. N. R. Tamarkin, F. K. Goodwin and J. Axelrod, *Life Sciences*, 9, 1397 (1970)
91. T. N. Chase, *In* The Torsion Dystonias. Supplement to Neurology (R. Eldridge, ed.), 20, p. 122 (1970)
92. H. Dekirmenjian and J. W. Maas, *Analyt. Biochem.*, 35, 113 (1970)
93. S. M. Schanberg, G. R. Breese, J. J. Schildkraut, E. K. Gordon and I. J. Kopin, *Biochem. Pharmac.*, 17, 2006 (1968)
94. G. Curzon, R. B. Godwin-Austen and B. D. Kantamaneni (in press)
95. G. Curzon, E. J. W. Gumpert and D. M. Sharpe, *Nature (New Biol.)*, 231, 189 (1971)
96. A. Carlsson, B. Falck, K. Fuxe and N. A. Hillarp, *Acta physiol. scand.*, 60, 112 (1964)
97. I. A. Pullar, J. M. Weddel, A. Hanieh, R. Ahmed and F. J. Gillingham, Abst. 2nd Internat. Meeting, Internat. Soc. for Neurochemistry, 328 (1969)
98. D. Joyce, *Br. J. Pharmac.*, 18, 370 (1962)
99. R. Maclean, W. J. Nicholson, C. M. B. Pare and R. S. Stacey, *Lancet*, ii, 205 (1965)
100. J. H. Dowson, *Lancet*, ii, 596 (1969)
101. H. R. Bourne, W. E. Bunney, R. W. Colburn, J. M. Davis, J. N. Davis, D. M. Shaw and A. J. Coppen, *Lancet*, ii, 805 (1968)
102. F. Grabarits, R. Chessick and H. Lal, *Biochem. Pharmac.*, 15, 127 (1966)
103. A. Williamson, Ph.D. Thesis, University of London (1969)
104. O. Hornykiewicz, *In* Comparative Neurochemistry (D. Richter, ed.), p. 379. Pergamon, Oxford (1964)
105. C. G. Gottfries, A. M. Rosengren and E. Rosengren, *Acta pharmac. tox.*, 23, 36 (1965)

106. A. Elbadawi, K. H. Hayashi and E. A. Schenk, *Histochemie*, 21, 21 (1970)
107. J. de Ajuriaguerra and G. Gauthier (eds), Monoamines et Noyaux Gris Centraux (in press)
108. D. B. Calne, Parkinsonsim: Physiology, Pharmacology and Treatment. Arnold, London (1970)
109. G. C. Cotzias, *Hospital Practice*, 35 (1969)
110. J. P. Martin, *Lancet*, i, 999 (1959)
111. A. Bertler and E. Rosengren, *Experientia*, 15, 10 (1959)
112. I. Sano, T. Gamo, Y. Kakimoto, K. Taniguchi, M. Takesada and K. Nishinuma, *Biochim. biophys. Acta*, 32, 586 (1959)
113. O. Hornykiewicz, *Wien. klin. Wschr.*, 75, 309 (1963)
114. H. Bernheimer, W. Birkmayer and O. Hornykiewicz, *Klin. Wschr.*, 39, 1056 (1961)
115. H. Bernheimer and O. Hornykiewicz, *Klin. Wschr.*, 43, 711 (1965)
116. O. Hornykiewicz, *In* Biochemical and Neurophysiological Correlation of Centrally Acting Drugs (E. Trabucchi, R. Paoletti and N. Canal. eds), p. 58. Macmillan, New York (1964)
117. R. B. Godwin-Austen, B. D. Kantamaneni and G. Curzon, *J. Neurol. Neurosurg. Psychiat.*, 34, 219 (1971)
118. H. C. Guldberg, J. W. Turner, A. Hanieh, G. W. Ashcroft, T. B. B. Crawford, W. L. M. Perry and F. J. Gillingham, *Confinia neurol.*, 29, 73 (1967)
119. G. S. Barolin, H. Bernheimer and O. Hornykiewicz, *Schweizer Archs. Neurol. Psychiat.*, 94, 241 (1964)
120. H. Bernheimer, W. Birkmayer and O. Hornykiewicz, *Klin. Wschr.*, 41, 465 (1963)
121. H. Bernheimer, W. Birkmayer and O. Hornykiewicz, *Wien. klin. Wschr.*, 74, 558 (1962)
122. G. G. S. Collins, M. Sandler, E. D. Williams and M. B. H. Youdim, *Nature (Lond.)*, 225, 817 (1970)
123. H. Bernheimer and O. Hornykiewicz, *Arch. Exp. Path. Pharmak.*, 243, 295 (1962)
124. C. Tretiakoff, Thesis, Paris (1919)
125. J. G. Greenfield and F. D. Bosanquet, *J. Neurol. Neurosurg. Psychiat.*, 16, 213 (1953)
126. N. E. Andén, A. Carlsson, A. Dahlström, K. Fuxe, N. A. Hillarp and K. Larsson, *Life Sciences*, 3, 523 (1964)
127. R. L. M. Faull and R. Laverty, *Expl. Neurol.*, 23, 332 (1969)
128. N. E. Andén, A. Dahlström, K. Fuxe and K. Larsson, *Am. J. Anat.*, 116, 329 (1965)
129. H. McLennan, *Experientia*, 21, 275 (1965)
130. L. J. Poirier and T. L. Sourkes, *Brain*, 88, 181 (1965)
131. T. L. Sourkes and L. Poirier, *Nature (Lond.)*, 207, 202 (1965)
132. L. J. Poirier, T. L. Sourkes, G. Bouvier, R. Boucher and S. Carabin, *Brain*, 89, 37 (1966)
133. L. J. Poirier, E. G. McGeer, L. Larochelle, P. L. McGeer, P. Bedard and R. Boucher, *Brain Res.*, 14, 147 (1969)

134. M. Goldstein, B. Anagnoste, A. F. Battista, W. S. Owen and S. Nakatani, *J. Neurochem.*, 16, 645 (1969)

135. U. Ungerstedt, *In* 6-Hydroxydopamine and catecholamine neurons (T. Malmfors and H. Thoenen, eds), p. 101. North Holland (1971)

136. U. Ungerstedt, *Eur. J. Pharmac.*, 5, 107 (1968)

137. J. M. Foley and D. Baxter, *J. Neuropath. exp. Neurol.*, 17, 586 (1958)

138. R. D. Lillie, *J. Histochem. Cytochem.*, 3, 453 (1955)

139. R. D. Lillie and H. Yamada, *Okajimas Folia Anat. Jap.*, 36, 155 (1960)

140. C. D. Marsden, *Q. Jl. microsc. Sci.*, 102, 407, 467 (1961)

141. J. H. Fellman, *J. Neurol. Neurosurg. Psychiat.*, 21, 58 (1958)

142. C. Vanderwende and M. T. Spoerlein, *Life Sciences*, 6, 386 (1963)

143. C. Vanderwende, *Archs Int. Pharmacodyn.*, 152, 433 (1964)

144. M. Bazelon, G. M. Fenichel and J. Randall, *Neurology, Minneap.*, 17, 512 (1967)

145. M. H. Van Woert, K. N. Prasad and D. C. Borg, *J. Neurochem.*, 14, 707 (1967)

146. T. Ishii and R. L. Friede, *Am. J. Anat.*, 122, 139 (1968)

147. S. H. Pomerantz, *J. biol. Chem.*, 241, 161 (1966)

148. A. Pullman and B. Pullman, *Biochim. biophys. Acta*, 54, 384 (1961)

149. G. C. Cotzias, P. S. Papavasiliou, M. H. Van Woert and A. Sakamoto, *Fedn. Proc.*, 23, Part 1, 713 (1964)

150. B. Commoner, J. Townsend and G. E. Pake, *Nature (Lond.)*, 174, 689 (1954)

151. G. Curzon, *Int. Rev. Neurobiol.*, 10, 323 (1967)

152. U. K. Rinne and V. Sonninen, Abst. 9th Int. Cong. Neurol., 169 (1969)

153. H. Weil-Malherbe and J. M. Van Buren, *J. Lab. clin. Med.*, 74, 305 (1969)

154. G. L. Mattock, D. L. Wilson and A. Hoffer, *Nature (Lond.)*, 213, 1189 (1967)

155. F. Bischoff and A. Torres, *Clin. Chem.*, 8, 370 (1962)

156. J. Braham, I. Sarova-Pinhas, M. Crispin, R. Golan, N. Levin and A. Szeinberg, *Brit. med. J.*, ii, 552 (1969)

157. E. Honos, A. D. Ericsson and D. S. McCann, *Life Sciences*, 9, 159 (1970)

158. A. Barbeau, G. Jasmin and Y. Duchastel, *Neurology, Minneap.*, 13, 56 (1963)

159. R. H. Resnick, S. J. Gray, J. P. Koch and W. H. Timberlake, *Proc. Soc. exp. Biol. Med.*, 110, 77 (1962)

160. S. O'Reilly, S. Loncin and B. Cooksey, *Neurology, Minneap.*, 15, 980 (1965)

161. A. Barbeau, A. J. de Groot, J. G. Joly, D. Raymond-Tremblay and J. Donaldson, *Rev. Can. Biol.*, 22, 469 (1963)

162. U. K. Rinne and V. Sonninen, *Nature (Lond.)*, 216, 489 (1967)

163. A. A. Boulton, R. J. Pollitt and J. R. Majer, *Nature (Lond.)*, 215, 132 (1967)

164. J. R. Stabenau, C. R. Creveling and J. Daly, Abst. 7th Cong. Coll. Int. Neuropsychopharmac., 417 (1970)
165. I. Smith and A. H. Kellow, *Nature (Lond.)*, 221, 1261 (1969)
166. F. A. Kuehl, W. J. A. Van den Heuvel and R. E. Ormond, *Nature (Lond.)*, 217, 136 (1968)
167. W. Birkmayer and O. Hornykiewicz, *Wien. klin. Wschr.*, 73, 787 (1961)
168. J. Hirschmann and A. Mayer, *Arzneimittel-Forsch.*, 14, 599 (1964)
169. F. Gerstenbrand, F. Pateisky and P. Prosenz, *Psychiat. Neurol.*, 146, 246 (1963)
170. A. J. Friedhoff, L. Hekimian, M. Alpert and E. Tobach, *J. Am. med. Ass.*, 184, 285 (1963)
171. W. Umbach and D. Baumann, *Arch. Psychiat. Nervkrankh*, 205, 281 (1964)
172. C. Fehling, *Acta Neurol. scand.*, 42, 367 (1966)
173. P. L. McGeer and L. R. Zeldowicz, *Can. med. Ass. J.*, 90, 463 (1964)
174. M. D. Yahr, R. C. Duvoisin, M. J. Schear, R. E. Barrett and M. M. Hoehn, *Archs. Neurol.*, 21, 343 (1969)
175. G. C. Cotzias, P. S. Papavasiliou and R. Gellene, *New Engl. J. Med.*, 280, 337 (1969)
176. R. B. Godwin-Austen, E. B. Tomlinson, C. C. Frears and H. W. L. Kok, *Lancet*, ii, 165 (1969)
177. D. B. Calne, A. S. D. Spiers, G. M. Stern, D. R. Laurence and P. Armitage, *Lancet*, i, 744 (1969)
178. A. Sadwin, *New Engl. J. Med.*, 280, 962 (1969)
179. D. B. Calne, G. M. Stern, D. R. Laurence, J. M. Sharkey and P. Armitage, *Lancet*, I, 744 (1969)
180. O. W. Sacks, M. Kohl, W. Schwartz and C. Messeloff, *Lancet*, i, 1006 (1970)
181. K. R. Hunter, G. M. Stern and J. Sharkey, *Lancet*, ii, 1366 (1970)
182. Anon. *Lancet*, i, 871 (1969)
183. Anon. *Br. med. J.*, i, 446 (1970)
184. R. M. Jenkins and R. H. Groh, *Lancet*, ii, 177 (1970)
185. A. R. Damasio, J. L. Antunes and C. Macedo, *Lancet*, ii, 611 (1970)
186. L. Rivera-Calimlim, C. A. Dujovne, J. P. Morgan, L. Lasagna and J. R. Bianchine, *Br. med. J.*, ii, 93 (1970)
187. G. Bartholini, R. Tissot and A. Pletscher, *Brain Res.*, 27, 163 (1971)
188. N. E. Andén, K. Fuxe, B. Hamberger and T. Hökfelt, *Acta physiol. scand.*, 67, 306 (1966)
189. U. Ungerstedt and G. Arbuthnott, *Brain Res.*, 24, 485 (1970)
190. U. Ungerstedt, *In* Monoamines et Noyaux Gris Centraux (J. de Ajuriaguerra and G. Gauthier, eds) (in press)
191. K. Y. Ng, T. N. Chase, R. W. Colburn and I. J. Kopin, *Science*, 170, 76 (1970)
192. D. B. Calne, F. Karoum, C. R. J. Ruthven and M. Sandler, *Br. J. Pharmac.*, 37, 57 (1969)
193. I. Kuruma, G. Bartholini and A. Pletscher, *Eur. J. Pharmac.*, 10, 189 (1970)

194. G. Bartholini, I. Kuruma and A. Pletscher, *Brit. J. Pharmac.*, 40, 461 (1970)
195. R. J. Wurtman, C. Chou and C. Rose, *J. Pharmac.*, 174, 351 (1970)
196. T. L. Sourkes, *Biochem. Med.*, 3, 321 (1970)
197. T. L. Sourkes, *Nature (Lond.)*, 229, 413 (1971)
198. M. Sandler, B. L. Goodwin and C. R. J. Ruthven, *Nature (Lond.)*, 229, 414 (1971)
199. A. Pletscher, *Archs. Neurol.*, 20, 187 (1969)
200. C. Owman and E. J. Rosengren, *J. Neurochem.*, 14, 547 (1967)
201. J. Siegfried, R. Klaiber, E. Perret and W. H. Ziegler, *Dt. med. Wschr.*, 94, 2678 (1969)
202. G. Bartholini and A. Pletscher, *J. Pharmac.*, 161, 14 (1968)
203. J. Constantinidis, G. Bartholini, F. Geissbuhler and R. Tissot, *Experientia*, 26, 381 (1970)
204. L. Butcher, J. Engel and K. Fuxe, *J. Pharm. Pharmac.*, 22, 313 (1970)
205. J. D. Utley and A. Carlsson, *Acta Pharmac. Tox.*, 23, 189 (1965)
206. R. M. Pinder, *Nature (Lond.)*, 228, 358 (1970)
207. J. Braham, *Brit. med. J.*, ii, 540 (1970)
208. L. Butcher and J. Engel, *Brain Res.*, 15, 233 (1969)
209. J. T. Coyle and S. H. Snyder, *Science*, 166, 899 (1969)
210. K. Fuxe, M. Goldstein and A. Ljungdahl, *Life Sciences*, 9, 811 (1970)
211. K. M. Taylor and S. H. Snyder, *Science*, 168, 1487 (1970)
212. R. S. Schwab, A. C. England, D. C. Poskanzer and R. R. Young, *J. Am. med. Ass.*, 208, 1168 (1969)
213. R. B. Godwin-Austen, C. C. Frears, S. Bergmann, J. D. Parkes and R. P. Knill-Jones, *Lancet*, ii, 383 (1970)
214. T. H. Svensson and U. Strömberg, *J. Pharm. Pharmac.*, 22, 639 (1970)
215. A. Pletscher, *In* Monoamines et Noyaux Gris Centraux (J. de Ajuriaguerra and G. Gauthier, eds) (in press)
216. J. D. Parkes, R. C. H. Baxter, G. Curzon, R. P. Knill-Jones, P. J. Knott, C. D. Marsden, R. Tattersall and D. Vollum, *Lancet*, 1, 1083 (1971)
217. A. M. Ernst, *Acta physiol. Pharmacol. Neerl.*, 15, 141 (1969)
218. G. C. Cotzias, P. S. Papavasiliou, C. Fehling, B. Kaufman and I. Mena, *New Engl. J. Med.*, 282, 31 (1970)
219. G. C. Cotzias, S. Düby, J. Z. Ginos, A. Steck and P. S. Papavasiliou, *New Engl. J. Med.*, 283, 1289 (1970)
220. P. Glow, *J. Neurol. Neurosurg. Psychiat.*, 22, 11 (1959)
221. G. Steg, *Acta physiol. scand. Suppl.*, 225 (1964)
222. B. E. Roos and G. Steg, *Life Sciences*, 3, 351 (1964)
223. A. Carlsson, *Prog. Brain Res.*, 8, 9 (1964)
224. A. Bertler, C. G. Gottfries, I. Nordenfelt and E. Rosengren, *Med. Exptl.*, 9, 17 (1963)
225. W. A. Lishman, *In* Biochemical Aspects of Neurological Disorders (J. N. Cumings and M. Kremer, eds), p. 62. Blackwell, Oxford (1968)

226. A. Carlsson and M. Lindqvist, *Acta pharmac. tox.*, **20**, 140 (1963)
227. N. E. Andén, B. E. Roos and B. Werdinius, *Life Sciences*, **3**, 149 (1964)
228. H. Nybäck, G. Sedvall and I. J. Kopin, *Life Sciences*, **6**, 2307 (1967)
229. G. Bartholini and A. Pletscher, *Experientia*, **25**, 919 (1969)
230. M. Da Prada and A. Pletscher, *Experientia*, **22**, 465 (1966)
231. R. O'Keeffe, D. F. Sharman and M. Vogt, *Br. J. Pharmac.*, **38**, 287 (1970)
232. K. Pind and A. Faurbye, *Acta Psychiat. scand.*, **46**, 323 (1970)
233. E. Christensen, J. E. Moller and A. Faurbye, *Acta Psychiat. scand.*, **46**, 14 (1970)
234. A. Villeneuve and Z. Böszörményi, *Lancet*, i, 353 (1970)
235. H. Hippius and G. Logemann, *Arzneimittel-Forsch.*, **20**, 894 (1970)
236. I. Munkvad, H. Pakkenberg and A. Randrup, *Brain Behav. and Evol.*, **1**, 89 (1968)
237. J. M. Van Rossum, *Int. Rev. Neurobiol.*, **12**, 307 (1970)
238. I. Mena, O. Marin, S. Fuenzalida, *Neurology, Minneap.*, **17**, 128 (1967)
239. R. H. Flinn, P. A. Neal, W. H. Reinhart, J. M. Dallavalle, W. B. Fulton and A. H. Dooley, *Publ. Hlth. Bull. (U.S.)*, No. 247 (1940)
240. L. Van Bogaert and M. J. Dallemagne, *Mschr. Psychiat. Neurol.*, **111**, 60 (1945-46)
241. A. Pentschew, F. F. Ebner and R. M. Kovatch, *J. Neuropathol. exptl. Neurol.*, **32**, 488 (1963)
242. J. H. Scherer, *J. comp. Neurol.*, **71**, 9 (1939)
243. G. C. Cotzias, *J. Neurosurg.*, **24**, 170 (1966)
244. N. H. Neff, R. E. Barrett and E. Costa, *Experientia*, **25**, 1140 (1969)
245. F. Seitelberger, H. Petsche, H. Bernheimer and O. Hornykiewicz, *Naturwissenschaften*, **51**, 314 (1964)
246. I. Mena, J. Court, S. Fuenzalida, P. S. Papavasiliou and G. Cotzias, *New Engl. J. Med.*, **282**, 5 (1970)
247. G. M. Yuill, *Lancet*, i, 44 (1971)
248. A. Barbeau, *Lancet*, ii, 1066 (1969)
249. H. C. Klawans, G. W. Paulson and A. Barbeau, *Lancet*, ii, 1185 (1970)
250. T. L. Sourkes, D. Pivnicki, W. T. Brown, M. H. W. Distler, G. F. Murphy, I. Sankoff and S. Saint Cyr, *Psychiat. Neurol., Basel*, **149**, 7 (1965)
251. C. M. Williams, S. Maury and R. F. Kibler, *J. Neurochem.*, **6**, 254 (1961)
252. U. K. Rinne, V. Sonninen and J. Palo, *Psychiat. Neurol., Basel*, **151**, 321 (1966)
253. A. Barbeau, *Neurology, Minneap.*, **10**, 446 (1960)
254. G. Curzon and I. Wald, *Clin. Chim. Acta*, **8**, 893 (1963)
255. G. W. Bruyn, *In* Handbook of Clinical Neurology (P. J. Vinken and G. W. Bruyn, eds), **6**, 298. North Holland, Amsterdam (1968)
256. O. Hornykiewicz, *In* Monoamines et Noyaux Gris Central (J. de Ajuriaguerra and G. Gauthier, eds) (in press)
257. E. J. W. Gumpert, D. M. Sharpe and G. Curzon (in press)

258. N. H. Cohen, *J. nerv. ment. Dis.*, 134, 62 (1962)
259. H. Pakkenberg, *Acta neurol. scand.*, 44, 391 (1968)
260. M. A. Dalby, *Br. med. J.*, ii, 422 (1969)
261. W. A. G. MacCallum, *Br. med. J.*, i, 760 (1970)
262. R. Fog and H. Pakkenberg, *Acta neurol. scand.*, 46, 249 (1970)
263. G. Curzon, B. D. Kantamaneni, E. J. W. Gumpert and D. M. Sharpe (in press)
264. D. K. Clark, C. H. Markham and W. G. Clark, Abst. 2nd Int. Cong. Neurogenetics, 40 (1967)
265. M. Sandler and M. B. H. Youdim, *Nature (Lond.)*, 217, 771 (1968)
266. I. J. Kopin and V. K. Weise, *Biochem. Pharmac.*, 17, 1461 (1968)
267. C. A. Soutar, *Br. med. J.*, iv, 55 (1970)
268. W. Birkmayer and M. Mentasti, *Arch. Psychiat. Nervkrankh.*, 210, 29 (1967)
269. S. Spector, A. Sjoerdsma and S. Udenfriend, *J. Pharmac.*, 147, 86 (1965)
270. C. H. Markham, W. G. Clark and W. D. Winters, *Life Sciences*, 9, 697 (1963)
271. T. L. Sourkes, G. F. Murphy, I. Sankoff, M. H. Wiseman-Distler and S. Saint-Cyr, *J. Neurochem.*, 10, 947 (1963)
272. C. C. Porter, D. E. Titus, B. E. Sanders and E. V. C. Smith, *Science*, 126, 1014 (1957)
273. G. Curzon, *Biochem. J.*, 79, 656 (1961)
274. R. P. P. Warner and I. Sternlieb, *J. Lab. clin. Med.*, 67, 934 (1966)
275. J. P. Morgan, T. J. Preziosi and J. R. Bianchine, *Lancet*, ii, 659 (1970)
276. A. Barbeau and H. Friesen, *Lancet*, i, 1180 (1970)
277. M. S. Ebadi, R. Bostad and R. J. Pellegrino, *J. Neurol. Neurosurg. Psychiat.*, 32, 393 (1969)
278. M. S. Ebadi, R. L. Russell and E. E. McCoy, *J. Neurochem.*, 15, 659 (1968)
279. M. Coleman, *In* The Torsion Dystonias (R. Eldridge, ed.), *Supplement to Neurology, Minneap.*, 20, 114 (1970)
280. M. Bazelon, A. Barnet, A. Lodge and S. S. Shelburne, *Brain*, 11, 397 (1968)
281. M. Bazelon, R. S. Paine, V. A. Cowie, P. Hunt, J. C. Houck and D. Mahanand, *Lancet*, i, 1130 (1967)
282. F. Rosner, B. H. Ong, R. S. Paine and D. Mahanand, *Lancet*, i, 1191 (1965)
283. J. Tu and H. Zellwerger, *Lancet*, ii, 715 (1965)
284. B. Frame, *Archs. intern. Med.*, 116, 424 (1965)
285. M. Sandler, F. Karoum and C. R. J. Ruthven, *Lancet*, ii, 770 (1970)
286. H. Stevens, *Archs. Neurol.*, 12, 311 (1965)
287. W. E. Bunney and J. M. Davis, *Archs gen. Psychiat.*, 13, 483 (1965)
288. O. Lingjaerde, *Acta psychiat. scand.*, 39, Suppl. 170 (1963)
289. P. O. Ganrot, E. Rosengren and C. G. Gottfries, *Experientia*, 18, 260 (1962)
290. C. M. B. Pare, *Biochem. J.*, 121, 36P (1971)

291. G. Curzon, *In* Biochemical Aspects of Neurological Disorders. 3rd series (J. N. Cumings and M. Kremer, eds), p. 82. Blackwell, Oxford (1968)
292. R. I. Katz, T. N. Chase and I. J. Kopin, *Science*, 162, 466 (1968)
293. H. Corrodi, K. Fuxe and M. Schou, *Life Sciences*, 8, 643 (1969)
294. M. H. Sheard and G. K. Aghajanian, *Life Sciences*, 9, 285 (1970)
295. M. I. Paul, B. R. Ditzion and D. S. Janowsky, *Lancet*, i, 88 (1970)
296. Y. H. Abdullah and K. Hamadah, *Lancet*, i, 378 (1970)
297. D. Eccleston, R. Loose, I. A. Pullar and R. F. Sugden, *Lancet*, ii, 612 (1970)
298. G. A. Robison, A. J. Coppen, P. C. Whybrow and A. J. Prange, *Lancet*, ii, 1028 (1970)
299. J. Häggendahl and M. Lindquist, *Acta physiol. scand.*, 60, 351 (1964)
300. S. S. Kety, *Science*, 132, 1861 (1960)
301. A. J. Coppen, *Br. J. Psychiat.*, 113, 1237 (1967)
302. A. J. Mandell and C. E. Spooner, *Science*, 162, 1442 (1969)
303. J. M. Davis, *Int. Rev. Neurobiol.*, 12, 145 (1970)
304. C. M. B. Pare and M. Sandler, *J. Neurol. Neurosurg. Psychiat.*, 22, 247 (1959)
305. H. M. Van Praag and B. Leijnse, *Psychopharmacologia*, 4, 1 (1963)
306. J. J. Burgermeister, P. Dick, G. Garrone, M. Guggisberg and M. Tissot, *Pr. med.*, 71, 1116 (1963)
307. A. J. Coppen, *In* Brain Chemistry and Mental Disease (B. T. Ho and W. M. McIsaac, eds), p. 123. Plenum Press, New York and London (1971)
308. D. M. Shaw, F. E. Camps and E. G. Eccleston, *Br. J. Psychiat.*, 113, 1407 (1967)
309. C. M. B. Pare, D. P. H. Yeung, K. Price and R. S. Stacey, *Lancet*, ii, 133 (1969)
310. A. Coppen, D. M. Shaw and J. P. Farrell, *Lancet*, i, 79 (1963)
311. C. M. B. Pare, *Lancet*, ii, 527 (1963)
312. A. Coppen, D. M. Shaw, B. Herzberg and R. Maggs, *Lancet*, ii, 1178 (1967)
313. A. Glassman and S. R. Platman, *J. Psychiat. Res.*, 7, 63 (1969)
314. W. G. Dewhurst, *Nature (Lond.)*, 218, 1130 (1968)
315. H. Weil-Malherbe, *Lancet*, ii, 219 (1968)
316. W. G. Dewhurst, *Lancet*, ii, 514 (1968)
317. W. G. Dewhurst, *Br. J. Psychiat.*, 116, 569 (1970)
318. G. Curzon, *Br. J. Psychiat.*, 116, 571 (1970)
319. A. Coppen, D. M. Shaw, A. Malleson, E. Eccleston and G. Gundy, *Br. J. Psychiat.*, 111, 993 (1965)
320. W. G. Dewhurst, *In* Studies in Psychiatry (M. Shepherd and D. L. Davies, eds), p. 289. Oxford (1968)
321. N. S. Kline, W. Sacks and G. M. Simpson, *Am. J. Psychiat.*, 121, 379 (1964)
322. A. T. B. Moir and D. Eccleston, *J. Neurochem.*, 15, 1093 (1968)
323. A. Coppen and R. Noguera, *Lancet*, i, 1111 (1970)
324. B. J. Carroll, R. M. Mowbray and B. Davies, *Lancet*, i, 967 (1970)

325. D. M. Shaw, *Lancet*, i, 1111 (1970)
326. W. H. Wunner, J. Bell and H. N. Munro, *Biochem. J.*, 101, 417 (1966)
327. G. Curzon and P. K. Bridges, *J. Neurol. Neurosurg. Psychiat.*, 33, 698 (1970)
328. W. E. Knox and V. H. Auerbach, *Br. J. exp. Path.*, 32, 462 (1951)
329. J. L. Gibbons and P. R. McHugh, *J. Psychiat. Res.*, 1, 162 (1962)
330. D. T. Fullerton, F. J. Wenzel, F. N. Lohrenz and H. Fahs, *Archs gen. Psychiat.*, 19, 674 (1968)
331. D. T. Fullerton, F. J. Wenzel, F. N. Lohrenz and H. Fahs, *Archs gen. Psychiat.*, 19, 682 (1968)
332. D. J. McClure, *J. psychosom. Res.*, 10, 189 (1966)
333. P. K. Bridges and M. T. Jones, *Br. J. Psychiat.*, 112, 1257 (1966)
334. R. J. Doig, R. V. Mummery, M. R. Willis and A. Elkes, *Br. J. Psychiat.*, 112, 1263 (1966)
335. M. S. Knapp, P. M. Keane and J. G. Wright, *Br. med. J.*, ii, 27 (1967)
336. P. W. P. Butler and G. M. Besser, *Lancet*, i, 1234 (1968)
337. B. J. Carroll, *Br. med. J.*, 3, 27 (1969)
338. E. J. Sachar, *Archs gen. Psychiat.*, 17, 544 (1967)
339. B. W. L. Brooksbank and A. Coppen, *Br. J. Psychiat.*, 113, 395 (1967)
340. I. P. Lapin and G. F. Oxenkrug, *Lancet*, i, 132 (1969)
341. G. Curzon, *Br. J. Psychiat.*, 115, 1367 (1969)
342. G. Curzon and A. R. Green, *Life Sciences*, 7, 657 (1969)
343. G. Curzon and A. R. Green, *Br. J. Pharmac.*, 37, 689 (1969)
344. A. R. Green and G. Curzon, *Nature (Lond.)*, 220, 1095 (1968)
345. T. L. Sourkes, K. Missala and M. Oravec, *J. Neurochem.*, 17, 111 (1970)
346. U. Scapagnini, P. Preziosi and A. de Schaepdryêr, *Pharmac. Res. Commun.*, 1, 63 (1969)
347. G. Nistico and P. Preziosi, *Pharmac. Res. Commun.*, 1, 363 (1969)
348. W. Kostowski, E. Giacalone, S. Garattini and L. Valzelli, *Eur. J. Pharmac.*, 4, 37 (1968)
349. J. F. Brody, *Psychopharmacologia*, 17, 14, (1970)
350. R. Rodnight, *Int. Rev. Neurobiol.*, 3, 251 (1961)
351. D. P. Rose, *Clin. Sci.*, 31, 265 (1966)
352. G. Nistico and P. Preziosi, *Lancet*, ii, 213 (1970)
353. P. A. Toseland and S. A. Price, *Br. med. J.*, i, 777 (1969)
354. M. J. Baumblatt and F. Winston, *Lancet*, i, 832 (1970)
355. A. R. Green, M. H. Joseph and G. Curzon, *Lancet*, i, 1288 (1970)
356. H. Weil-Malherbe and R. Ström-Olsen, *J. ment. Sci.*, 104, 696 (1958)
357. J. Dawson and A. Bone, *Br. J. Psychiat.*, 109, 629 (1963)
358. R. Takahashi, Y. Nagao, K. Tsuchiya, M. Takamizawa, T. Kobayashi, M. Toru, K. Kobayashi and T. Kariya, *J. Psychiat. Res.*, 6, 185 (1968)
359. F. H. Messiha, D. Agallianos and C. Clower, *Nature (Lond.)*, 225, 868 (1970)
360. J. Häggendal and B. Werdinius, *Acta physiol. scand.*, 66, 223 (1966)

361. J. W. Maas, T. Fawcett and H. Dekirmenjian, *Arch. gen. Psychiat.*, 19, 129 (1968)
362. R. Takahashi, H. Utena, Y. Machiyama, M. Kurihara, T. Otsuka, T. Nakamura and H. Kanamura, *Life Sciences*, 7, 1219 (1968)
363. R. Takahashi, Abst. 7th Meeting, Coll. Int. Neuropsychopharmac., 425 (1970)
364. A. Carlsson, M. Lindquist and T. Magnusson, *Nature (Lond.)*, 180, 1200 (1957)
365. R. Degwitz, R. Frowein, C. Kulenkampff and V. Mohs, *Klin. Wschr.*, 38, 120 (1960)
366. V. C. G. Ingvarsson, *Arzneimittel-Forsch.*, 15, 849 (1965)
367. N. Mattusek, H. Pohlmeier and E. Ruther, *Klin. Wschr.*, 44, 727 (1966)
368. F. K. Goodwin, H. K. Brodie, D. L. Murphy and W. H. Bunney, *Lancet*, i, 908 (1970)
369. D. L. Murphy, H. K. H. Brodie, F. K. Goodwin and W. E. Bunney, *Nature (Lond.)*, 229, 135 (1971)
370. W. E. Bunney, D. L. Murphy, F. K. Goodwin and G. F. Borge, *Lancet*, i, 1022 (1970)
371. J. R. Bueno and H. Himwich, *Psychosomatics*, 8, 82 (1967)
372. F. P. Miller and R. P. Maickel, *Life Sciences*, 8, 487 (1969)
373. A. J. Mandell, *In* Biochemistry of Brain and Memory (S. P. Datta, ed.). Plenum Press, New York (in press)
374. J. R. Smythies, *Neurosciences, Res. Prog. Bull.*, 8, No. 1 (1970)
375. K. Kunz and M. Vojtechovsky, Abst. 7th Meeting. Coll. Int. Neuropsychopharmac., 259 (1970)
376. D. W. Woolley and E. Shaw, *Br. med. J.*, ii, 122 (1954)
377. J. A. Rosecrans, R. A. Lovell and D. X. Freedman, *Biochem. Pharmac.*, 16, 2011 (1967)
378. G. K. Aghajanian, W. E. Foote and M. H. Sheard, *J. Pharmac.*, 171, 178 (1970)
379. H. Osmond, J. Harley-Mason and J. R. Smythies, *J. ment. Sci.*, 98, 309 (1952)
380. A. Hoffer and H. Osmond, *J. nerv. ment. Dis.*, 128, 18 (1959)
381. R. G. Heath, S. Martens, B. E. Leach, M. Cohen and C. Angel, *Am. J. Psychiat.*, 114, 14 (1957)
382. M. K. Horwitt, *Science*, 124, 429 (1956)
383. S. Kety, *Science*, 129, 1590 (1959)
384. H. Tanimukai and H. E. Himwich, *In* Modern Trends in Psychological Medicine (J. H. Price, ed.), 2, p. 78. Butterworth, London (1970)
385. W. Pollin, P. V. Cardon and S. S. Kety, *Science*, 133, 104 (1961)
386. G. G. Brune and H. E. Himwich, *J. nerv. ment. Dis.*, 134, 447 (1962)
387. F. Alexander, G. C. Curtis, H. Sprince and A. P. Crosley, *J. nerv. ment. Dis.*, 137, 135 (1963)
388. A. J. Friedhoff and E. Van Winkle, *Nature (Lond.)*, 194, 897 (1962)
389. R. E. Bourdillon, C. A. Clarke, A. P. Ridges, P. M. Sheppard, P. Harper and S. A. Leslie, *Nature (Lond.)*, 208, 453 (1965)
390. A. A. Boulton and C. A. Felton, *Nature (Lond.)*, 211, 1404 (1966)

391. C. R. Creveling and J. W. Daly, *Nature (Lond.)*, 216, 190 (1967)
392. Anonymous, *Lancet*, ii, 848 (1966)
393. P. H. Connell, Amphetamine Psychosis. Chapman and Hall, London (1958)
394. J. Axelrod, *Neurosciences res. Prog. Bull.*, 8, 16 (1970)
395. W. E. Foote, M. H. Sheard and G. K. Aghajanian, *Nature (Lond.)*, 222, 567 (1969)
396. J. Barchas, F. Da Costa and S. Spector, *Nature (Lond.)*, 214, 919 (1967)
397. P. K. Gessner and I. H. Page, *Am. J. Physiol.*, 203, 167 (1962)
398. S. Szara, *In* Amines and Schizophrenia (H. F. Himwich, ed.), p. 441. Pergamon, London (1967)
399. J. Axelrod, *J. Pharmac.*, 138, 28 (1962)
400. H. Tanimukai, *J. Chromatog.*, 30, 155 (1967)
401. H. Tanimukai, R. Ginther, J. Spaide, J. R. Bueno and H. E. Himwich, *Life Sciences*, 6, 1697 (1967)
402. A. Faurbye and K. Pind, *Nature (Lond.)*, 220, 489 (1968)
403. H. E. Himwich, N. Narasimhachari, B. Heller, J. Spaide, L. Haskovec, M. Fujimori and K. Tabushi, *In* Biochemistry of Brain and Memory (S. P. Datta, ed.). Plenum Press, New York (in press)
404. H. H. Berlet, J. Spaide, H. Kohl, C. Bull and H. E. Himwich, *J. nerv. ment. Dis.*, 140, 297 (1965)
405. C. M. B. Pare, M. Sandler and R. S. Stacey, *Lancet*, i, 551 (1957)
406. C. M. B. Pare, M. Sandler and R. S. Stacey, *Archs. Dis. Childh.*, 34, 422 (1959)
407. C. M. McKean, S. M. Schanberg and N. J. Giarman, *Science*, 157, 213 (1967)
408. L. S. Penrose, *Lancet*, ii, 192 (1935)
409. T. A. Munro, *Ann. Eugen.*, 14, 60 (1947)
410. R. T. C. Pratt, D. Gardiner, G. Curzon, M. F. Piercy and J. N. Cumings, *Br. J. Psychiat.*, 109, 624 (1963)
411. E. Geller and A. Yuwiler, *J. Neurochem.*, 14, 725 (1967)
412. P. S. V. Ramanamurthy and S. G. Srikantia, *J. Neurochem.*, 17, 27 (1970)
413. J. H. Menkes, *Pediatrics*, 23, 348 (1959)
414. C. Gopalan and S. G. Srikantia, *Lancet*, i, 954 (1960)
415. K. Yamaguchi, M. Schimoyama and R. K. Gholson, *Biochim. biophys. Acta*, 146, 102 (1967)
416. L. A. Hersov and R. Rodnight, *J. Neurol. Neurosurg. Psychiat.*, 23, 40 (1960)
417. M. D. Milne, M. A. Crawford, C. B. Girao and L. W. Loughridge, *Q. Jl. Med.*, 29, 407 (1960)
418. H. Green and J. L. Sawyer, *Proc. Soc. exp. Biol. Med.*, 104, 153 (1960)
419. R. D. Eastham and J. Jancar, Clinical Pathology in Mental Retardation. Wright, Bristol (1968)
420. P. H. Wender, *Lancet*, ii, 1012 (1969)
421. A. Pletscher, *Br. J. Pharmac.*, 32, 1 (1968)
422. H. S. Sudak and J. W. Maas, *Science*, 146, 418 (1964)

423. C. G. Gottfries, I. Gottfries and B. E. Roos, *Br. J. Psychiat.*, 115, 563 (1969)

424. C. G. Gottfries, I. Gottfries and B. E. Roos, *Acta psychiat. scand.*, 46, 99 (1970)

425. A. M. Ostfeld, The Common Headache Syndrome, Thomas Springfield, Illinois (1962)

426. R. W. Kimball and A. P. Friedman, *Recent Advances in Biol. Psych.*, 3, 200 (1961)

427. D. A. Curran and J. W. Lance, *J. Neurol. Neurosurg. Psychiat.*, 27, 463 (1964)

428. C. A. Keele, *In* Background to Migraine, 1st Migraine Symposium (R. A. Smith, ed.), p. 126. Heinemann, London (1967)

429. F. Sicuteri, A. Testi and B. Anselmi, *Int. Archs. Allergy*, 19, 55 (1961)

430. F. Sicuteri, *Triangle (En.)*, 6, 116 (1963)

431. D. A. Curran, H. Hinterberger and J. W. Lance, *Brain*, 88, 997 (1965)

432. G. Curzon, P. Theaker and B. Phillips, *J. Neurol. Neurosurg. Psychiat.*, 29, 85 (1966)

433. D. A. Campbell, K. M. Hay and E. M. Tonks, *Br. med. J.*, ii, 1424 (1951)

434. G. Bertaccini and G. Baronio, *Archs. int. Pharmacodyn.*, 155, 57 (1965)

435. V. Erspamer and G. Bertaccini, *Archs. int. Pharmacodyn.*, 137, 6 (1962)

436. E. Bülbring and R. C. Y. Lin, *J. Physiol.*, 140, 381 (1958)

437. B. Adams, *Lancet*, i, 207 (1960)

438. A. M. Ostfeld, *J. Am. Med. Ass.*, 174, 1188 (1960)

439. R. W. Kimball, A. P. Friedman and E. Vallejo, *Neurology, Minneap.*, 10, 107 (1960)

440. M. Anthony, H. Hinterberger and J. W. Lance, *Archs. Neurol.*, 16, 544 (1967)

441. H. Hinterberger, M. Anthony and M. K. Vagholkar, *Clin. Sci.*, 34, 271 (1968)

442. G. Curzon, M. Barrie and M. I. P. Wilkinson, *J. Neurol. Neurosurg. Psychiat.*, 32, 555 (1969)

443. S. Campus, F. Fabris, A. Rappelli, L. Gastaldi, V. Gai and G. Nattero, *Boll. Soc. ital. biol. sper.*, 43, 1844 (1967)

444. E. Hanington, M. Horn and M. Wilkinson, *In* Background to Migraine, 3rd Migraine Symposium (A. L. Cochrane, ed.), p. 113. Heinemann, London (1970)

445. E. Hanington, *Br. med. J.*, ii, 550 (1967)

446. O. Sjaastad and P. Stensrud, *Acta Neurol. scand.*, 47, 120 (1971)

447. M. B. H. Youdim, S. Bonham-Carter, M. Sandler, E. Hanington and M. Wilkinson, *Nature (Lond.)*, 230, 127 (1971)

448. I. Smith, A. H. Kellow, P. E. Mullen and E. Hanington, *Nature (Lond.)*, 230, 246 (1971)

449. M. Barrie and A. Jowett, *Brain*, 90, 785 (1967)

CHAPTER 6

Biochemical Neurological Disease in Children

L. I. WOOLF

6.1 INTRODUCTION

Biochemical disease involves a departure from the normal in some body component, e.g. an enzyme, a structural protein or a membrane transport mechanism. Some biochemical diseases are almost entirely environmental in origin, e.g. lead encephalopathy, but at present attention is largely directed to genetically determined conditions—the inborn errors of metabolism and other molecular diseases. In some cases it is the interaction between genotype and external environment which brings about the signs and symptoms, in others, such as the gangliosidoses, no modification of the external environment can appreciably alter the course of the disease.

Structural genes are coded for the polypeptides which compose the body's proteins. Substitution of one purine or pyrimidine base by another on the DNA constituting a structural gene results in a change in the polypeptide, e.g. a different amino acid residue at a particular point on the chain. Base substitution on the DNA does not necessarily have this result—since the genetic code is degenerate, base substitution can result in a triplet coded for the same amino acid(though not necessarily the same transfer RNA) or it may result in a chain terminator triplet leading to cutting short the normal polypeptide chain. Other mutation mechanisms exist, they also lead to production of a structurally abnormal protein or failure to produce normal amounts of the protein. If the protein in question is an enzyme, substitution of one amino acid for another may have little effect on its catalytic properties if the substitution is far from the active site, but, if near the active site, such substitution may affect affinity for substrate, cofactor or product, turnover rate, pH dependency, stability and sensitivity to inhibitors. Very often the result is complete loss of enzymic properties. Membrane transport mechanisms depend on proteins that, to some extent, resemble enzymes and the effects of mutation of the relevant genes are similar.

If the mutant gene is on an autosome, most often the individual will have a normal allele on the homologous chromosome and will be able to biosynthesize the normal enzyme etc. at half the normal rate. Very often, such a heterozygote suffers no ill effects and his heterozygosity can be detected, if at all, only by refined biochemical techniques. However, a homozygote for the mutant gene will lack the enzyme or membrane transport mechanism either wholly or, where the mutant gene is coded for a modified or reduced amount of enzyme etc., partly. This deficiency can bring about disease. Enzymic activity is partly determined by such factors as membrane attachment and metabolic paths involving feed-back control loops—the activity of an enzyme can be modified by a mutation not directly affecting the structural gene or genes coded for the enzyme.

Deficiency in a transport mechanism will, in most of the conditions so far studied, result in failure of the renal tubules to reabsorb specific substances from the glomerular filtrate or failure to absorb specific substances from the gut. The clinical effects vary with the substance and site involved but these conditions naturally do not affect the foetus and are often harmless after birth. On the other hand, a deficiency of a mechanism transporting an essential nutrient into all the cells would probably be incompatible with even brief intra-uterine life and it is not surprising that such inborn errors of metabolism have not yet been recognized.

The clinical effects of an inborn error of metabolism, and the time course of any disease caused, depend on the nature of the defect and, to some extent, the external environment. Absence of L-xylulose reductase causes accumulation of L-xylulose which is excreted in the urine [1]. Pentosuria is, as far as is known, a completely harmless biochemical abnormality, L-xylulose being non-toxic and xylitol not being an essential substance. In contrast, absence of hexosaminidase-A prevents the degradation of gangliosides beyond the stage of G_{M2}—monosialoceramide trihexoside—and this, being non-diffusible, steadily accumulates in the neurones in the course of their metabolism, interfering with their functions and causing Tay-Sachs' disease [2].

The mechanism by which deficiency of some intraneuronal enzymes bring about neurological disease is easy to understand even where not all the steps are as yet clear. In the case where the defective enzyme is normally found only in, say, the liver, the link with neurological disease can be more obscure. This problem of pathogenesis is now one of the major areas of research in inborn errors of metabolism.

Lack of an enzyme causes a metabolic block, i.e. the normal substrate of the missing enzyme accumulates. If the substrate is non-diffusible, intracellular accumulation occurs in the various tissues at a rate related to the normal rate of degradation or other metabolic change of the substrate in the respective tissues. If the substrate is diffusible, it will tend to distribute itself among the body fluids and tissues, though not necessarily evenly, and the total body content of the substrate will rise, often enormously. A non-diffusible substrate will in general start to accumulate in the tissues before birth, but a diffusible substrate crosses the placenta and, provided the mother does not entirely lack the enzyme, is metabolized in the maternal tissues. Few substances are metabolized by a single route even though this may normally account for almost the whole metabolism of the substance. If the main path is blocked by lack of the relevant enzyme, the consequent rise in concentration of the substrate causes normally minor side reactions to proceed at an appreciable rate, in some cases producing large amounts of what are normally very minor metabolites. The most fruitful theory of pathogenesis, in those neurological diseases where a non-C.N.S. enzyme is deficient, is that the substrate of the missing enzyme or one of the abnormal metabolites is toxic when present in high concentration, affecting the C.N.S. In other cases it seems probable that a diffusible product of the normal enzymic reaction is necessary for normal brain function and is lacking to some extent in the inborn error of metabolism.

As in so much else, our knowledge of inborn errors of metabolism is dependent on the development of appropriate techniques. Paper chromatography of amino acids was introduced in 1944 and, as a direct consequence, we now know of about 70 disorders of amino acid metabolism compared with the four or five recognized before then. Techniques in the fields of carbohydrate, lipid, mucopolysaccharide, purine, pyrimidine, vitamin and mineral metabolism have advanced less rapidly, though the pace is increasing, and we know of fewer metabolic disorders in each of these fields. All inborn errors of metabolism are rare and, unless they are associated with some clear clinical entity leading to intensive laboratory investigation, are unlikely to come to light. It is natural, therefore, to concentrate the search for such conditions by investigating people selected for some distinctive clinical feature, e.g. the severely mentally retarded or children with progressive cerebral dysfunction. Many aminoacidopathies were first found in mentally retarded children and there is a natural tendency in each condition to consider the biochemical and clinical features to be causally related. In some cases, e.g. typical phenylketonuria or leucinosis (maple syrup urine disease), this is clearly so, in others, such as cystathioninuria or hyperprolinaemia, the association is probably fortuitous. The discovery of clinically normal individuals with, say, histidinaemia does not exclude the possibility that the neurological features in the cases first described were caused by the biochemical abnormality—it would be necessary to determine the frequency of occurrence of the metabolic error in the sick and the well before a conclusion could be reached; for several rare conditions this is not yet possible. The general principles are best illustrated by considering a few specific conditions: galactosaemia, fructose intolerance, homocystinuria, phenylketonuria, leucinosis (maple syrup urine disease), disorders of the urea cycle, hyperglycinaemia, Hartnup disease, hyperuricaemia with neurological signs (Lesch-Nyhan syndrome) and Leigh's encephalopathy.

6.2 GENETICS

In the great majority of cases, a heterozygote for a mutant gene will show no clinical abnormality and only subtle biochemical differences from normal, i.e. almost all inborn errors of metabolism are inherited as recessive characters, either autosomal or sex-linked. In the few dominantly inherited conditions either the residual enzyme or transport mechanism, generally 50% of normal, is not adequate to meet normal metabolic demands (e.g. renal glucosuria in which the maximum rate of renal tubular reabsorption of glucose is not sufficient to prevent some spill over) or some feedback control of enzyme activity is lacking, e.g. in acute intermittent porphyria where the amount of δ-aminolaevulinic synthetase in the liver may be seven times the normal on occasions.

If we assume that between 1/60 and 1/300 of the total genes at a given locus have undergone mutation in a given population, then the former figure would correspond to one affected homozygote in 3,600 live births and the latter to one in 90,000; the social consequences would be very different. Inborn errors of metabolism causing neurological disease have a low or very low overall incidence, though one or other may be more frequent in a particular geographical area and/or ethnic group. These pockets of high incidence of diseases which are lethal or severely disabling are best explained by balanced polymorphisms but, with one or two exceptions, the nature of the balancing heterozygote advantage is unknown. Of the conditions considered here, phenylketonuria is the least rare with an incidence of between 1 : 14,000 and 1 : 20,000 live births in Britain and North America. The distribution is however uneven, the incidence in Southern Ireland and West Scotland, and in those of Irish or West Scottish descent, being 1 : 4,000, possibily even higher in Yemenite Jews, but only 1 : 60,000 in Japan and virtually zero among Ashkenazi Jews [3, 4, 5]. At the other extreme, only a single case of valinaemia has as yet been described.

When a child is affected with a biochemical neurological disease, the parents and other relatives often seek advice on the chances of further children being affected. The genetic counsellor must be certain of the diagnosis (including, in some cases, the biochemical variant involved) and mode of inheritance if he is to perform the difficult and delicate task of advising the parents. In the case of siblings and other relatives of a child with a recessively inherited condition, the question arises of their own and their spouses' carrier status; for a growing number of conditions more or less reliable tests for heterozygosity are available. These tests depend on direct enzyme assay in biopsy specimens, leucocytes or fibroblasts grown in tissue culture, on the results of loading doses of the substrate of the deficient enzyme or, in some X-linked conditions, on the demonstration of two clones of cells. Recently amniocentesis has added a new weapon: examination of cells in the amniotic fluid obtained at, say, the 14th week can, in a growing number of conditions, reveal whether the foetus lacks the relevant enzyme, i.e. whether the infant, if born to term, would suffer from the disease.

6.3 GALACTOSAEMIA [6, 7]

6.3.1 Normal metabolism of galactose [8]

Galactose is normally phosphorylated by ATP acting with galactokinase (EC 2.7.1.6) to give galactose-1-phosphate (Gal-1-P). Gal-1-P reacts with uridine-diphosphoglucose (UDPG) to give uridine-diphosphogalactose (UDPGal) and glucose-1-phosphate (G-1-P), the reaction being catalysed by Gal-1-P-uridyl transferase (EC 2.7.7.12). UDPGal is acted on by epimerase (EC 5.1.3.2) to yield UDPG which can form glycogen or take part in other reactions as a reactive form of glucose.

$$\text{Galactose} \underset{1}{\overset{\rightarrow}{}} \text{Gal-1-P} \underset{2}{\overset{\rightleftharpoons}{}} \text{UDPGal} \underset{3}{\overset{\rightleftharpoons}{}} \text{UDPG}$$

All three enzymes are present in many if not all cells, including erythrocytes, though most galactose is metabolized in the liver.

6.3.2 The metabolic defect in galactosaemia

In galactosaemia Gal-1-P-uridyl transferase (EC 2.7.7.12) is absent or inactive; therefore reaction 2 cannot proceed and Gal-1-P accumulates in the tissues [9, 10]. Although reaction 1 is formally irreversible, accumulation of Gal-1-P tends to inhibit galactokinase, leading to accumulation of galactose, and Gal-1-P, if not metabolized by other paths, is slowly converted to galactose and inorganic phosphate. The characteristic biochemical picture is of high concentrations of galactose in plasma and urine (sometimes 1,000 mg/100 ml or more) and a high intracellular concentration of Gal-1-P, e.g. 100 mg per 100 ml packed erythrocytes.

A number of secondary reactions occur as a consequence of the high concentrations of galactose and Gal-1-P in the body fluids and tissues. Some galactose is reduced to galactitol by aldose reductase and NADPH; galactitol is not metabolized but tends to accumulate in certain tissues, notably the brain (e.g. 20 μmole per g), lens of the eye (e.g. 2.5 μmole per g) and skeletal muscle (e.g. 16 μmole per g) as well as being excreted in the urine (say 200 mg per 100 ml) [11]. Other metabolic pathways are known though their relative importance (and even the existence of some) has been questioned. Gal-1-P reacts with UTP in the presence of a UDPGal pyrophosphorylase to yield UDPGal [12]

$$Gal\text{-}1\text{-}P + UTP \rightleftharpoons UDPGal + PP$$

The enzyme is present in very low concentrations at birth, but the amount in liver and brain increases with time and this reaction may account for up to 15% of normal galactose metabolism. The existence of a pentose shunt,

$$Gal\text{-}1\text{-}P \rightleftharpoons Gal\text{-}6\text{-}P \rightarrow 6\text{-}P\text{-galactonic acid} \rightarrow D\text{-xylulose}$$

has been claimed [13], but doubt has been thrown on the existence of a specific Gal-6-P dehydrogenase [14].

Gal-1-P is acted on by phosphoglucomutase to produce Gal-6-P [15]. The affinity of Gal-1-P for the enzyme is high, but the turnover rate is only 1/400 of the conversion of glucose-1-phosphate to glucose-6-phosphate; in consequence Gal-1-P is a potent competitive inhibitor of phosphoglucomutase [9, 16, 17]. There is some evidence that other enzymes are inhibited by Gal-1-P. The inhibition of phosphoglucomutase may be the cause of the hypoglucosaemia since this enzyme is necessary for the release of glucose from glycogen.

6.3.3 Clinical consequences and treatment

Onset of symptoms is usually very early, the infant failing to thrive within a few weeks or months of birth. Vomiting and/or diarrhoea and jaundice are commonly seen. Some neonates present with a fulminating form of the disease and die in liver failure within a few weeks. The survivors usually have some degree of hepatic cirrhosis, bilateral cataracts and renal tubular dysfunction.

Mental retardation is the only neurological feature described. Usually this is only moderately severe, e.g. I.Q. 40 to 60. This may be because in galactosaemia the brain is a less important target organ than, say, the liver or may be because only the less severely affected survive. The pathogenesis of the mental retardation is uncertain. No morphological abnormality of the brain has been found at autopsy. This is in contrast to the chick which, if fed a high galactose diet, undergoes clinically and histologically demonstrable damage to the basal ganglia [18, 19]. If damage to the infant's liver leads to a high enough concentration of free bilirubin in the blood, kernicterus may develop with its characteristic clinical features. Although the concentration of glucose in the blood is rather low, the symptoms and signs of galactosaemia do not resemble hypoglycaemia. It seems probable that Gal-1-P accumulating within the brain cells is the toxic substance, though the mechanism of its action is unknown.

Gal-1-P is very probably also the toxic substance responsible for the renal tubular dysfunction—perhaps by interfering with the bioenergetics of the epithelial cells; this may also be the mechanism of liver damage. Gal-1-P, once formed within a cell, does not readily cross the plasma membrane, hence the intracellular accumulation of Gal-1-P in galactosaemia, even *in utero* if the mother drinks milk during pregnancy and galactose is therefore present in the maternal and foetal circulations. This accounts for the low birth weight of galactosaemics and for those patients born with evidence of liver damage and cataracts.

The cataracts in galactosaemia seem to be associated with the accumulation of galactitol in the lens [11]. Galactitol is formed from galactose within the lens fibres and diffuses out only slowly; the resulting osmotic effect may disrupt the fibres. It is also possible that, in the reduction of galactose to galactitol, the oxidation-reduction balance (e.g. content of reduced gluta-thione) is altered, resulting in damage to the lens fibre.

Treatment with a diet free from sources of galactose, if started in earliest infancy, usually completely prevents the hepatic cirrhosis, cataracts, and renal tubular dysfunction which are otherwise inevitable. The I.Q. usually stays within the normal range though in a proportion of cases, in spite of effective treatment instituted early, the child is to some extent retarded. These cases pull the mean I.Q. of treated cases down to 91 compared to 110 for their unaffected siblings [20]. The school performance seems, at least in some cases, to be poorer than is suggested by the I.Q., particularly in mathematics and spatial relations, and some children show ill-defined "behaviour disorders" [20]. These findings, and the children of lower I.Q., may reflect prenatal damage to the brain by Gal-1-P. The mother of a galactosaemic child should take a galactose-free diet during subsequent pregnancies.

6.3.4 Variant forms of galactosaemia

In the so-called "negro variant" of galactosaemia, clinical manifestations are confined to infancy and are sometimes mild or completely absent. The adult, given a test dose of ^{14}C-galactose, produces $^{14}CO_2$ at the same rate as a normal individual and about eight times as fast as a typical galactosaemic [21]. Yet the erythrocytes contain no Gal-1-P uridyl transferase. Much speculation of alternative metabolic paths was ended by the demonstration that liver biopsy specimens from these individuals appeared to metabolize galactose by the normal route at about 75% of the normal rate [21]. Individuals have also been described with normal erythrocyte Gal-1-P uridyl transferase but very marked galactose intolerance [22]. It seems probable that the hepatic and erythrocyte enzymes are, to some extent, under separate genetic control.

The Duarte gene [23] does not lead to disease but to a qualitatively altered erythrocyte Gal-1-P uridyl transferase with about half the normal activity and different electrophoretic properties. Other genes coded for qualitatively different Gal-1-P uridyl transferases are known; some lead to disease, e.g. when the enzyme has low stability.

In the "Swiss variant", better termed galactokinase deficiency, reaction 1 is blocked [24]. Hence galactose accumulates but Gal-1-P does not. Galactose and galactitol are excreted in the urine accompanied by some glucose, presumably from competition for renal tubular reabsorption sites. There is no mental retardation or other evidence of neurological disease. The liver and kidneys are unaffected. Affected individuals develop, as the only clinical manifestation, cataracts indistinguishable from those of galactosaemia.

6.4 FRUCTOSE INTOLERANCE

6.4.1 Metabolism of fructose

This normally proceeds as follows:

$$
\begin{array}{llll}
& & & \text{Glyceraldehyde} \\
\text{Fructose} \xrightarrow{1} & \text{Fructose-1-P} \xrightarrow{2} & & + \\
& & & \text{Dihydroxyacetone} \quad\Big)\, 3 \\
\text{Fructose-6-P} \xleftarrow{5} & \text{Fructose-1,6-diP} \xrightleftharpoons{4} & & + \\
{}_{6}\Updownarrow & & & \text{Glyceraldehyde-3-P} \\
\text{Glucose-6-P} \xrightarrow{7} & \text{Glucose} & &
\end{array}
$$

Reactions 1 to 7 take place in the liver and form the major route by which dietary fructose is metabolized; other, minor, reactions take place in other tissues. Reaction 1 is catalysed by fructose kinase (EC 2.7.1.4) and reaction 2 by fructose-1-phosphate aldolase.

In fructose intolerance, liver fructose-1-phosphate aldolase is inactive [25, 26], an altered enzyme with a much higher K_m being biosynthesized (at least in some cases [27]), and, in consequence, after ingesting fructose or oligosaccharides hydrolysed to fructose in the gut, fructose-1-phosphate accumulates intracellularly. Fructose-1-phosphate inhibits the conversion of glycogen to glucose; the mechanism is not known but inhibition of phosphorylase and sequestration of inorganic phosphate have both been suggested. There is, in consequence, a profound fall in blood glucose concentration, reaching a minimum about one hour after ingestion of fructose [28]. Since the brain can, for practical purposes, use only glucose, this hypoglucosaemia may cause seizures or loss of consciousness.

An individual with fructose intolerance who knowingly or unknowingly ingests fructose or sucrose almost immediately has alarming symptoms including nausea, severe abdominal pain and sometimes loss of consciousness [29]. These are too rapid in onset to be caused by hypoglucosaemia and probably reflect an effect of fructose on the mucosa of the gut similar to its effect on liver and kidney cells. In the cells of the liver, kidney and, probably, gut, fructose is converted to fructose-1-phosphate which inhibits utilization of the cell's stores of glycogen, i.e. its main source of energy. This leads to cellular dysfunction and, eventually, cell damage. The effects of giving a formula containing sucrose to a neonate or infant lacking fructose-1-phosphate aldolase are failure to thrive, hepatomegaly, jaundice and generalized renal tubular dysfunction [30]. Some die in infancy, but the survivors are often normal. Some cases diagnosed as familial tyrosinaemia may, in reality, have fructose intolerance with very marked hepatic and renal damage leading to death in liver failure or hepatic cirrhosis and the Fanconi syndrome [31].

Treatment consists in giving a diet free from fructose and any fructose-yielding saccharide. Sorbitol must also be avoided. As well as sugar, sweetmeats, cake, honey etc., all fruits and many vegetables must be forbidden. Those who survive infancy develop an aversion from such foods; they have remarkably good teeth. The effect of such dietary restriction is complete normality unless there are already irreversible effects such as brain damage from hypoglucosaemia or hepatic cirrhosis.

Essential fructosuria is an unrelated and completely harmless condition caused by deficiency of fructokinase [32].

6.5 HOMOCYSTINURIA

6.5.1 Methionine metabolism

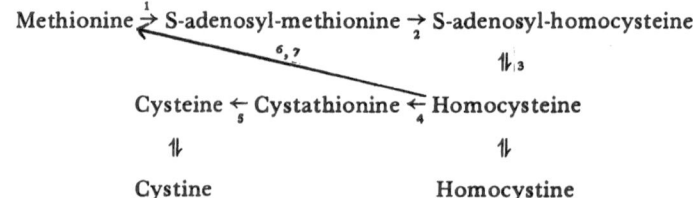

Reaction 4 is catalysed by cystathionine synthase (EC 4.2.1.13), an enzyme widely distributed in the tissues. In homocystinuria, cystathionine synthase is virtually completely absent or inactive in all tissues examined: liver, brain and fibroblasts grown in tissue culture [33]. In some cases 1 to 2% of the normal enzymic activity can be demonstrated, in others no enzymic activity has been found [34]. As a result of the metabolic block, homocysteine accumulates and is partly converted to homocystine, partly to homocysteine-cysteine mixed disulphide and partly S-methylated to methionine by reactions 6 and 7 with, respectively, N^5-methyltetrahydrofolic acid and betaine as methyl donors. In infancy methionine and homocysteine are present in high concentrations in the plasma while homocystine and homocysteine-cysteine mixed disulphide are excreted in the urine; later the concentration of methionine in the plasma drops. Cystathionine is normally present in highest concentration in the cells of the brain, though traces are found elsewhere and in the urine; in homocystinuria no cystathionine can usually be demonstrated in the brain or urine [35]. The body's cysteine and cystine are also largely biosynthesized from methionine, though some is obtained from cysteine and cystine in dietary proteins; in homocystinuria, cysteine/cystine becomes an essential amino acid.

6.5.2 Clinical effects

Between 50 and 60% show mental retardation varying in degree from mild to profound [36]. Epileptic seizures are common in the more severely retarded. There is a generalized disorder of connective tissue causing ectopia lentis, arachnodactyly, unduly tall stature (patients resemble those with Marfan's syndrome) and, probably, some abnormality of the walls of blood vessels. There is also a marked tendency to develop thromboses and, by some tests, the platelets are unusually sticky. These thromboses may lead to pulmonary embolism, the commonest cause of death, or may occur in coronary or cerebral vessels; many homocystinurics die in childhood from one of these causes.

Children with homocystinuria are clinically normal at birth, the various features of the disease appearing over the years.

Ectopia lentis may appear at any time between one month and
eleven years after birth, arachnodactyly and tall stature around
puberty. There occurs, in some cases, dramatically sudden
neurological deterioration; e.g. a boy aged 2½ years and only
very slightly retarded was, by 3½ years of age, a complete
ament having lost all his previous motor skills, ability to
communicate, social training etc. and suffering very frequent
seizures. He died of pulmonary embolism and, at necropsy, no
gross morphological abnormality of the brain was found. There
appears to be a defect in myelination in some cases. Although
the brain lacks cystathionine in homocystinuria, this can be
excluded as the cause of the neurological disease since the
low-methionine diet prevents neurological deterioration but
cannot increase the cystathionine content of the brain. The
normal function of brain cystathionine is obscure.

6.5.3 Treatment

Treatment with a diet low in methionine was introduced in
1966 [37, 38, 39] and is effective in reducing the
concentrations of methionine, homocysteine etc. in the blood
and other body fluids (homocystine and homocysteine are not
normal dietary components). The principles are the same as for
the treatment of phenylketonuria (see below). The diet must
contain adequate amounts of cystine/cysteine, though the
physical growth of homocystinurics suggests that the normal
diet supplies adequate amounts of these amino acids, essential
for homocystinurics. If this treatment is started soon after
birth, the physical signs of homocystinuria do not appear and
the children develop normally. If started later, further
deterioration may be prevented (the treatment is too new for
proper assessment) and the platelets lose their abnormal
stickiness.

Cystathionine synthase has pyridoxal phosphate as cofactor;
a radically different form of treatment was introduced in 1967:
giving pyridoxine at a dosage level of 50 to 200 mg per
day [40]. The concentrations of methionine and homocysteine
in the blood, and of homocystine and homocysteine-cysteine
mixed disulphide in the urine, fell sharply on such treatment in

some cases, about 50% of those investigated [41]. The clinical effects of this simple treatment were, in those patients who responded biochemically, as good as those of the low-methionine diet. These pyridoxine-responsive patients were those who, on liver biopsy or fibroblast culture, showed some residual cystathionine synthase activity—1 to 2% of normal before pyridoxine treatment and 3 to 4% after [33]. It seems that 3% of the normal amount of cystathionine synthase is sufficient to metabolize all the homocysteine normally met with. The response to a methionine load, however, remains abnormal. It seems probable that pyridoxal phosphate derived from pyridoxine increases the stability of the enzyme.

6.6 Phenylketonuria [42, 43]

6.6.1 Phenylalanine metabolism

This normally proceeds as follows:

Phenylalanine $\underset{1}{\rightarrow}$ Tyrosine $\underset{2}{\rightleftharpoons}$ p-Hydroxyphenylpyruvic Acid

$$\downarrow 3$$

$CO_2 + H_2O \underset{5}{\leftarrow} \underset{4}{\leftarrow}$ Homogentisic Acid

Reaction 1, the substitution of a hydroxyl group for hydrogen in the *para* position, involves an enzyme, phenylalanine hydroxylase (EC 1.14.3.1), acting with tetrahydrobiopterin and molecular oxygen to yield tyrosine, quinonoid dihydrobiopterin and water [44]. Catalase and another, unidentified, protein are necessary for full enzymic activity—the reaction mechanism and the structure of phenylalanine hydroxylase are not yet fully understood. A second enzyme, dihydropteridine reductase, catalyses the reduction by NADH of the quinonoid dihydrobiopterin to tetrahydrobiopterin.

In phenylketonuria (typical or "classical" variety) the phenylalanine hydroxylating system is inactive, all the evidence pointing to lack of phenylalanine hydroxylase [45]. As a consequence, phenylalanine accumulates in the tissues and body fluids, reaching concentrations as high as 120 mg per 100 ml plasma (normal ~0.9). The concentration of tyrosine is about

0.6 mg per 100 ml plasma (normal ~1), but it is uncertain to what extent this is the result of failure to synthesize tyrosine rather than an effect of high concentrations of phenylalanine on plasma levels of other amino acids in general [46]. Certainly, the normal diet contains enough tyrosine (an essential amino acid in phenylketonuria) for the body's needs.

The high concentration of phenylalanine in the tissues causes an increase in the rate of reactions such as transamination and decarboxylation which normally account for only 2 to 3% of phenylalanine metabolism (Figure 6.1). In consequence, con-

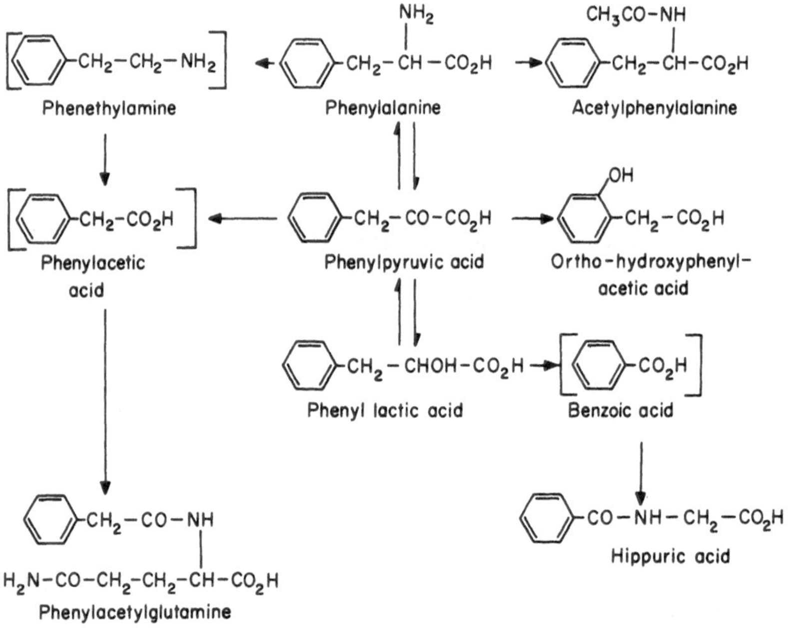

Figure 6.1. Metabolism of phenylalanine in phenylketonuria. Square brackets enclose substances not excreted in the urine. (Courtesy Blackwell, Oxford.)

siderable amounts of phenylpyruvic acid, phenyllactic acid, phenylacetylglutamine, o-hydroxyphenylacetic acid and N-acetylphenylalanine, as well as some minor metabolites, are formed in phenylketonuria and excreted in the urine. There are also disturbances of tyrosine and tryptophan metabolism leading to increased excretion of p-hydroxyphenyllactic acid,

p-hydroxyphenylpyruvic acid, indolyllactic acid, indolylpyruvic acid, indolylacetic acid (free and conjugated) and indoxyl sulphate [47, 48]. The indoxyl sulphate and indolylacetic acid are related to inhibition by phenylalanine of tryptophan absorption from the gut (cf. the Hartnup syndrome), the other substances appear to be truly endogenous.

Phenylketonurics are normal at birth but deteriorate during the first year of life [49]. The most obvious clinical feature of typical phenylketonuria is profound mental retardation, the I.Q. of two-thirds of patients being below 30 and the I.Q. of 98% being below 60 [50]. There are other neurological features: 25% suffer from epilepsy after the age of one year, minor seizures, major seizures or both. Between 90 and 95% of phenylketonurics show an abnormality of the E.E.G., usually a diffuse, irregular spike and wave pattern, in some cases three per second, and, in some younger children, hypsarhythmia [51]. Behavioural abnormalities are seen in almost all—a failure to relate to people, hyperkinesis in some of the less retarded, and meaningless, repetitive gestures in the more severely retarded [52]. An odd shuffling gait is common, particularly in the older patients.

There are few characteristic features outside the C.N.S. The head tends to be small. Hypopigmentation is not very pronounced, but there is on the average less melanin in hair and skin of phenylketonurics than in their age-matched sibs [53]. A few patients suffer from severe eczema. Life expectancy is the same as for other retardates of similar I.Q.

6.6.2 Pathology

Morphologically the brain shows few abnormalities apart from a moderate deficiency of myelin, most easily demonstrated by lipid analysis [54]. In a few brains areas of sudanophil demyelination are seen: these contain cholesterol esters. Leucodystrophy in late adolescence or early adult life is a feature of phenylketonuria seen in a minority [55].

6.6.3 Treatment

This is with a diet low in phenylalanine [42, 43, 49, 56, 57]. The diet must contain enough phenylalanine for synthesis of the body's proteins and also enough additional tyrosine to replace the normal dietary phenylalanine. Several preparations are commercially available. Treatment must always be under strict biochemical control. With these precautions, treated children grow and physically develop normally. If the diet is instituted in early infancy, before any clinical features have appeared, the infant's mind develops normally: the I.Q., once the child is old enough for testing, is normal (mean 95, range 60-130), there are no behavioural disorders, no seizures and the E.E.G. is normal [58]. If started later, after signs of brain damage have appeared, there is usually, though not always, marked improvement within days of starting the diet [59-62]; the behaviour improves dramatically, seizures may stop completely or become much less frequent, and the E.E.G. becomes more nearly normal. Not surprisingly, the I.Q. responds much more slowly, taking perhaps four years to rise by 30 points and, in some cases, showing no significant rise at all. However, even when formal tests show no rise in I.Q., dietary treatment may be worth while for the behavioural improvement.

6.6.4 Pathogenesis

The problem of pathogenesis has received more attention in the case of phenylketonuria than in most other inborn errors of metabolism. As soon as the intoxication theory was put forward, and supporting evidence in the results of dietary treatment accumulated, the search began. Early hypotheses incriminated one or other of the "abnormal" metabolites of phenylalanine, e.g. phenylacetic acid [63], known to affect the C.N.S., o-tyramine [64] (which probably does not occur). Several of these metabolites can inhibit such enzymes as DOPA-decarboxylase, tryptophan hydroxylase and glutamic decarboxylase of brain [65]. In fact, the concentrations of serotonin, noradrenaline and adrenaline in the blood are low in phenylketonuria [65, 66] and some theories of pathogenesis have considered that lack of these and other neurotransmitter substances at the synapses, caused by inhibition of the relevant enzyme, was the cause of the neurological disease. This was difficult to combine with the demonstrable deficiencies in myelination. It has been shown that, in myelin, it is the protein component which is primarily affected [67] and also that high concentrations of phenylalanine in the blood hinder the entry of tryptophan, tyrosine and possibly other amino acids into brain cells [68]. The synthesis of protein in brain cells is thereby inhibited, polyribosomes being few or unstable [69]. It seems reasonable to suggest that this accounts for the lack of proteolipid protein and hence of myelin. Since the inhibition of protein synthesis continues as long as the concentration of phenylalanine is elevated, the normal metabolism of brain cells must be severely affected, but capable of returning to normal as soon as the concentration of phenylalanine in the blood drops. This theory accounts satisfactorily both for the rapid response in behaviour, E.E.G. etc. when the low-phenylalanine diet is started after infancy and for the residual neurological deficit related to the lack of myelin.

6.6.5 Screening

Because treatment is most effective if started in earliest infancy, it is necessary to make the diagnosis of phenyl-ketonuria before any clinical signs appear, i.e. from the biochemical changes. Every newborn infant must be tested and, therefore, the test used must be inexpensive, simple and reliable [70, 71]. The available methods are determination of phenylalanine concentration in the blood, o-hydroxyphenyl-acetic acid in urine or phenylpyruvic acid in urine. The third method, once widely used, has now been largely abandoned; the first and, to a lesser extent, the second are used on a very large scale in many countries. Sometimes tests for other conditions, such as homocystinuria, galactosaemia and maple syrup urine disease, are combined with the test for phenylketonuria.

6.6.6 Other varieties of phenylalaninaemia

Since 1951 it has been recognized that some atypical individuals showing the biochemical features of phenyl-ketonuria have normal intelligence and no neurological abnormalities [72]. In at least some of these the concentration of phenylalanine in the blood is lower than in typical phenylketonuria and they metabolize an injected load of phenylalanine faster [73].

A probably different variety was detected in screening programmes: infants whose blood phenylalanine level rose to 10-50 mg per 100 ml then, after some months, fell to 3-15 mg per 100 ml. This has been termed "time-variable phenyl-alaninaemia"; it seems to be rarely associated with mental retardation [70, 74]. Both these varieties together with typical phenylketonuria are given the generic name phenylalanin-aemia [73].

6.7 MAPLE SYRUP URINE DISEASE (LEUCINOSIS)

6.7.1 Metabolism of valine, isoleucine and leucine [75]

The three branched chain amino acids are normally metabolized as shown in Figure 6.2. Each amino acid is converted to the corresponding α-keto acid by a transaminase specific for that amino acid. A solitary case of valinaemia is known, caused by lack of valine transaminase [76]; the patient is mentally retarded. The three α-keto acids are decarboxylated by two (or possibly three) enzyme systems, one specific for α-keto-isovaleric acid, the other acting on α-keto-isocaproic and α-keto-β-methylvaleric acids [77, 78]. The reaction is complex, proceeding in three distinct steps [78] and requiring co-enzyme A, thiamine pyrophosphate, lipoic acid and NAD^+. The end products are the co-enzyme A thio-esters of the branched chain fatty acids.

$R.CO.CO_2H$ + Thiamine pyrophosphate $\xrightarrow{1}$ [R.CHO-Thiamine
pyrophosphate] + CO_2

[R.CHO-Thiamine pyrophosphate] + lipoic acid $\xrightarrow{2}$ [R.CO-S-lipoic-SH] +
Thiamine pyrophosphate

[R.CO.S-lipoic-SH] + CoA $\xrightarrow{3}$ R.CO.S-CoA + Dihydrolipoic acid

Dihydrolipoic acid + NAD^+ $\xrightarrow{4}$ Lipoic acid + NADH + H^+

Three different protein molecules are probably involved: a more or less specific decarboxylase catalysing reaction 1, a lipoic acid reductase transacetylase catalysing reactions 2 and 3, and lipoamide-oxido-reductase catalysing reaction 4, the three proteins being combined in a multi-enzyme particle. In leucinosis, the oxidative decarboxylation of the three branched-chain α-keto acids, but not that of other α-keto acids, is blocked by inactivity of the two (or, possibly, three) decarboxylases [79, 80, 81] (Figure 6.2); leucocytes have 1 to 3% of the normal enzymic activity [82]. There is unresolved argument as to whether the primary defect is lack of the decarboxylase acting on α-keto-isocaproic and α-keto-β-methyl-valeric acids, α-keto-isovaleric decarboxylase being inhibited by the accumulation of the other two branched chain α-keto acids, or whether the gene mutation causes diminished production of both (or all three) decarboxylases [83].

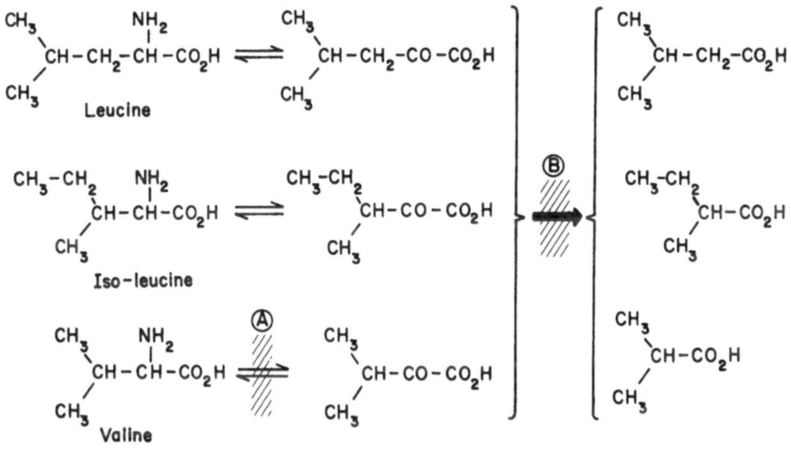

Figure 6.2. Metabolism of leucine, isoleucine and valine. The metabolic block in hypervalinaemia is marked "A", that in maple syrup urine disease "B". At least two different decarboxylases are involved. (Courtesy Blackwell, Oxford.)

As a consequence of the enzyme block, the three α-keto acids accumulate in the tissues and body fluids. The transamination step is reversible, hence the concentrations of leucine and isoleucine in the body fluids rise to about 10 to 15 times normal and that of valine to four to five times normal. The α-keto acids also undergo other reactions, including reduction to the α-hydroxy acids, some of the products being excreted and giving the urine the characteristic odour resembling maple syrup.

6.7.2. Clinical features

Affected infants are normal at birth but, after a few days, cease to suck, show lethargy and go rapidly downhill. They lose the Moro reflex, show diminished consciousness, have periods of coma, are hypertonic, show rigidity and, sometimes, opisthotonos. Some have seizures—in all the E.E.G. is grossly abnormal. The cerebral degeneration is rapidly progressive and they die, usually in respiratory failure, after a few weeks or months. Rarely, some live for almost two years; at the other extreme, in the first few cases described, the infants died within two weeks of birth.

6.7.3 Pathology and pathogenesis

The brain shows a gross deficiency of myelination, in some cases presenting as status spongiosus with small vacuoles throughout the white matter which has hardly any myelin [85]. There is no evidence of demyelination, it appears rather that myelination was abruptly halted very soon after birth.

Leucine resembles phenylalanine in hindering polyribosome formation, and therefore protein synthesis, in brain cells. The basic pathogenesis appears to be similar, though leucine is evidently far more toxic than phenylalanine.

6.7.4 Treatment

This is with a diet low in valine, leucine and isoleucine [86]. Since all three are essential amino acids, the diet presents more difficulties than does the low-phenylalanine diet. However, at least six children with leucinosis have now been successfully treated; the concentrations of valine, leucine and isoleucine in the blood were kept in the normal range and the children survived and thrived more or less normally, in most cases showing no intellectual defect or other evidence of neurological disease while good biochemical control was maintained [87]. If the concentrations of valine, isoleucine and leucine in the blood rose at any time, e.g. during a febrile illness, the child quickly became ataxic and this was equally quickly reversed when the body chemistry returned to normal. In a serious relapse, the most effective treatment was peritoneal dialysis or exchange transfusion [87].

6.7.5 Variant forms of leucinosis

As a very rare variant, in some cases biochemical and clinical abnormalities appear only during infections [88]. At most times the blood levels of leucine, isoleucine, valine and the corresponding α-keto acids are normal, but during febrile illnesses they rise and the urine acquires the characteristic smell of maple syrup. At these times the children become comatose or show other signs of C.N.S. involvement and some die. Peritoneal dialysis during acute episodes is effective and no other treatment is necessary. In the two families so far investigated [89], the leucocytes of the affected children had 12% in one family, and 6% in the other, of the normal capacity for decarboxylating the three branched chain α-keto acids; this activity is virtually zero in the typical form.

A second variant form [90] is characterized by mental retardation (I.Q. ~50) and no other evidence of neurological disease. The serum and urine levels of leucine, isoleucine, valine and the corresponding α-keto acids are in the leucinosis range continuously, not merely during infections. The leucocytes contained 15 to 25% of the normal activities of the branched chain α-keto acid decarboxylases.

In yet another variant [91], the clinical course was relatively mild, a developmental quotient of 37 and a diffusely abnormal E.E.G. being the only features, and the concentrations of valine, leucine and isoleucine in the blood were five times the normal. On giving extra thiamine, 10 mg per day, the body chemistry quickly became normal, the features of leucinosis reappearing when thiamine was withdrawn. On the high thiamine intake the leucocytes had 40% of the normal ability to oxidize leucine.

6.8 UREA CYCLE DISORDERS

6.8.1 Ammonia metabolism

Ammonia is one end product of the metabolism of all the amino acids and of most other nitrogenous substances. It is a very toxic substance, relatively low concentrations in the blood causing serious neurological signs. Ammonia is converted to non-toxic urea by the Krebs-Henseleit urea cycle (Figure 6.3), this conversion occurring mainly in the liver but also in brain and many other tissues. Four different enzymic defects of the urea cycle have been described: in hyperammonaemia type II, carbamyl phosphate synthase (reaction 1) is deficient [92], in hyperammonaemia type I, ornithine-carbamyl transferase (reaction 2) is deficient [93]; in citrullinaemia, argininosuccinate synthase (reaction 3) is deficient [94]; in argininosuccinic aciduria, argininosuccinase (reaction 4) is deficient [95].

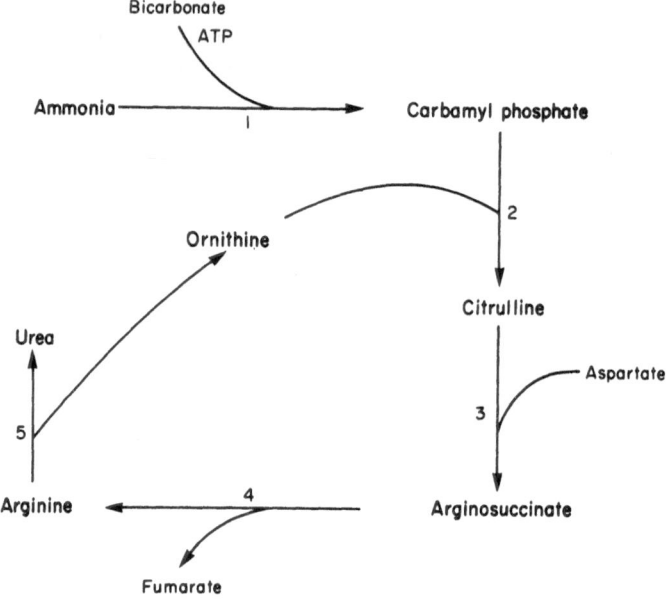

Figure 6.3. Conversion of ammonia to urea by the Krebs-Henseleit cycle (also known as the urea or ornithine cycle). (Courtesy Blackwell, Oxford.)

Deficiency of one of these enzymes causes accumulation of its substrate and also, to a lesser extent, accumulation of the substrates of preceding enzymes in the Krebs-Henseleit cycle. Thus, in argininosuccinic aciduria, not only is the concentration of argininosuccinic acid in urine and C.S.F. markedly elevated, but the concentrations of citrulline and ammonia in the blood are also raised. A raised concentration of ammonia in the blood is characteristic of all four conditions and probably largely accounts for the clinical features. On the other hand, the concentrations of urea in blood and urine are normal; the enzyme block is apparently incomplete in all four conditions as seen, perhaps because a complete block of the urea cycle in the foetus would be lethal.

6.8.2 Clinical features

The infant, sometimes in the first week after birth, has attacks of vomiting, dehydration, apathy, lethargy or coma. Convulsions appear, the E.E.G. becomes diffusely abnormal and the child shows severe mental retardation, ataxia and intention tremor. In some cases of argininosuccinic aciduria there are also abnormalities of the skin and hair (trichorexis nodosa).

Hyperammonaemia type I is one of the very few aminoacidopathies in which the heterozygote shows a clinical abnormality. During pregnancy the mother of a child later shown to have this disease suffered severe headaches and attacks of migraine and the concentration of ammonia in her blood was slightly elevated [96].

6.8.3 Treatment

A diet low in protein reduces ammonia production and is the only treatment at present available. It reduces seizure frequency; it may prevent mental retardation if given from earliest infancy. In the case of argininosuccinic aciduria, additional arginine must be added to the low protein diet, otherwise the children deteriorate, arginine being an essential amino acid in this condition.

6.9 GLYCINAEMIA AND METHYLMALONIC ACIDAEMIA

Three conditions show certain similarities and can be considered together: ketotic glycinaemia [97], non-ketotic glycinaemia [98] and methylmalonic acidaemia [99]. In all three the concentration of glycine in the blood is from 12 to 70 mg per 100 ml (normal $\leqslant$ 2 mg per 100 ml) and the concentration of glycine in the urine is from 4,000 to 8,000 mg per g creatinine (normal $\leqslant 400$). Hyperglycinaemia has also been found in a boy with hyperammonaemia type II [100]. Glycinuria and iminoglycinuria, on the other hand, are unrelated to these three conditions and reflect defective renal tubular reabsorption of glycine and, in the case of iminoglycinuria, of proline and hydroxyproline [101].

6.9.1 Metabolism of glycine

The metabolism of glycine is complex but a major pathway is:

Glycine + Tetrahydrofolic acid → Hydroxymethyltetrahydrofolic
$$\text{acid} + CO_2 + NH_3$$
Glycine + Hydroxymethyltetrahydrofolic acid ⇌ Serine + Tetrahydrofolic acid

Both reactions are catalysed by serine hydroxymethyltransferase (EC 2.1.2.1). In non-ketotic glycinaemia this enzyme is partly or completely inactive and glycine therefore accumulates [102].

A second metabolic path leads to oxalic acid:

$$\text{Glycine} \curvearrowright \text{Glyoxylate} \rightarrow \text{Oxalate}$$

In some patients with non-ketotic glycinaemia (including one patient shown to lack serine hydroxymethyltransferase) hypo-oxaluria has been found [98] though oxalic acid excretion is normal in others and, in some cases, hypo-oxaluria is intermittent.

6.9.2 Methylmalonic acid metabolism

Methylmalonic acid is produced and catabolized as follows:

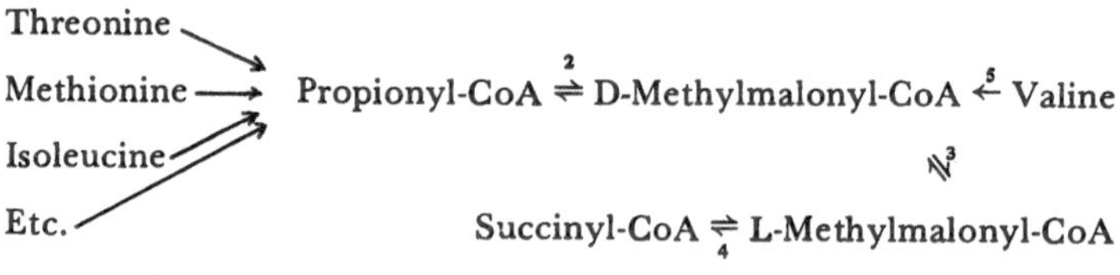

Threonine
Methionine ⟶ Propionyl-CoA $\overset{2}{\rightleftharpoons}$ D-Methylmalonyl-CoA $\overset{5}{\leftarrow}$ Valine
Isoleucine
Etc.   Succinyl-CoA $\rightleftharpoons$ L-Methylmalonyl-CoA
                                              4

The reactions marked 1 and 5 all go through several steps. Reaction 2 is catalysed by propionyl CoA carboxylase

(EC 6.4.1.3) which has biotin as a cofactor. Reaction 3 is catalysed by methylmalonyl-CoA racemase (EC 5.1.99.1) and reaction 4 by methylmalonyl-CoA mutase (EC 5.4.99.2) which has deoxyadenosyl-B_{12} as cofactor.

In vitamin B_{12} deficiency, methylmalonic acid is excreted in the urine [103]. However, there also exists methylmalonic acidaemia as an inborn error of metabolism, distinct from vitamin B_{12} deficiency, with higher concentrations of methylmalonic acid in blood and urine [99, 104]. The blood and urine contain excess glycine—up to 12 mg per 100 ml blood and up to 4,000 mg per g creatinine in urine [99, 104-107]. The site of the metabolic block is reaction 4, methylmalonic acidaemia is caused by lack or inactivity of methylmalonyl-CoA mutase [108, 109]. Although there is no deficiency of vitamin B_{12}, giving large doses causes a decrease in methylmalonic acid excretion in some cases (B_{12}-responsive) [110]. Liver biopsy specimens from B_{12}-responsive patients converted methylmalonyl-CoA to succinyl-CoA at $\sim 10\%$ of the normal rate, rising to normal with added B_{12} cofactor; specimens from B_{12}-unresponsive patients did not convert any methylmalonyl-CoA to succinyl-CoA with or without added B_{12} cofactor [111].

In ketotic glycinaemia, propionyl-CoA carboxylase is absent or inactive and, in consequence, propionic acid cannot be converted to D-methylmalonic acid [112]. Patients do not accumulate propionic acid, except in traces, but the concentration of glycine in the blood rises to 70 mg per 100 ml and that in the urine to 6,000 mg per g creatinine. No methylmalonic acid is detectable in blood or urine.

In both ketotic glycinaemia and methylmalonic acidaemia there is marked intermittent acidosis and ketosis, but the urinary ketones are butanone, pentanones, and hexanones rather than the more usual acetone [113]. The origin of these higher ketones is unknown. There is no ketosis or acidosis in non-ketotic glycinaemia. There is no explanation of the high concentrations of glycine found in blood and urine in ketotic glycinaemia and methylmalonic acidaemia. The metabolism of glycine does not seem to touch that of methylmalonic acid or propionic acid.

6.9.3 Clinical features [114]

In all three conditions the first signs commonly appear within 48 h of birth. The infant ceases to suck, becomes drowsy and may have convulsions. At this time marked ketosis appears in ketotic glycinaemia and methylmalonic acidaemia. Most affected infants go rapidly downhill and die within a few days or weeks of birth. In some cases the onset of symptoms is later, up to four months of age, and the disease runs a slower course with survival for several years. The survivors show mental and physical retardation (I.Q. ~50), seizures, E.E.G. abnormalities, spasticity and opisthotonos. They also show neutropenia, thrombocytopenia, osteoporosis and, in the cases of ketotic glycinaemia and methylmalonic acidaemia, attacks of lethargy and vomiting accompanying ketosis and acidosis.

6.9.4 Effect of amino acids. Treatment

In non-ketotic glycinaemia, glycine and serine are toxic [115]. Treatment with a diet low in these two amino acids is effective in restoring the body chemistry to normal; treated infants survive and the neurological signs decrease.

In ketotic glycinaemia, glycine is without any toxic effect. Isoleucine, methionine and threonine, which yield propionic acid, are very toxic. Administration of one of these three amino acids rapidly causes ketosis, acidosis, lethargy and convulsions. Leucine and valine, which are not metabolized through propionic acid, are as toxic as isoleucine, threonine and methionine—all other amino acids are non-toxic [114]. The toxicity of leucine and valine is not understood.

In methylmalonic acidaemia, leucine, valine, isoleucine, methionine and threonine are toxic and all other amino acids (including glycine) are non-toxic, as is found in ketotic glycinaemia [99]. There is no explanation of the effect of leucine.

Treatment of both ketotic glycinaemia and methylmalonic acidaemia is with a diet low in the five toxic amino acids. On this treatment children survive and thrive, though it is too soon for assessment of the effect on the C.N.S.

6.10 HARTNUP DISEASE

There exist, in the cell membranes of the epithelial cells lining the proximal renal tubules, a number of different mechanisms each responsible for reabsorbing a specific substance or group of related substances from the glomerular filtrate. These different mechanisms probably reflect different protein molecules in the membrane, each having an affinity for a specific substrate or group of substrates and behaving in several ways like enzymes but with the property of transporting their substrates through the membranes rather than chemically altering them [116]. One of these mechanisms reabsorbs ornithine, arginine, lysine and, in a different way, cystine; a second reabsorbs glycine, proline and hydroxyproline; a third reabsorbs glutamic and aspartic acids; a fourth reabsorbs tryptophan, alanine, asparagine, citrulline, glutamine, histidine, isoleucine, leucine, phenylalanine, serine, threonine, tyrosine and valine. Between them these four mechanisms account for the reabsorption of all the α-amino acids of plasma except methionine which may have a fifth mechanism to itself [117]. In reality the picture is more complex: there may be more than one reabsorptive mechanism for a given amino acid; glycine and histidine behave anomalously and seem to have weak affinities for several of the carriers; cystine excretion in, e.g., cystinuria is not understood—it is linked to the excretion of lysine, arginine and ornithine but cystine may not be reabsorbed by the same carrier as these three.

In Hartnup disease [118] there is a defect in the reabsorption of the fourth group of amino acids and these 13 mono-amino mono-carboxylic acids are excreted in the urine in large amounts [119]. The concentrations in plasma are low. A similar defect occurs in the jejunal mucosa in most of the reported cases—greatly reduced absorption of tryptophan from the gut has been demonstrated [120] and there is evidence of reduced absorption of the other 12 amino acids involved [121]. A variant lacking the jejunal defect has been reported [117]. The failure to absorb tryptophan from the gut results in relatively large amounts of this amino acid entering the colon and being acted on by the colonic flora [120]. Considerable amounts of indole and indolylacetic acid, among other derivatives, are formed in the gut, absorbed and metabolized by "detoxication mechanisms" in the liver and elsewhere. The urinary content of indican (indoxyl sulphate from indole), indolylacetyl-glucuronide and indolylacetylglutamine (both from indolyl-acetic acid) among other indole derivatives is considerably above normal, at any rate at times [121a].

6.10.1 Clinical features

Some subjects with the biochemical error suffer no clinical effects. However, cerebellar ataxia occurred in 11 out of 16 cases and 15 suffered from photosensitive dermatitis [122]. Other clinical features seen in different patients include attacks of nystagmus, fainting, unexplained pains, delirium with hallucinations, disturbed behaviour, emotional lability and E.E.G. disturbances. Mental retardation has been reported in some but it is not certain whether this is a chance association. The ataxic episodes, which are the most constant neurological finding, are transitory and become less severe and less frequent as the child gets older. The dermatitis is seen only on exposed areas and is worse in summer than winter. Clinically, Hartnup disease resembles pellagra, but the former is familial, being inherited as an autosomal recessive character, whereas pellagra is dietary in origin.

Patients with Hartnup disease are slightly but significantly shorter than their age-matched sibs.

6.10.2 Pathogenesis

The metabolism of tryptophan is complex, but approximately one-sixtieth of the tryptophan ingested is normally converted to nicotinamide and this is a major source of the vitamin. In Hartnup disease, absorption of tryptophan from the gut is diminished, reducing the amount available for biosynthesis of nicotinamide, and the renal tubular defect causes urinary loss of tryptophan, still further reducing the body's store. More important than these is the effect of indole produced in the colon [123]: indole inhibits the enzymes tryptophan-pyrrolase (EC 1.13.1.12) and kynurenine formamidase (EC 3.5.1.9) both of which are necessary for the conversion of tryptophan to nicotinamide. It has been shown that, in Hartnup disease, urinary excretion of kynurenine and nicotinamide derivatives increased after intravenously administered tryptophan but actually decreased when the tryptophan was given by mouth [123]. Apart from height, the clinical features of Hartnup disease, so closely resembling pellagra, can be explained by a deficiency of nicotinamide brought about by decreased amounts of available tryptophan and the toxic effects of indole, and possibly other substances, absorbed from the gut. The relatively poor growth [124] probably reflects the poor absorption of a number of essential amino acids from the gut and their loss in the urine.

6.10.3 Treatment

Logically, Hartnup disease should be treated with nicotinamide, at least 15 to 35 mg per day, to replace that normally formed from dietary tryptophan. During acute exacerbations, consideration might be given to reducing the bacterial flora in the gut by giving, e.g., neomycin and nystatin. The slightly diminished stature could be corrected in childhood by giving a high protein diet, but with the risk of increased production of toxic substances in the gut. Monoamine oxidase inhibitors should be avoided at all times since they prevent conversion of the very toxic substance tryptamine, which is probably produced in the gut in Hartnup disease, to the far less toxic indolylacetic acid [120].

6.11 JUVENILE HYPERURICAEMIA WITH CHOREO-ATHETOSIS (LESCH-NYHAN SYNDROME)

6.11.1 Purine metabolism

The normal pathway of purine anabolism and catabolism is shown in Figure 6.4 with many intermediate steps omitted. Reactions 2 and 3, of phosphoribosylpyrophosphate with guanine and hypoxanthine to produce guanylic acid and inosinic acid, respectively, are catalysed by a single enzyme—hypoxanthine-guanine phosphoribosyltransferase. The reaction

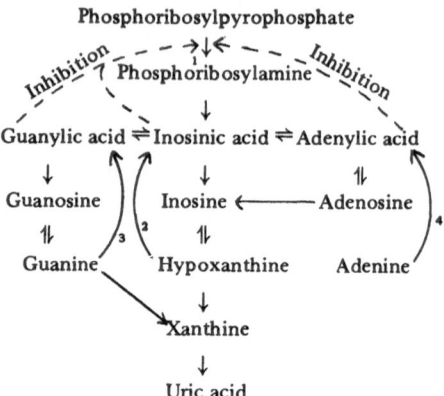

Figure 6.4. Normal anabolism and catabolism of purines. (Abridged. After Seegmiller [127].)

of adenine with phosphoribosylpyrophosphate to produce adenylic acid, reaction 4, is catalysed by a different enzyme, adenine phosphoribosyltransferase. The products of these reactions, guanylic, inosinic and adenylic acids, inhibit reaction 1, normally the rate-limiting step in purine bio-synthesis, and so form a negative feed-back regulator of this rate.

In the Lesch-Nyhan syndrome, hypoxanthine-guanine phos-phoribosyltransferase is virtually absent [125], an unstable variant enzyme being present, and, in consequence, guanylic and inosinic acids are not formed from guanine and hypoxanthine. The feed-back inhibition is therefore deficient and the rate of purine biosynthesis is elevated [126]. Uric acid is produced at five to six times the normal rate and at three times the rate, corrected for body weight, found in adults with gout. The concentration of uric acid in the blood lies between 8 and 15 mg per 100 ml (normal: 5.6 ± 1.1; gouty subjects: 9.2 ± 1.1).

Drugs affecting purine metabolism act aberrantly in the Lesch-Nyhan syndrome [127]. Azathioprine and 6-mercapto-purine do not affect purine synthesis; allopurinol reduces uric acid production but causes an equivalent increase in oxypurines; probenecid increases urinary excretion of uric acid and decreases its concentration in the blood. None of these drugs has any clinical effect on the course of the disease.

Fibroblasts grown in tissue culture show the lack of hypoxanthine-guanine phosphoribosyltransferase (present in normal fibroblasts) and the consequent biochemical changes, including greatly increased production of purines [125, 126]. These fibroblasts do not grow well unless the medium contains either adenine or additional folic acid (50 times the normal requirement). The fibroblasts do not show any marked deficiency of the purine nucleotides but do show a four-fold increase in the concentration of phosphoribosylpyrophosphate.

6.11.2 Clinical and genetic features [128, 129, 130]

Affected infants are mostly normal at birth though some show slight hypotonia. At 4-6 months there is motor retardation and difficulty with mucus. About one year of age, choreo-athetotic movements and some spasticity appear and gradually worsen. Affected children thrash about and may need restraint; in some cases seizures and/or opisthotonos appear. At about two to three years, they begin biting their cheeks, lips and fingers, producing severe mutilations with large defects of their lips and, in some, amputated phalanges. They also scratch and tear at their noses and faces, producing further serious mutilations. They appear completely conscious of the pain they suffer during these episodes of self-mutilation, yet unable to stop. As well as self-aggression, they attack others with violence or insults. The I.Q. is usually in the range 20-70.

In spite of the high concentration of uric acid in the blood, arthritis is rare, though not unknown. Gouty nephropathy does, however, occur. Most patients die in late childhood or adolescence with renal colic, uncontrollable vomiting or in seizures.

Some patients suffer from megaloblastic anaemia which does not respond to folic acid but does respond to administration of adenine.

Only boys are affected but the disease is carried by the female; a single mutant gene on the X-chromosome is responsible and fibroblasts from the mothers of affected boys show, when grown in tissue culture, two cell populations, one possessing hypoxanthine-guanine phosphoribosyltransferase and the other lacking the enzyme.

6.11.3 Pathogenesis. Relationship to gout

Neuropathy is so rare in gout that uric acid intoxication is very unlikely as a cause of the neurological signs in the Lesch-Nyhan syndrome [132]. The missing enzyme, hypoxanthine-guanine phosphoribosyltransferase, is normally found in the basal ganglia of the brain in higher concentration than anywhere else in the body [132, 133]. The clinical features can be related to disease of the basal ganglia and it seems probable that this enzyme plays some vital role there. Hypoxanthine and xanthine concentrations in the C.S.F. are three to four times normal but, as with uric acid, it seems doubtful that these oxypurines are toxic [127].

In $\geqslant 95\%$ of the sufferers from gout, the activity of hypoxanthine-guanine phosphoribosyltransferase is normal, but in a minority ($\leqslant 5\%$) this activity is low [133]. These patients have a tendency to early development of arthritis and nephropathy. About one-third of them, those in whom the activity of the enzyme is lowest, show some neurological abnormalities, particularly mental retardation. This type of gout is related to variant forms of hypoxanthine-guanine phosphoribosyltransferase, a different variant in each family, the activity being up to 1% of normal [127]. In some families, the variant enzyme shows different activities towards hypoxanthine and guanine.

6.12 LEIGH'S ENCEPHALOPATHY

6.12.1 Pyruvate carboxylase

One of the major reactions of pyruvate is with CO_2 to produce oxalacetic acid

$$CH_3.CO.CO_2H + CO_2 \rightarrow HO_2C.CH_2.CO.CO_2H$$

The reaction is catalysed by pyruvate carboxylase, an enzyme requiring biotin and found in liver, kidney and, in smaller amounts, brain and adipose tissue [134]. Oxalacetic acid enters the citric acid cycle and, via phosphoenolpyruvate, is converted to glucose.

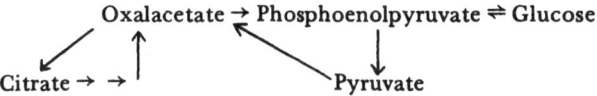

Pyruvate carboxylase stands at the cross-roads in gluconeogenesis, i.e. the conversion of amino acids to carbohydrate.

In Leigh's encephalopathy, pyruvate carboxylase is virtually absent from the liver [135, 136]. As a consequence, the concentration of pyruvic acid [137] in the blood rises (up to 5 mg per 100 ml) and this leads to lactic acidaemia [138] (30 mg per 100 ml or more), hyperalaninaemia (up to 12 mg per 100 ml) lactic aciduria and increased excretion of alanine [139], the three substances being interconvertible.

$$CH_3.CHOH.CO_2H \rightleftharpoons CH_3.CO.CO_2H \rightleftharpoons CH_3.CH(NH_2).CO_2H$$

In some cases there is a generalized aminoaciduria, possibly renal in origin [138]. Affected children show fasting hypoglycaemia, though the responses to glucose loads, adrenaline and glucagon are normal.

Treatment with lipoic acid decreases the concentrations of pyruvic and lactic acids in the blood [137], perhaps by increasing the oxidative decarboxylation of pyruvic acid to acetyl-CoA.

6.12.2 Clinical features [136-140]

Affected children are normal at birth but, before six months of age, show signs of mental retardation and failure to gain weight normally. Mental development slows down and comes to a halt and they show progressive hypotonia. A fluctuating course with relapses and remissions is common. Patients have attacks of vomiting, sweating, sighing and hyperpnoea; while many patients have acidosis, hyperventilation is also seen in non-acidotic patients [139]. Other, less constant, features include ataxia, pyramidal signs, ptosis, an expressionless facies and depressed tendon reflexes. Posterior nerve roots and peripheral nerves are also involved. Death occurs, usually in respiratory failure, between 7 months and 15 years of age, depending on the rate of progression of the disease.

At autopsy, multiple areas of necrosis are found in the grey matter of the central part of the brain and in the spinal cord [141]. Leigh compared these changes to Wernicke's encephalopathy, though with a different distribution. This suggested either thiamine deficiency or inability to utilize thiamine normally, but treatment with thiamine or thiamine pyrophosphate has no effect on the course of the disease [142]. Lipoic acid, like thiamine pyrophosphate involved in the oxidative decarboxylation of pyruvic acid, has been given to some patients [137]; the concentration of pyruvic acid in the blood fell and clinical improvement was claimed. Others have tried lipoic acid treatment with less success—the pyruvic acid content of the blood fell, but there was no effect on the clinical course of the disease [136]. It is now known that the enzymes decarboxylating pyruvic acid are normal and that the metabolic error results from a lack of pyruvate carboxylase.

REFERENCES

1. H. H. Hiatt, *In* The Metabolic Basis of Inherited Disease (J. B. Stanbury, J. B. Wyngaarden and D. S. Fredrickson, eds), p. 109. McGraw-Hill, New York and London (1966)
2. S. O'Kada and J. S. O'Brien, *Science,* 160, 1002 (1968)
3. C. O. Carter and L. I. Woolf, *Ann. Hum. Genet.,* 25, 57 (1961)
4. K. Tanaka, E. Matsunaga, Y. Handa, T. Murata and K. Takehara, *Jap. J. Hum. Genet.,* 6, 65 (1961)
5. B. E. Cohen, A. Szeinberg, H. Boichis and E. Bodonyi, *Pediatrics, Springfield,* 32, 1069 (1963)
6. L. I. Woolf, *Adv. Clin. Chem.,* 5, 1 (1962)
7. D. Y.-Y. Hsia (ed.), Galactosemia. Charles C. Thomas, Springfield, Illinois (1969)
8. H. M. Kalckar, B. Braganca and A. Munch-Petersen, *Nature (Lond.),* 172, 1038 (1953)
9. V. Schwarz, L. Golberg, G. M. Komrower and A. Holzel, *Biochem. J.,* 62, 34 (1956)
10. E. P. Anderson, H. M. Kalckar and K. J. Isselbacher, *Science,* 125, 113 (1957)
11. W. W. Wells, *In* Galactosemia (D. Y.-Y. Hsia, ed.), p. 227. Charles C. Thomas, Springfield, Illinois (1969)
12. K. J. Isselbacher, *J. Biol. Chem.,* 232, 429 (1958)
13. P. Cuatrecasas and S. Segal, *Science,* 153, 549 (1966)
14. E. Beutler, *Science,* 156, 1516 (1967)

15. T. Inouye, M. Tannenbaum and D. Y.-Y. Hsia, *Nature (Lond.)*, 193, 67 (1962)
16. J. B. Sidbury, Jr., Am. Chem. Soc., 132nd Meeting, New York, N.Y., p. 27C (1957)
17. V. Ginsburg and E. F. Neufeld, Am. Chem. Soc., 132nd Meeting, New York, N.Y., p. 27C (1957)
18. H. Dam, *Proc. Soc. Exptl. Biol. Med.*, 55, 57 (1944)
19. R. H. Rigdon, J. R. Couch, C. R. Creger and T. M. Ferguson, *Experientia*, 19, 349 (1963)
20. H. L. Nadler, T. Inouye and D. Y.-Y. Hsia, *In* Galactosemia (D. Y.-Y. Hsia, ed.), p. 127. Charles C. Thomas, Springfield, Illinois (1969)
21. S. Segal. *In* Galactosemia (D. Y. Y. Hsia, ed.), p. 176. Charles C. Thomas, Springfield, Illinois (1969)
22. V. Schwarz, A. R. Wells, A. Holzel, G. M. Komrower and I. M. N. Simpson, *Ann. Hum. Genet.*, 25, 179 (1961)
23. C. K. Mathai and E. Beutler, *Science*, 154, 1179 (1966)
24. R. Gitzelmann, *Lancet*, 2, 670 (1965)
25. H. G. Hers and G. Joassin, *Enzymol. biol. et clin.*, 1, 4 (1961)
26. E. R. Froesch, *In* Genetic Defects of Biologically Active Proteins (F. Linneweh, ed.), p. 242. Urban and Schwarzenberg, Munich (1962)
27. Y. Nordmann, F. Schapira and J. C. Dreyfus, *Society for the Study of Inborn Errors of Metabolism*, Symposium No. 6, 99 (1969)
28. E. R. Froesch, H. P. Wolf, H. Baitsch, A. Prader and A. Labhart, *Amer. J. Med.*, 34, 151 (1963)
29. R. A. Chambers and R. T. C. Pratt, *Lancet*, 2, 340 (1956)
30. E. R. Froesch, A. Prader, A. Labhart, H. W. Stuber and H. P. Wolf, *Schweiz. med. Wchnschr.*, 87, 1168 (1957)
31. S. Halvorsen and L. R. Gjessing, *In* Phenylketonuria and Some Other Inborn Errors of Amino Acid Metabolism (H. Bickel, F. P. Hudson and L. I. Woolf, eds), p. 301. Georg Thieme Verlag, Stuttgart (1971)
32. F. Schapira, G. Schapira and J.-C. Dreyfus, *Enzymol. biol. et clin.*, 1, 170 (1961/1962)
33. S. H. Mudd, W. A. Edwards, P. M. Loeb, M. S. Brown and L. Laster, *J. Clin. Invest.*, 49, 1762 (1970)
34. F. J. van Sprang, *In* Phenylketonuria and Some Other Inborn Errors of Amino Acid Metabolism (H. Bickel, F. P. Hudson and L. I. Woolf, eds), p. 325. Georg Thieme Verlag, Stuttgart (1971)
35. T. Gerritsen and H. A. Waisman, *Pediatrics*, 33, 413 (1964)
36. R. N. Schimke, V. A. McKusick, T. Huang and A. D. Pollack, *J. Amer. Med. Ass.*, 193, 87 (1965)
37. G. M. Komrower, A. M. Lambert, D. C. Cusworth and R. G. Westall, *Archs Dis. Childh.*, 41, 666 (1966)
38. D. P. Brenton, D. C. Cusworth, C. E. Dent and E. E. Jones, *Quart. J. Med.*, 35, 325 (1966)
39. T. L. Perry, H. G. Dunn, S. Hansen, L. McDougall and P. D. Warrington, *Pediatrics*, 37, 502 (1966)

40. G. W. Barber and G. L. Spaeth, *Lancet*, 1, 337 (1967)
41. N. A. J. Carson, *In* Phenylketonuria and Some Other Inborn Errors of Amino Acid Metabolism (H. Bickel, F. P. Hudson and L. I. Woolf, eds), p. 289. Georg Thieme Verlag, Stuttgart (1971)
42. L. I. Woolf, *Adv. Clin. Chem.*, 6, 97 (1963)
43. H. Bickel, F. P. Hudson and L. I. Woolf (eds), Phenylketonuria and Some Other Inborn Errors of Amino Acid Metabolism. Georg Thieme Verlag, Stuttgart (1971)
44. S. Kaufman, *J. Biol. Chem.*, 239, 332 (1964)
45. S. Kaufman, *Science*, 128, 1506 (1958)
46. V. G. Patton, D. N. Wade and L. I. Woolf. Unpublished observations
47. M. D. Armstrong and K. S. Robinson, *Arch. Biochem. Biophys.*, 52, 287 (1954)
48. S. P. Bessman and K. Tada, *Metab. Clin. Exptl.*, 9, 377 (1960)
49. L. I. Woolf, *In* Mental Retardation (J. Wortis, ed.), p. 29. Grune and Stratton, New York and London (1970)
50. W. E. Knox, *In* The Metabolic Basis of Inherited Disease (J. B. Stanbury, J. B. Wyngaarden and D. S. Fredrickson, eds), p. 321. McGraw-Hill, Inc., New York (1960)
51. N. L. Low, J. F. Bosma and M. D. Armstrong, *A.M.A. Arch. Neurol. Psychiat.*, 77, 359 (1957)
52. B. S. Sutherland, H. K. Berry and H. C. Shirkey, *J. Pediat.*, 57, 521 (1960)
53. V. Cowie and L. S. Penrose, *Ann. Eugenics*, 15, 297 (1949-1951)
54. L. Crome, V. Tymms and L. I. Woolf, *J. Neurol. Neurosurg. Psychiat.*, 25, 143 (1962)
55. L. Crome, *J. Neurol. Neurosurg. Psychiat.*, 25, 149 (1962)
56. L. I. Woolf and D. G. Vulliamy, *Archs Dis. Childh.*, 26, 487 (1951)
57. Medical Research Council Conference on Phenylketonuria, *Brit. Med. J.*, 1, 1691 (1963)
58. A. Lütcke, *In* Phenylketonuria and Some Other Inborn Errors of Amino Acid Metabolism (H. Bickel, F. P. Hudson and L. I. Woolf (eds), p. 269. Georg Thieme Verlag, Stuttgart (1971)
59. R. O. Fisch, F. Torres, H. J. Gravem, C. S. Greenwood and J. A. Anderson, *Neurology, Minneap.*, 19, 659 (1969)
60. I. M. Hackney, W. B. Hanley, W. Davidson and L. Lindsao, *J. Pediat.*, 72, 646 (1968)
61. L. I. Woolf, R. Griffiths and A. Moncrieff, *Brit. Med. J.*, 1, 57 (1955)
62. L. I. Woolf, R. Griffiths, A. Moncrieff, S. Coates and F. Dillistone, *Archs Dis. Childh.*, 33, 31 (1958)
63. L. I. Woolf, *Biochem. J.*, 49, ix (1951)
64. C. Mitoma, H. S. Posner, D. F. Bogdanski and S. Udenfriend, *J. Pharmacol. Exptl. Therap.*, 120, 188 (1957)
65. A. N. Davison and M. Sandler, *Nature (Lond.)*, 181, 186 (1958)
66. H. Weil-Malherbe, *In* Biochemistry of the Developing Nervous Systems: Proceedings of the First International Neurochemistry Symposium, Oxford, 1954 (H. Waelsch, ed.), p. 458. Academic Press, New York (1955)

67. H. C. Agrawal, A. H. Bone and A. N. Davison, *In* Phenylketonuria and Some Other Inborn Errors of Amino Acid Metabolism (H. Bickel, F. P. Hudson and L. I. Woolf, eds), p. 121. Georg Thieme Verlag, Stuttgart (1971)

68. C. M. McKean, D. M. Boggs and N. A. Peterson, *J. Neurochem.*, 15, 235 (1968)

69. K. Aoki and F. L. Siegel, *Science*, 168, 129 (1970)

70. L. I. Woolf, *In* Phenylketonuria and Allied Metabolic Diseases (J. A. Anderson and K. F. Swaiman, eds), p. 50. U.S. Government Printing Office, Washington, D.C. (1967)

71. Medical Research Council Working Party on Phenylketonuria, *Brit. Med. J.*, 4, 7 (1968)

72. V. A. Cowie, *Lancet*, 1, 272 (1951)

73. L. I. Woolf, *In* Phenylketonuria and Some Other Inborn Errors of Amino Acid Metabolism (H. Bickel, F. P. Hudson and L. I. Woolf, eds), p. 103. Georg Thieme Verlag, Stuttgart (1971)

74. M. E. O'Flynn, P. Tillman and D. Y.-Y. Hsia, *Amer. J. Dis. Child.*, 113, 22 (1967)

75. J. Dancis and M. Levitz, *In* The Metabolic Basis of Inherited Disease (J. B. Stanbury, J. B. Wyngaarden and D. S. Fredrickson, eds), p. 353. McGraw Hill, Inc., New York (1966)

76. J. Dancis, J. Hutzler, K. Tada, Y. Wada, T. Morikawa and T. Arakawa, *Pediatrics*, 39, 813 (1967)

77. J. A. Bowden and J. L. Connelly, *J. Biol. Chem.*, 243, 3526 (1968)

78. W. Goedde and W. Keller, *In* Amino Acid Metabolism and Genetic Variation (W. L. Nyhan, ed.), p. 191. McGraw-Hill, New York and London (1967)

79. J. H. Menkes, *Pediatrics*, 23, 348 (1959)

80. D. Y. MacKenzie and L. I. Woolf, *Brit. Med. J.*, 1, 90 (1959)

81. J. Dancis, M. Levitz, S. Miller and R. G. Westall, *Brit. Med. J.*, 1, 91, (1959)

82. J. Dancis, J. Hutzler and M. Levitz, *J. Pediat.*, 66, 595 (1965)

83. S. E. Snyderman, *In* Amino Acid Metabolism and Genetic Variation (W. L. Nyhan, ed.), p. 171. McGraw-Hill, New York and London (1967)

84. J. Dancis, M. Levitz and R. G. Westall, *Pediatrics*, 25, 72 (1960)

85. L. Crome, G. Dutton and C. F. Ross, *J. Path. Bact.*, 81, 379 (1961)

86. R. G. Westall, *Archs Dis. Childh.*, 38, 485 (1963)

87. S. E. Snyderman, *In* Phenylketonuria and Some Other Inborn Errors of Amino Acid Metabolism (H. Bickel, F. P. Hudson and L. I. Woolf, eds), p. 283. Georg Thieme Verlag, Stuttgart (1971)

88. R. Kiil and T. Rokkones, *Acta. Paediat.*, 53, 356 (1964)

89. J. Dancis, J. Hutzler and T. Rokkones, *New Engl. J. Med.*, 276, 84 (1967)

90. J. D. Schulman, T. L. Lustberg, J. L. Kennedy, M. Museles and J. E. Seegmiller, *Amer. J. Med.*, 49, 118 (1970)

91. C. R. Scriver, S. Mackenzie, C. L. Clow and E. Delvin, *Lancet*, 1, 310 (1971)

92. J. M. Freeman, J. F. Nicholson, W. S. Masland, L. P. Rowland and S. Carter, *J. Pediat.*, **65**, 1093 (1964)
93. A. Russell, B. Levin, V. G. Oberholzer and L. Sinclair, *Lancet*, **2**, 699 (1962)
94. W. C. McMurray, J. C. Rathbun, F. Mohyaddin and S. J. Koegler, *Pediatrics*, **32**, 347 (1963)
95. S. Tomlinson and R. G. Westall, *Clin. Sci.*, **26**, 261 (1964)
96. A. Russell, *Society for the Study of Inborn Errors of Metabolism*, Symposium No 6, 134 (1969)
97. B. Childs, W. L. Nyhan, M. Borden, L. Bard and R. E. Cooke, *Pediatrics*, **27**, 522 (1961)
98. T. Gerritsen, E. Kaveggia and H. A. Waisman, *Pediatrics*, **36**, 882 (1965)
99. V. G. Oberholzer, B. Levin, E. A. Burgess and W. F. Young, *Archs Dis. Childh.*, **42**, 492 (1967)
100. M. L. Efron, *In* Amino Acid Metabolism and Genetic Variation (W. L. Nyhan, ed.), p. 219. McGraw-Hill, New York and London (1967)
101. G. R. Fraser, A. I. Friedmann, V. M. Patton, D. N. Wade and L. I. Woolf, *Humangenetik*, **6**, 362 (1968)
102. T. Ando, W. L. Nyhan, T. Gerritsen, L. Gong, D. C. Heiner and P. F. Bray, *Pediat. Res.*, **2**, 254 (1968)
103. D. Gompertz, J. Hywell, J. Ones and J. P. Knowles, *Lancet*, **1**, 424 (1967)
104. G. Morrow, III, L. A. Barness, V. H. Auerbach, A. M. DiGeorge, T. Ando and W. L. Nyhan, *J. Pediat.*, **74**, 680 (1969)
105. O. Stokke, L. Eldjarn, K. R. Norum, J. Steen-Johnsen and S. Halvorsen, *Scand. J. clin. Lab. Invest.*, **20**, 313 (1967)
106. G. Morrow, III, L. A. Barness, V. H. Auerbach and A. M. DiGeorge, Soc. Pediat. Res. (Abst.) Atlantic City, May 3-4, 20 (1968)
107. B. Lindblad, B. S. Lindblad, P. Olin, B. Svanberg and R. Zetterström, *Acta Paediat. Scand.*, **57**, 417 (1968)
108. V. H. Auerbach, G. Morrow, III, A. M. DiGeorge and L. A. Barness, FEBS (Abst) Madrid, April 7-11, 103 (1969)
109. G. Morrow, III, L. A. Barness, G. J. Cardinale, R. H. Abeles and J. G. Flaks, *Proc. Nat. Acad. Sci.*, **63**, 191 (1969)
110. L. E. Rosenberg, A. Lilljeqvist and Y. E. Hsia, *Science*, **162**, 805 (1968)
111. V. H. Auerbach, G. Morrow, III, A. M. DiGeorge and L. A. Barness, *In* Phenylketonuria and Some Other Inborn Errors of Amino Acid Metabolism (H. Bickel, F. P. Hudson and L. I. Woolf, eds), p. 314. Georg Thieme Verlag, Stuttgart (1971)
112. Y. E. Hsia, K. J. Scully and L. E. Rosenberg, *Lancet*, **1**, 757 (1967)
113. J. H. Menkes, *J. Pediat.*, **69**, 413 (1966)
114. W. L. Nyhan, T. Ando and T. Gerritsen, *In* Amino Acid Metabolism and Genetic Variation (W. L. Nyhan, ed.), p. 255. McGraw-Hill, New York and London (1967)
115. J. H. P. Jonxis, F. A. Hommes and C. J. de Groot, *In* Phenylketonuria and Some Other Inborn Errors of Amino Acid

Metabolism (H. Bickel, F. P. Hudson and L. I. Woolf, eds), p. 307. Georg Thieme Verlag, Stuttgart (1971)

116. L. I. Woolf, Renal Tubular Dysfunction. Thomas, Springfield, Ill. (1966)

117. C. R. Scriver, *In* Amino Acid Metabolism and Genetic Variation (W. L. Nyhan, ed.), p. 327. McGraw-Hill, New York and London (1967)

118. D. N. Baron, C. E. Dent, H. Harris, E. W. Hart and J. B. Jepson, *Lancet*, 2, 421 (1956)

119. D. F. Evered, *Biochem.. J.*, 62, 416 (1956)

120. M. D. Milne, M. A. Crawford, C. B. Girao and L. W. Loughridge, *Quart. J Med.*, 29, 407 (1960)

121. C. R. Scriver, *New Engl. J. Med.*, 273, 530 (1965)

121a. K. N. F. Shaw, D. Redlich, S. W. Wright and J. B. Jepson, *Fed. Proc.*, 194, 134 (1960)

122. K. Halvorsen and S. Halvorsen, *Pediatrics*, 31, 29 (1963)

123. P. de Laey, C. Hooft, J. Timmermans and J. Snoeck, *Ann. Paediat.*, 202, 145 (1964)

124. J. E. Colliss, A. J. Levi and M. D. Milne, *Brit. Med. J.*, 1, 590 (1963)

125. J. E. Seegmiller, F. M. Rosenbloom and W. N. Kelley, *Science*, 155, 1682 (1967)

126. F. M. Rosenbloom, J. F. Henderson, I. C. Caldwell, W. N. Kelley and J. E. Seegmiller, *J. Biol. Chem.*, 243, 1166 (1968)

127. J. E. Seegmiller, *FEBS Symposium*, 19, 325 (1969)

128. W. Catel and J. Schmidt, *Dt. Med. Wschr.*, 84, 2145 (1959)

129. I. D. Riley, *Archs Dis. Childh.*, 35, 293 (1960)

130. M. Lesch and W. L. Nyhan, *Amer. J. Med.*, 36, 561 (1964)

131. F. M. Rosenbloom, W. N. Kelley, J. F. Henderson and J. Seegmiller, *Lancet*, 2, 305 (1967)

132. F. M. Rosenbloom, W. N. Kelley, J. Miller, J. F. Henderson and J. E. Seegmiller, *J. Amer. Med. Ass.* 202, 103 (1967)

133. W. N. Kelley, M. L. Greene, F. M. Rosenbloom, J. F. Henderson and J. E. Seegmiller, *Ann. Int. Med.*, 70, 155 (1969)

134. M. F. Utter, *FEBS Symposium*, 19, 91 (1969)

135. F. A. Hommes, A. H. Polman and T. Reerink, *Archs Dis. Childh.*, 43, 423 (1968)

136. C. J. de Groot, F. A. Hommes and J. H. P. Jonxis, *Society for the Study of Inborn Errors of Metabolism*, Symposium No. 6, 77 (1969)

137. B. E. Clayton, R. H. Dobbs and A. D. Patrick, *Archs Dis. Childh.*, 42, 467 (1967)

138. H. E. Worsley, R. W. Brookfield, J. S. Elwood, R. L. Noble and W. H. Taylor, *Archs Dis. Childh.*, 40, 492 (1965)

139. H. G. Dunn and C. L. Dolman, *Neurology, Minneap.*, 19, 536 (1969)

140. D. Leigh, *J. Neurol. Neurosurg. Psychiat.*, 14, 216 (1951)

141. L. C. Crome and J. Stern, Pathology of Mental Retardation, p. 314. Churchill, London (1967)

142. A. H. Greenhouse and S. A. Schneck, *Neurology, Minneap.*, 18, 1 (1968)

Index